THE CLINICAL POTENTIAL OF INTERFERONS

Executive Committee

JAPAN MEDICAL RESEARCH FOUNDATION PUBLICATION NO. 15

THE CLINICAL POTENTIAL OF INTERFERONS
Treatment of Viral Diseases and Malignant Tumors

Proceedings of the International Conference on Clinical
Potentials of Interferons in Viral Diseases and Malignant Tumors,
held December 2-4, 1980

Edited by
REISAKU KONO
JAN VILČEK

UNIVERSITY OF TOKYO PRESS

JAPAN MEDICAL RESEARCH FOUNDATION
PUBLICATION NO. 15

Published by
UNIVERSITY OF TOKYO PRESS
UTP 3047–67670–5149
ISBN 0–86008–313–6

Printed in Japan.

Foreword

The development of modern medicine has contributed to clarifying the etiology and treatment of various diseases as well as to improving public health and welfare. However, there are many diseases of unknown etiology, for which there is no known treatment, which still leave large numbers of patients in a chronic incurable state. In order to promote research on the etiology and treatment of such intractable diseases, non-governmental funding, as well as governmental support, is very important. The Japan Medical Research Foundation has been in existence since October 1973 in order to meet this need with aid from non-governmental financial sources.

The increased supply of interferon has made it possible to treat patients with virus diseases or malignancies with this drug on a trial basis, and so experience with interferon therapy is accumulating. Therefore, I firmly believe it useful for investigators from many parts of world to exchange their experiences and knowledge and to discuss matters of mutual interest in this symposium. Four sessions constitute this symposium: their topics are Production and Purification of Human Interferons, Clinical Applications, Safety Control, and Future Problems and General Discussion. This symposium was held under the auspices of the Japan Medical Research Foundation, and I am hopeful that the publication of its proceedings will make its work available to a wide scientific readership.

February 10, 1982

Masayoshi YAMAMOTO

President
Japan Medical Research Foundation

Preface

This book is the exciting outcome of the International Conference on Clinical Potentials of Interferon in Viral Diseases and Malignant Tumors, held December 2–4, 1980 at the Oiso Prince Hotel, Japan.

I wish to express my sincere appreciation to all the members of the Organizing and Executive Committee: Dr. Yasuichi Nagano, Dr. Yoshimi Kawade, Dr. Tsunataro Kishida, Dr. Noboru Kobayashi, Dr. Seiya Kohno, Dr. Shigeyasu Kobayashi, Dr. Tsuguo Kuwata, Dr. Thomas Merigan, Dr. Yoshio Sakurai, Dr. Masanori Shimoyama, Dr. Akira Shishido, Dr. Yukio Uchida, Dr. Jan Vilček, and Dr. Shudo Yamazaki.

I would like to thank president M. Yamamoto and the rest of the staff at the Japan Medical Research Foundation for promoting the conference on which the papers in the book are based. And also I am particularly grateful to the organizations whose financial support facilitated the editing of the book.

I believe that this is the first book that concentrates on the clinical application of interferon. In this sense, it is unique and will be welcomed by the medical circles of the world.

February 10, 1982

Reisaku KONO
Chairman of the Symposium

Contents

ix

II. CLINICAL APPLICATIONS

III. SAFETY CONTROL

IV. FUTURE PROBLEM AND GENERAL DISCUSSIONS

Note on Usage

In the interest of economy and consistency, the word "interferon" has been abbreviated in IFN throughout this volume, with one exception: in the paper by Pestka *et al.* (pp. 369–380), it is abbreviated as IF.

Opening Remarks

Distinguished guests and colleagues from many countries:

It is an honor and privilege for me to say a few worlds in opening this Conference on the Clinical Potentials of Interferons in Viral Diseases and Malignant Tumors. On behalf of the Organizing Committee, first of all, I cordially welcome all the participants in the meeting.

Since this conference is sponsored by the Japan Medical Research Foundation, I think it is necessary to give a brief description of the foundation. It was established in October 1973, under the auspices of the Ministry of Welfare and Public Health, and its aim is to promote research on etiology and pathogenesis and to find effective treatments for various chronic intractable diseases that have attracted public attention in recent years.

One of the main activities of the Foundation is sponsoring international symposia or workshops on particular diseases or on special problems of medical importance, inviting eminent foreign researchers in the field and subsidizing their travel to Japan. All invited participants from both in and outside of Japan get together in closed or semi-closed conditions to discuss the topic, and the proceedings of the presentations and discussions are published within a year by the Foundation.

The first symposium, in 1974, which I also chaired, was on slow virus infections. From the beginning I have participated, as a virologist, on the Planning Committee. The clinical application of interferon is a most pertinent and attractive subject for an international conference sponsored by the foundation. The time is ripe to consider this subject, since the increased supply of interferon has made it possible to treat patients with virus diseases or malignancies in many countries on a trial basis, and so experience in interferon therapy is accumulating. I believe that Japanese experiences with fibroblast interferon will be of interest and valuable to the foreign participants; the results of our trial treatments have not been reported systematically before.

The clinical application of interferon has just begun, and hence there are still vast unknown areas at the moment. Therefore, I firmly believe it useful for investigators from many parts of the world to exchange their experiences and knowledge and discuss matters of mutual interest in the next three days. The number of participants are 18 from outside of Japan and 215 from this country. The organization and the program were constructed over a year's time by the members of the Executive Committee consisting of scientists from Japan and abroad. I am particularly grateful to Dr. Vilček and Dr. Merigan who participated as members of the committee and gave us valuable suggestions and help.

Finally, I would like to express our sincere appreciation to the Japan Medical Research Foundation and other organizations for their generous sponsorship of this Conference and to all of you distinguished participants from many countries. We hope all the foreign participants will also enjoy their stay here in Oiso and other places in Japan.

December 2, 1980

Reisaku KONO
Chairman of the Organizing Committe

THE CLINICAL POTENTIAL
OF INTERFERONS

The Status of Interferon Research

Jan VILČEK

Department of Microbiology, New York University School of Medicine, New York, NY 10016 U.S.A.

The field interferon research has grown tremendously since its humble beginnings over 20 years ago. It is, of course, impossible to summarize all the recent exciting developments in one short paper. Several hundred pages would probably be necessary to relay the important and new information emerging from the many interferon research centers throughout the world.

My paper will discuss only a few selected areas of recent progress. For obvious reasons, many examples of advances in interferon research I have selected for this paper are related to studies done in my own laboratory. This will give me the opportunity to present some of our recent work, particularly in the area of gamma (immune) interferon research. However, this disproportionate emphasis on some areas is not meant to imply that there are not many other branches of interferon research deserving credit. For example, a great deal of important progress has been attained in studies on the molecular mechanisms of interferon action. No attempt will be made to review these studies in this paper, although they clearly represent one of the most important areas of interferon research.

PURIFICATION OF INTERFERONS AND GENE CLONING

After two decades of unsuccessful attempts, several types of interferon (IFN) have been purified to homogeneity. It has thus become possible to establish the amino acid composition and partial amino acid sequence of some human and mouse IFNs.

When N-terminal amino acid sequences of HuIFN-β derived from human fibroblasts[1] and of a subspecies of HuIFN-α isolated from cultures of lymphoblastoid cells[2] were compared, no homology was found. These structural dif-

3

ferences are in good agreement with the known physicochemical,[3,4] biological,[5] and antigenic[6] differences of these two major species of human IFN (Table 1). In contrast, partial homology was found between the N-terminal amino acid sequences of two larger subspecies of mouse IFN and human IFN-β.[7] Even stronger homology was found between a small subspecies of mouse IFN and human IFN-α from lymphoblastoid cells.[7] These results are in good agreement with earlier findings of partial antigenic homology between certain IFN species in the mouse and man.[8,9] The findings indicate that some structural homology between corresponding IFN species has been preserved during evolution. Available evidence suggests that the structure of alpha interferons has remained more highly conserved than that of beta interferons.

Table 1. Some distinguishing properties of human alpha (leukocyte), beta (fibroblast), and gamma (immune) interferons.

Property	IFN-α	IFN-β	IFN-γ
Activity in bovine EBTr cells	High	Very low	Undetectable
Stability at pH 2	Stable	Stable	Unstable
Stability after 0.1 % SDS	Stable	Partially stable	Unstable
Binding to Concanavalin A-Sepharose	Mostly unbound	Complete	Complete
Apparent molecular weight	15,000–22,000	24,000	58,000
Approximate isoelectric point	5.0 to 7.0	6.5	8.6
Number of known subspecies	≥ 8	≥ 2	?

Direct analysis of purified IFNs is not the only source of information about the structure of IFN molecules. Even more useful information has been obtained as a result of IFN gene cloning—an area that only about one year ago appeared to belong to the realm of science fiction. The first successful cloning of an IFN DNA sequence was accomplished in Japan by Taniguchi et al.[10] employing mRNA isolated from induced human fibroblasts as the starting material. This work resulted in the elucidation of the nucleotide sequence of the cloned DNA and of the complete amino acid sequence deduced from it. The N-terminal amino acid sequence derived from the sequence analysis of cloned DNA[11] matched completely the sequence derived by Knight et al.[1] from the analysis of purified IFN-β.

Only a few months later Nagata et al.[12] reported the cloning of IFN-α cDNA made with mRNA isolated from induced human buffy coat cells. Comparison of the cloned IFN-α and IFN-β DNA sequences revealed that both IFNs are composed of 166 amino acids.[13] Of these, 48 appeared in the same position in both molecules, suggesting that the two IFNs have evolved from a common ancestral gene. The fact that the amino acid composition of more than two-thirds of the alpha and beta interferon molecules was different agrees well with the earlier described antigenic specificity of these two species of human IFN.[6] On the other hand, considerable structural homology can be found in the two molecules, particularly in the middle portions and near the C-terminal ends.[13] It is very likely that the conserved regions of the two molecules are important for biological activity.

A somewhat unexpected result of gene cloning experiments was the demonstration that IFN-α is comprised of numerous subspecies, each of them apparently coded for by separate structural genes.[14,15] IFN-α subspecies differ from each other in approximately 10–30% of amino acid residues, i.e., they are much more closely related to each other than to IFN-β. Although the exact number of IFN-α subspecies is not yet known, at least 8 have been identified so far. In contrast, only 2 subspecies of IFN-β have been tentatively recognized in recent experiments (ref. 16; M. Revel, personal communication).

Another surprising recent finding is the apparent absence of major carbohydrate residues in several subspecies of HuIFN-α.[17] This finding virtually shatters the 20-year-old belief that all IFNs are glycoproteins. However, it still seems fairly certain that IFN-β and IFN-γ are usually glycosylated (Table 1).

More information about the structure of IFNs has been accumulated within the last year than in the preceding two decades. Thus, for the first time it will be possible to launch meaningful structure-function studies with pure, homogeneous IFN preparations. The availability of large quantities of pure IFN-α and IFN-β synthesized in bacteria from cloned DNA sequences will undoubtedly facilitate future IFN research.

GAMMA INTERFERON RESEARCH

Compared to its more fortunate alpha and beta relatives, IFN-γ still suffers the fate of a poor Cinderella. But one day in the not so distant future Cinderella's prince will come—be it through the intervention of a fairy godmother or, perhaps, by gene cloning! In fact, there may already have been found at least one fairy godmother with the un-fairy-tale-like name of 12-0-tetradecanoylphorbol-13-acetate (TPA).

One of the major problems in IFN-γ research has been the lack of efficient, reproducible methods for its production. Without sufficient quantities of high-titered starting material, purification has remained an insurmountable task. Development of efficient production methods is also a prerequisite for successful cloning of the IFN cDNA.

Several methods of IFN-γ production have been described since Wheelock's original demonstration[18] that production of an "interferon-like" material could be stimulated in human lymphocytes by contact with phytohemagglutinin (PHA). All described methods of IFN-γ production are based on the stimulation of cultured lymphocytes with mitogens, e.g., lectins,[18] antilymphocytic serum,[19] or staphylococcal enterotoxin A.[20] Unfortunately, the yields of IFN produced with any of these mitogenes are generally quite variable.

TPA was shown to enhance the mitogenic activity of some lectins in lymphocyte cultures.[21,22] Furthermore, treatment of human lymphoblastoid cells with TPA was shown to enhance "spontaneous" IFN production.[23] These findings prompted us to examine the effect of TPA on PHA-induced production of IFN-γ in human lymphocyte cultures. Treatment with TPA resulted in a marked enhancement of IFN yields[24,25] in white blood cell cultures stimulated with PHA and many other T-cell mitogens.

Another important improvement in the methodology of IFN-γ production has come from the use of white blood cell concentrates generated as a by-product of plateletpheresis. Such plateletpheresis "residues" provide a rich source of human lymphocytes, which, for reasons that are not entirely understood, appear to represent a more efficient source of IFN-γ than mononuclear cells obtained from buffy coats. In our laboratory, mononuclear cells are routinely isolated from plateletpheresis residues by ficoll-hypaque centrifugation. Cultures are then seeded in serum-free RPMI 1640 medium and IFN-γ production is induced by combined treatment with TPA and PHA. Details of this procedure are described elsewhere (ref. 25; Y. K. Yip, manuscript in preparation).

This method has made possible the production of enough IFN-γ for partial physicochemical characterization.[25] Results obtained so far indicate that HuIFN-γ is likely to be a glycoprotein since virtually all activity was retained on Concanavalin A-Sepharose columns and subsequently eluted with a buffer containing α-methyl-D-mannopyranoside. This property is useful for differentiation between IFN-α, IFN-β and IFN-γ (Table 1). The apparent molecular weight determined by gel filtration on Biogel P-100 or P-200 columns was $58,000 \pm 3,000$. This result is in quite good agreement with an earlier report by Falcoff,[19] who had studied the properties of HuIFN-γ stimulated with antilymphocyte serum. In contrast, Langford et al.,[20] working with staphylococcal enterotoxin A-induced IFN, observed two components with apparent molecular weights of 40,000–46,000 and 65,000–70,000. Whether the molecular weights determined by gel filtration under nondenaturing conditions reflect the true molecular size of IFN-γ is not yet clear. It is well known that aggregation of IFN molecules can occur unless all noncovalent interactions are prevented. Unfortunately, the bulk of IFN-γ activity is irreversibly destroyed on exposure to sodium dodecyl sulfate, precluding a more conclusive analysis of molecular size of this IFN (Y. K. Yip et al., manuscript in preparation).

On isoelectric focusing of HuIFN-γ, the bulk of activity was recovered from a single peak with the PI of approximately 8.5.[25] This unusually high isolectric point, also observed by Langford et al.,[20] might explain the characteristic instability of IFN-γ on exposure to low pH. This property might facilitate the separation of IFN-γ from most other proteins in the crude material.

A relatively simple 3-step procedure resulted in a 1,000-fold purification of IFN-γ (to a specific activity greater than 10^7 units per mg of protein) with about 40% final recovery of IFN activity.[25] This accomplishment gives some reason for optimism about prospects for the complete purification of HuIFN-γ in the not too distant future. Availability of this IFN in pure form would allow direct analysis of the amino acid composition and sequence—much as was possible in the recent studies with some other IFN species.

In the meantime, some progress has been made in the characterization of HuIFN-γ mRNA.[26] It is hoped that this work will ultimately lead to the cloning of complementary DNA, making possible a rapid elucidation of the complete structure of this interferon. Cloning might also provide the ultimate means for the production of ample quantities of IFN-γ.

It thus appears that progress is being made towards the goal of a better understanding of IFN-γ structure and function. Sufficient quantities of highly purified material should soon become available to re-examine some fascinating observations made with relatively crude IFN-γ preparations, e.g., the reported potent cell growth inhibitory[27] and anti-tumor effects.[28,29] Will IFN-γ indeed prove to be more potent as an immunoregulatory substance and less potent as an antiviral agent than the other IFNs? Answers to these questions should be available in the not too distant future.

ROLE OF INTERFERON IN HOST RESISTANCE TO TUMORS

In recent years the major interest in IFN has shifted from its role as an antiviral agent to its potential as an antitumor substance. This change has occurred gradually as a result of several related developments, the roots of which can be traced back to demonstration of the inhibitory effect of IFNs on cell division, first reported in 1962 by Paucker et al.[30] This report was received with a great deal of skepticism, with most critics ascribing the cell growth inhibitory effect to impurities present in the crude IFN preparation.

In subsequent years several reports have been published on the inhibition of Friend leukemia in mice by IFN and IFN inducers.[31,32] The observed inhibitory effects on Friend leukemia were originally ascribed to an inhibition of the causative virus. However, an extension of these studies by Gresser and Bourali showed that treatment of mice with exogenous IFN also inhibited the growth of transplantable tumors, not known to be of viral origin.[33] Gradually it has become clear that the antitumor effects of IFN in transplantable tumors in mice definitely cannot be mediated by an inhibitory action on virus replication alone. The results obtained in experimental studies on mice undoubtedly had a strong influence on the pioneering clinical studies in tumor patients initiated by Strander and Cantell and their colleagues.[34]

Recent studies have corroborated and greatly extended earlier observations on the inhibitory action of interferon on cell growth (reviewed in ref. 35). However, not all antitumor effects of IFN in animals could be explained by a direct effect on tumor cell growth. It has become evident that at least some of these effects were due to a stimulation of cellular immune responses by IFN and, specifically, to an activation of cytotoxic lymphocytes[36-38] and macrophages.[39]

It appears that among the cytotoxic lymphocytes a critical role is being played by natural killer (NK) cells. First of all, the cytotoxicity of NK cells is strongly activatable by treatment with IFN.[38,40] Moreover, it appears that NK cells also become potent IFN producers when they are brought into contact with tumor cells.[40] Thus, IFN appears to represent an important autoregulatory mechanism in NK cells (Fig. 1).

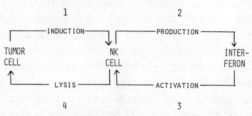

Fig. 1.   Proposed interrelationships among tumor cells, natural killer (NK) cells, and IFN. Numbers designate the sequence of events.

That this mechanism probably operates in the intact organism was recently demonstrated in an ingenious series of experiments by Minato et al.[41] These investigators employed athymic nude mice injected with various tumor cells. Human HeLa cells and hamster BHK cells readily produced tumors in the nude mice, but lost the ability to form tumors when they had been persistently infected with mumps or vesicular stomatitis virus. However, injection of mice with a potent anti-mouse IFN serum rendered nude mice susceptible to heterotransplantation with the persistently infected HeLa and BHK cells. This result indicated that IFN production, presumably induced by the viruses released from the persistently infected cells, was responsible for tumor rejection in the nude mice.

Somewhat unexpected was the finding that nude mice treated with anti-interferon serum also became more susceptible to tumor formation by HeLa or BHK cells which did not carry persistent virus infections.[41] This result suggests that IFN induction in response to tumor cells alone plays a role in host defense against the invading tumor. A related recent study in mice showed that the magnitude of IFN response to injected tumor cells correlates closely with the level of NK cell activity, supporting the existence of a close relationship between IFN and NK cells *in vivo*.[42]

These studies clearly established the role of the IFN system as a natural defense mechanism against tumors. Together with the demonstrated effects of IFN on cell division, these results provide some rational basis for the use of IFN in cancer therapy. However, in order to be able to predict the outcome of IFN therapy in cancer more accurately, we need to learn more about the interrelationship of IFN with various host defense mechanisms.

CONCLUSION

It is clear that IFN research is in a state of vigorous, excellent health. There has been rapid accumulation of new information about the structure and diversity of IFNs. These studies are now being followed by an analysis of the genetic control of IFN synthesis. With the aid of the available IFN DNA probes it is now possible not only to determine the number of related structural genes in a cell, but also to analyze their chromosomal localization. It is therefore likely that the controversies over the question of which chromosomes carry structural genes for IFN will soon be resolved, at least for IFN-α and IFN-β which cross-hybridize with the available probes.

With the newly available tools of recombinant DNA research it should now also be possible to make more rapid progress in our understanding of the process of IFN induction. Structural analysis of DNA sequences upstream from the coding sequences for the signal polypeptide might provide molecular clues for the mechanism of the unique event of IFN induction. Progress in this area would be most welcome as our understanding of how viruses or polynucleotides and other inducers turn on IFN production is still quite rudimentary.[43]

While progress in certain areas of IFN research is likely to be predictable, it is the promise of finding unexpected answers and the serendipitous discovery of new phenomena that make IFN research (and probably any other *good* research) truly exciting. Some time ago nobody could have "planned" the discovery of the role of 2', 5'-oligoadenylate as a major regulatory molecule involved in IFN action.[44] Equally unexpected was the emergence of the central role played by IFN in the regulation of NK cell cytotoxicity.[38,40,42] The large number of subspecies in the IFN-α family discovered by gene cloning[14,15] could not have been predicted from data available only a few months ago. Though unpredictable, this new information ultimately will not only contribute to our wealth of basic knowledge, but should also make it possible to use IFN in the prophylaxis and treatment of virus infections and tumors in a more intelligent, rational, and predictable way.

The organizers of this conference should be congratulated for bringing together leading scientists and clinicians from Japan and other parts of the world. The very rapid recent progress in IFN research makes it likely that at least some of the "clinical potentials of interferons in viral diseases and malignant tumors" will be realized in the near future.

REFERENCES

1. Knight, E., Jr., Hunkapiller, M. W., Korant, B. D., Hardy, R. W. F., and Hood, L. E.: Human fibroblast interferon: Amino acid analysis and amino terminal amino acid sequence. *Science*, **207**: 525–526, 1980.
2. Zoon, K. C., Smith, M. E., Bridgen, P. J., Anfinsen, C. B., Hunkapiller, M. W., and Hood, L. E.: Amino terminal sequence of the major component of human lymphoblastoid interferon. *Science*, **207**: 527–528, 1980.
3. Stewart, W. E., II, De Somer, P., Edy, V. G., Paucker, K., Berg, K., and Ogburn, C. A.: Distinct molecular species of human interferons: Requirement for stabilization and reactivation of human leukocyte and fibroblast interferons. *J. Gen. Virol.*, **26**: 327–331, 1975.
4. Vilček, J., Havell, E. A., and Yamazaki, S.: Antigenic, physicochemical, and biological characterization of human interferons. *Ann. N. Y. Acad. Sci.*, **284**: 703–710, 1977.
5. Gresser, I., Bandu, M.-T., Brouty-Boye, D., and Tovey, M.: Pronounced antiviral activity of human interferon on bovine and porcine cells. *Nature*, **251**: 543–545, 1974.
6. Havell, E. A., Berman, B., Ogburn, C., Berg, K., Paucker, K., and Vilček, J.: Two antigenically distinct species of human interferon. *Proc. Natl. Acad. Sci. U.S.A.*, **72**: 2185–2187, 1975.
7. Taira, H., Broeze, R. J., Jayaram, B. M., Lengyel, P., Hunkapiller, M. W., and Hood, L. E.: Mouse interferons: Amino terminal amino acid sequences of various species. *Science*, **207**: 528–530, 1980.
8. Havell, E. A.: Isolation of a subspecies of murine interferon antigenically related to human leukocyte interferon. *Virology*, **92**: 324–330, 1979.
9. Yamamoto, Y. and Kawade, Y.: Antigenicity of mouse interferons: Distinct antigenicity of the two L cell interferon species. *Virology*, **103**: 80–88, 1980.
10. Taniguchi, T., Sakai, M., Fujii-Kuriyama, Y., Muramatsu, M., Kobayashi, S., and Sudo, T.: Construction and identification of a bacterial plasmid containing the human fibroblast interferon gene sequence. *Proc. Japan. Acad.*, **55** (B): 464–469, 1979.
11. Taniguchi, T., Ohno, S., Fujii-Kuriyama, Y., and Muramatsu, M.: The nucleotide sequence of human fibroblast interferon cDNA. *Gene*, **10**: 11–15, 1980.
12. Nagata, S., Taira, H., Johnsrud, L., Hall, A., Streuli, M., Escodi, J., Cantell, K., and Weissmann, C.: Synthesis in *E. coli* of a polypeptide with human leukocyte interferon activity. *Nature*, **284**: 316–320, 1980.
13. Taniguchi, T., Mantei, N., Schwarzstein, M., Nagata, S., Muramatsu, M., and Weissmann, C.: Human leukocyte and fibroblast interferons are structurally related. *Nature*, **285**: 547–549, 1980.
14. Nagata, S., Mantei, N., and Weissmann, C.: The structure of the eight or more distinct chromosomal genes for human interferon-α. *Nature*, **287**: 401–408, 1980.
15. Goeddel, D. V., Leung, D. W., Dull, T. J., Gross, M., Lawn, R. M., McCandliss, R., Seeburg, P. H., Ullrich, A., Yelverton, E., and Gray, P. W.: The structure of eight distinct cloned human leukocyte interferon cDNAs. *Nature*, **290**: 20–26, 1981.

16. Sehgal, P. B. and Sagar, A. D.: Heterogeneity of poly (I). poly(C)-induced human fibroblast interferon mRNA species. *Nature*, **288**: 95–97, 1980.
17. Allen, G. and Fantes, K. H.: A family of structural genes for human lymphobastoid (leukocyte-type) interferon. *Nature*, **287**: 408–411, 1980.
18. Wheelock, E. F.: Interferon-like virus-inhibitor induced in human leukocytes by phytohemagglutinin. *Science*, **149**: 310–311, 1965.
19. Falcoff, R.: Some properties of virus and immune-induced human lymphocyte interferons. *J. Gen. Virol.*, **16**: 251–253, 1972.
20. Langford, M. P., Georgiades, J. A., Stanton, G. J., Dianzani, F., and Johnson, H. M.: Large-scale production and physicochemical characterization of human immune interferon. *Infect. Immun.*, **26**: 36–41, 1979.
21. Mastro, A. M. and Mueller, G. C.: Synergistic action of phorbol esters in mitogen activated bovine lymphocytes. *Exp. Cell Res.*, **88**: 40–46, 1974.
22. Wang, J. L., McClain, D. A., and Edelman, G. M.: Modulation of lymphocyte mitogenesis. *Proc. Natl. Acad. Sci. USA*, **72**: 1917–1921, 1975.
23. Klein, G. and Vilček, J.: Attempts to induce interferon production by IUDR-induction and EBV-superinfection in human lymphoma lines and their hybrids. *J. Gen. Virol.*, **46**: 111–117, 1980.
24. Vilček, J., Sulea, I. T., Volvovitz, F., and Yip, Y. K.: Characterization of interferons produced in cultures of human lymphocytes by stimulation with *Corynebacterium parvum* and phytohemagglutinin. In: A. L. De Weck, F. Kristensen and M. Landy (eds.), Biochemical Characterization of Lymphokines. Academic Press, 1980, p. 323.
25. Yip, Y. K., Pang, R. H. L., Urban, C., and Vilček, J.: Partial purification and characterization of human gamma (immune) interferon. *Proc. Natl. Acad. Sci. USA*, **78**: 1601–1605, 1981.
26. Taniguchi, T., Pang, R. H. L., Yip, Y. K., Henriksen, D., and Vilček, J.: Partial characterization of gamma (immune) interferon mRNA extracted from human lymphocytes. *Proc. Natl. Acad. Sci. USA*, **78**: 3469–3472, 1981.
27. Rubin, B. Y. and Gupta, S. L.: Differential efficacies of human type I and type II interferons as antiviral and antiproliferative agents. *Proc. Natl. Acad. Sci. USA*, **77**: 5928–5932, 1980.
28. Crane, J. L., Glasgow, L. A., Kern, E. R., and Younger, J. S.: Inhibition of murine osteogenic sarcomas by treatment with type I or type II interferon. *J. Nat. Cancer Inst.*, **61**: 871–874, 1978.
29. Fleischmann, W. R., Kleyn, K. M., and Baron, S.: Potentiation of antitumor effect of virus-induced interferon by mouse immune interferon preparations. *J. Nat. Cancer Inst.*, **65**: 963–966, 1980.
30. Paucker, K., Cantell, K., and Henle, W.: Quantitative studies on viral interference in suspended L cells. III. Effect of interfering viruses and interferon on the growth rate of cells. *Virology*, **17**: 324–334, 1962.
31. Gresser, I., Copey, J., Falcoff, E., and Fontaine, D.: Interferon and murine leukemia. I. Inhibitory effects of interferon preparations on development of Friend leukemia in mice. *Proc. Soc. Exp. Biol. Med.*, **124**: 84–91, 1967.
32. Wheelock, E. F.: Effect of statolon on Friend virus leukemia in mice. *Proc. Soc. Exp. Biol. Med.*, **124**: 855–858, 1967.
33. Gresser, I. and Bourali, C.: Exogenous interferon and inducers of interferon in the treatment of Balb/c mice inoculated with RC_{19} tumor cells. *Nature*, **223**: 844–845, 1969.
34. Strander, H., Cantell, K., Carstrom, G., and Jakobsson, P. A.: Clinical and laboratory investigations in man: Systemic administration of potent interferon to man. *J. Nat. Cancer Inst.*, **51**: 733–742, 1973.

35. Taylor-Papadimitriou, J.: Effects of interferons on cell growth and function. In: I. Gresser (ed.) Interferon 1980. Academic Press, London, 1980, p. 13.
36. Svet-Moldavsky, G. J. and Chernyakovskaya, I. Y.: Interferon and the interaction of allogeneic normal and immune lymphocytes with L cells. Nature, 215: 1299–1300, 1967.
37. Lindahl, P., Leary, P., and Gresser, I.: Enhancement by interferon of the specific cytotoxicity of sensitized lymphocytes. Proc. Natl. Acad. Sci. USA, 69: 721–725, 1972.
38. Gidlund, M., Orn, A., Wigzell, H., Senik, A., and Gresser, I.: Enhanced NK cell activity in mice injected with interferon and interferon inducers. Nature, 273: 759–761, 1978.
39. Schultz, R. M., Papamatheakis, J. D., and Chirigos, M. A.: Interferon: An inducer of macrophage activation by polyanions. Science, 197: 674–676, 1977.
40. Santoli, D., Trinchieri, G., and Koprowski, H.: Cell-mediated cytotoxicity against virus-infected target cells in humans. II. Interferon induction and activation of natural killer cells. J. Immunol., 121: 532–538, 1978.
41. Minato, N., Reid, L., Neighbour, A., Bloom, B. R., and Holland, J.: Interferon, NK cells and persistent virus infection. Ann. N. Y. Acad. Sci., 350: 42–54, 1980.
42. Djeu, J. Y., Huang, K.-Y., and Herberman, R. B.: Augmentation of mouse natural killer activity and induction of interferon by tumor cells in vivo. J. Exp. Med., 151: 781–789, 1980.
43. Vilček, J. and Kohase, M.: Regulation of interferon production: Cell culture studies. Tex. Rep. Biol. Med., 35: 57–62, 1977.
44. Kerr, I. M. and Brown, R. E.: ppA 2'p5'A2'p5'A: An inhibitor of protein synthesis synthesized with an enzyme fraction from interferon-treated cells. Proc. Natl. Acad. Sci. USA, 75: 256–260, 1978.

Discussion

Dr. OHTSUKI: What is the difference in molecular mechanism between alpha and gamma interferons?

Dr. VILČEK: I don't think anybody can answer this question with any degree of certainty. However, there are some differences that I mentioned in my talk and others that I didn't have a chance to mention. For instance, as I said, it was shown by Dr. Dianzani that the induction of the antiviral state is much slower with gamma interferon than with the other interferons, suggesting that perhaps the primary role of this interferon is not to function as an antiviral molecule, but to mediate some other activities. It can be shown that there is an induction of several new enzymes in cells treated with gamma interferon. For instance, there is induction of the 2'-5'(A)-synthetase, and I believe that it was also shown that there is induction of the kinase in cells treated with gamma interferon. But the relative proportions of the newly induced proteins are different in cells stimulated with gamma interferon and in cells stimulated with alpha interferon. I have the results of an experiment done in our laboratory that I did not show, which confirm a previous observation made in Dr. Baron's laboratory, showing that there is a cooperative effect between gamma interferon on the one hand and alpha or beta interferon on the other hand, which also suggests that the mechanism of action is somewhat different with the two types of interferon.

Dr. KAWADE: Have you conducted studies with the gamma interferon that are similar to your earlier studies with the alpha and beta interferons, on the action of the glycosylation inhibitor?

Dr. VILČEK: Yes, indeed. I didn't have time to show all the results, but we did show very clearly that tunicamycin as well as 2-deoxy-glucose cause a dose-dependent inhibition of gamma interferon production in our system. This probably confirms the conclusion that gamma interferon is a glycoprotein.

Dr. KAWADE: Carter *et al.* have used tunicamycin and reported that gamma interferon production is not inhibited. So your results would not coincide with theirs, is that correct?

Dr. VILČEK: That is correct.

Dr. KAWADE: My next question concerns the antiviral activity of gamma interferon. As you have already mentioned in your lecture, there are several reports of the high antiviral activity of gamma interferon. Have you carried out any comparisons of activity on the purified material that you obtained?

Dr. VILČEK: Not with the purified material. We did some preliminary experiments, but I would rather not tell you about this publicly. I'll tell you about the results privately.

Dr. KAWADE: Thank you.

Dr. BORDEN: Have you looked at the production of alpha and beta interferons as enhanced by TPA? Is this an effect unique to gamma interferons, in terms of TPA augmentation of interferon production, or does it also apply to alpha and beta with Poly I : C, NDV, etc.?

Dr. VILČEK: Thank you for bringing up this question. In fact, both alpha and beta interferon synthesis, in several systems that we studied, is inhibited by TPA. This is an additional advantage, in my opinion, because you obtain much more homogeneous starting material. Many investigators find that their crude preparations of gamma interferon are contaminated by alpha or beta interferon. We don't find this, and I believe that this is because of the use of TPA.

Dr. BORDEN: Do you have some speculations as to the cellular mechanisms involved with augmentation of gamma production and depression of alpha and beta?

Dr. VILČEK: TPA is one of the few molecules that exerts more biological effects than interferon. There are hundreds of various effects of TPA described in the literature, including the enhancement of the synthesis of some proteins and the inhibition of the synthesis of other proteins. Probably all of these effects are the result of interaction with the cell membrane, but I don't think I care to speculate on the mechanism any further.

Dr. TOVEY: Your method of producing gamma interferon with TPA is certainly a very efficient method, as we have found also since you reported this. There is one problem, though. You mentioned possible clinical trials. As you know, TPA is a tumor promoter, and also an extremely efficient inducer of EBV virus; and as most people are sero-positive for EB virus and indeed harbor latent virus, probably in their lymphocytes, may this not pose problems?

Dr. VILČEK: That is a very valid point. Before any clinical trials can even be planned, one would have to make sure that TPA is removed in the purification process. I don't believe this should be too difficult, because of the low molecular weight of

TPA compared to interferon, and most likely—although we have not checked it—TPA would be efficiently removed during a purification sequence such as the one that I showed.

Dr. TOVEY: What's probably more difficult is eliminating the induction of latent EBV and in fact there is a synergistic induction of EBV with PHA. PHA also induces latent EB virus.

Dr. REVEL: You mentioned that the gamma interferon works more slowly to establish the antiviral effect. Have you measured the kinetics of 2′-5′ oligo(A)synthetase induction to see if it is slower with gamma interferon than with the other interferons?

Dr. VILČEK: We have not done that, but Corrado Baglioni has a paper in press showing that the induction of 2′-5′(A) is much slower than with the other interferons.

Dr. BILLIAU: You mentioned that you did your titrations on trisomic cells. Is it correct that the immune interferon, the gamma type, also has a differential effect on trisomic cells? Are the titers higher on trisomic cells, in your hands?

Dr. VILČEK: We have not made a systematic comparison between many different diploid cells and cells with trisomy 21. We only compared one diploid cell, FS7, and one cell with trisomy 21, the GM-258 cell strain, and there is a clear difference between these two cell strains, in that the cell with trisomy 21 is much more sensitive. We have not done enough studies to be sure that this difference is really due to the extra chromosome 21.

Dr. BILLIAU: We also did some comparisons, although not extensive ones, but there is a large variability in different lines of diploid cells. The trisomic ones fell in between the other ones.

I.

PRODUCTION AND PURIFICATION OF HUMAN INTERFERONS

Preparation of Human Leukocyte Interferon for Clinical Use

H.-L. Kauppinen, V. Koistinen, G. Myllylä, S. Hirvonen, and K. Cantell

Finnish Red Cross Blood Transfusion Service, Kivihaantie 7 and Central Public Health Laboratory, Mannerheimintie 166, Helsinki, Finland

INTRODUCTION

Human leukocyte interferon (HuIFN-α) has been produced in our laboratories for clinical use for several years. The total production has increased yearly, due to the increased number of blood units utilized and the increased recovery of IFN. However, the number of blood units has not increased in the last 2 years, but optimization of the preparation procedures has resulted in more than a 2-fold increase of production of crude IFN per blood unit. This paper describes briefly the present method used in our laboratories.[1,2]

METHODS

Collection of Buffy Coats

The blood, about 450 ml, is collected into a double bag system. The primary bag contains 63 ml of CPD solution (Fenwal, R. 1632). The blood bags are centrifuged at 6,400 g for 4 min at 4°C. The plasma is pressed into a transfer bag. The tubing connecting the bags is cut. The buffy coat is harvested into a special siphon measuring a volume of 40 ml. Twenty-five buffy coats are pooled in a 1,000 ml flask fitted to the siphon. The pooled buffy coats are stored overnight at 4°C for production.

After harvesting the buffy coats, 80 ml of saline-adenine-glucose solution[3] is transferred from the satellite bag into the leukocyte-poor, packed red cell concentrate which is used clinically.

Purification of Leukocytes

The pooled buffy coats are purified in batches of 50 units by hemolyzing the

17

red cells with 8 liters of cold 0.83% NH_4Cl for 10 min. The suspension is centrifuged by continuous flow basket centriguge at 1,100–1,400 g at a flow rate of 300 ml per min. Three pools of 50 buffy coats are centrifuged successively in the same rotor. The cells are suspended in PBS (pH 7.4 with 25 μg of neomycin per ml, without calcium or magnesium) and harvested into one liter centrifuge bottles. The bottles are filled with cold NH_4Cl, kept for 10 min at 4° C, and centrifuged at 165–200 g for 25 min. The purified cells are resuspended in 100 ml of cold incubation medium and kept on a magnetic stirrer in an ice bath until used for culture.

Recovery of Leukocytes

The recovery of leukocytes from a buffy coat of 40 ml is 1.65×10^9 cells. A good half of these, i.e., 0.9×10^9 cells, are mononuclear cells. They comprise about 90% of the total amount of lymphocytes in the original blood unit.[4]

During the purification process 25–30% of the cells are lost, roughly equal proportions of mono- and polymorphonuclear cells. Practically all the cells are viable. The purified cell suspension contains around 1.15×10^9 leukocytes per buffy coat.

Incubation

Incubation of cells is carried out in wide-neck, round-bottom 6 liter flasks. The cells are suspended in medium to a concentration of 1×10^7 viable cells per ml. The medium consists of Eagle's minimum essential medium (MEM) without phosphates, and it is supplemented with 3 mg tricine, 25 μg of neomycin, and 1.8 mg of human "agamma serum" per ml. The pH of the medium is adjusted to 7.4–7.5. High-titer crude IFN is added to a final concentration of 100–200 IU per ml for priming of the cells.

The incubation flasks are half-filled with culture suspension. They are covered loosely with aluminum foil and incubated in a water bath at 37.5° C. The cells are kept in agitation by magnetic stirring. About 2 hours later Sendai virus is added to a final concentration of 100–150 HA per ml. IFN synthesis is detected 2 hours after induction and the maximum IFN activity is reached in 5 or 6 hours after induction. In routine practice the incubation is continued overnight. On the next morning cells and debris are removed by centrifugation. The supernatant, the crude IFN, is stored at 4° C for purification.

Cell Concentration

The cell concentration of 1×10^7 cells per ml used routinely is based on earlier studies[5] for optimum cell concentration for the highest IFN titer per ml. Recently, systematic studies were performed by carrying out production at different cell concentrations between 0.25 and 2×10^7 cells per ml. Several pools of 21.5–43 liters of crude IFN were prepared at different cell densities, and the samples of the pools assayed for IFN. The results showed that the titers were best at about 1×10^7 cells per ml. When IFN recovery was calculated as unit per cell, the maximum yield was achieved at the concentration of 0.25–0.5 $\times 10^7$ cells per ml. The highest cell concentration at which recovery of IFN was optimal appeared to be 0.5 $\times 10^7$ cells per ml. At this concentration about 10^7 IU of crude IFN were obtained per buffy coat.

Purification

A method has been developed for a large scale purification of IFN.[6,7] The proteins in crude IFN are precipitated with 0.5 M KSCN at pH 3.5 and the precipitate dissolved in 94% ethanol at —20°C in one-fifth of the volume of the original crude IFN. The pH of the supernatant is raised by steps while the impurities are precipitated into two fractions at pH 5.5 and 5.75. Finally, IFN is precipitated at pH 8. This precipitate is dissolved in 0.1 M phosphate buffer, pH 8.0, with 0.5 M KSCN.

The partially purified IFN achieved is concentrated by precipitating in two fractions. The first fraction, P-IF B, is precipitated at pH 5.1–4.7, and the second fraction, P-IF A, at pH 2.8. The precipitates are dissolved in 0.1 M phosphate buffer, pH 8.0, with 0.5 M KSCN and finally dialyzed against PBS, pH 7.3. The total recovery is 60–70%. The relative recovery and the purity of the two fractions depend on the pH at which P-IF B is removed. The specific activities of the preparations range between 1 and 5×10^6 IU/mg of protein. SDS-polyacrylamide gel electrophoresis shows that both fractions are heterogeneous and contain different proportions of distinct molecular forms of INF. Since no difference in the biological activity of these fractions has been found so far, they are routinely pooled in preparations for clinical use.

REFERENCES

1. Cantell, K., Hirvonen, S., Kauppinen, H.-L., and Myllylä, G.: Production of interferon in human leukocytes from normal donors with the use of Sendai virus. In: S. Pestka (ed.) Methods in Enzymology. Academic Press, New York, in press.
2. Cantell, K., Hirvonen, S., and Koistinen, V.: Partial purification of human leukocyte interferon on a large scale. In: S. Pestka (ed.), Methods in Enzymology. Academic Press, New York, in press.
3. Högman, C. F., Hedlund, K., and Zetterström, H.: Clinical usefulness of red cells preserved in protein-poor mediums. *N. Engl. J. Med.*, **299**: 1377–1382, 1978.
4. Kauppinen, H.-L. and Myllylä, G.: Efficient use of blood leukocytes for interferon production. In: A. Khan, N. O. Hill, and G. Dorn, (eds.), Interferon: Properties and Clinical Uses. Leland Fikes Foundation Press, Dallas, 1980, p. 1.
5. Cantell, K., Strander, H., Hadhazy, G., and Nevanlinna, H. R.: How much interferon can be prepared in human leukocyte suspensions. In: The Interferons. Academic Press, New York, 1968, p. 223.

6. Cantell, K., Hirvonen, S., Mogensen, K. E., and Pyhälä, L.: In: (ed.) C. Waymouth. The production and use of interferon for the treatment and prevention of human virus infections. Tissue Culture Association, Rockville, Md., 1974, p. 35.
7. Cantell, K. and Hirvonen, S.: Large scale production of human leukocyte interferon containing 10^8 units per ml. *J. Gen. Virol.*, **39**: 541–543, 1978.

Discussion

Dr. BILLIAU: When you increase the buffy coat harvest to 40 m, do you then have considerably more red cells than when you don't? Is this not disturbing? How far can you go, in other words?

Dr. KAUPPINEN: The amount of cells increase with increasing volume of buffy coat, thus more ammonium chloride is needed to hemolyse them, but not quite in same proportion. Earlier we used 6 volumes of ammonium chloride per one volume of buffy coat, but now we are using only 4 volumes that seems to be still enough to hemolyse the red cells.

Dr. FINTER: Could I ask what proportion of all the blood that is available to the Finnish Red Cross and to Dr. Cantell is processed for making interferon? You said you are processing 90,000 buffy coats per annum. How much more would it be possible to process in Finland?

Dr. KAUPPINEN: We get about 120,000 units of fresh blood in Finland, which are available for buffy coat harvesting without any further difficulties. But as you may think, the number of blood units varies from day to day. Some days we get so many that we cannot handle them all. Besides those 120,000 units we have over 200,000 blood units harvested in Finland, which are not available for interferon production unless we change our normal system of blood processing.

Dr. KOBAYASHI: Could I ask you about the contaminants originating in egg protein or Sendai virus protein in your preparation? What amount of egg protein or virus protein is there in your sample?

Dr. KAUPPINEN: Our P-1F preparation contains roughly 0.1% interferon. It does contain virus protein as well egg proteins. The amount of these is not known. They can be detected, since patients make antibodies against these proteins. So far, no allergic reactions have occurred.

Dr. KOBAYASHI: So now you have no anxiety over using your interferon, and neither will you in the future?

Dr. KAUPPINEN: Of course we are looking forward to getting more purified interferon and to being able to use monoclonal antibody. That will be the next step.

Preparation and Properties of Human Leukocyte Interferon

Akio MATSUO,* Takaaki FUJITA,* Saburo HAYASHI,* Tadakazu SUYAMA,* Jiro IMANISHI,[2]* and Tsunataro KISHIDA[2]*

*Research Laboratories, The Green Cross Corporation, 3-5-44, Miyakojima-Nakadori, Miyakojima-ku, Osaka, [2]*Department of Microbiology, Kyoto Prefectural University of Medicine, Kawaramachi, Kamikyo-ku, Kyoto 602, Japan

SUMMARY

An HuIFN-α preparation for clinical use, partially purified by chromatography on SP-Sephadex C-25 and gel filtration on Sephadex G-100, was separated into two molecular populations with peaks at about 21,500 and 15,000 daltons by SDS-polyacrylamide gel electrophoresis. On isoelectric focusing it migrated into a broad band of activity distributed from pH 5.0 to 7.0 with peaks at pI 5.4 and 5.8. It was resolved into two components by poly U or ConA-Sepharose chromatography. The two components separated by poly U-Sepharose chromatography were similar to those separated by ConA-Sepharose chromatography in the molecular weight. The poly U-nonbinding component of HuIFN-α did not bind to ConA-Sepharose, but the poly U-binding component was further separated into two components by ConA-Sepharose chromatography. There was no significant difference in the growth inhibition of Raji cells among the fractions obtained by ConA-Sepharose chromatography. These data suggest that the HuIFN-α preparation contains at least three molecular species: (1) the 15,000-dalton IFN species having neither a carbohydrate moiety nor an affinity to polynucleotide, (2) the 15,000-dalton species having an affinity to polynucleotide but no carbohydrate moiety, and (3) the 21,500-dalton species having both a carbo-hydrate moiety and an affinity to polynucleotide. The low molecular weight species seems to be slightly more acidic than the high molecular weight species.

INTRODUCTION

The clinical use of human leukocyte interferon (HuIFN-α) in the treatment of viral and malignant diseases has expanded rapidly during the past few years. In 1970 we began our work on the production and purification of HuIFN-α

21

and started to treat patients with various diseases systemically or topically. Some workers have reported that there are more than one molecular varieties of HuIFN-α.[2-10] There is some controversy about whether HuIFN-α contains a carbohydrate moiety.[11-15]

The primary purpose of this report is to describe a procedure for the further purification of HuIFN-α. Incidentally in our experiments we found of that HuIFN-α demonstrated different affinities to poly U and ConA because of the heterogeneity in molecular size and charge and these observation will also be described.

MATERIALS AND METHODS

Preparation of HuIFN-α

Human leukocytes were purified with 0.83 % ammonium chloride from buffy coats and adjusted to 10^7 viable cells/ml with Eagle's MEM supplemented with 5 % Plasmanate. After pretreatment of crude IFN at a concentration of 100 IU/ml for 2 hours at 37° C, it was kept standing for 2 days at pH 2 and 4° C to inactivate Sendai virus.

Purification of HuIFN-α

The outline of the purification procedure is shown in Fig. 1. We used SP-Sephadex C-25 for the concentration and partial purification of HuIFN-α with a modifications of Bodo's method[16] for the purification of Namalwa inter-

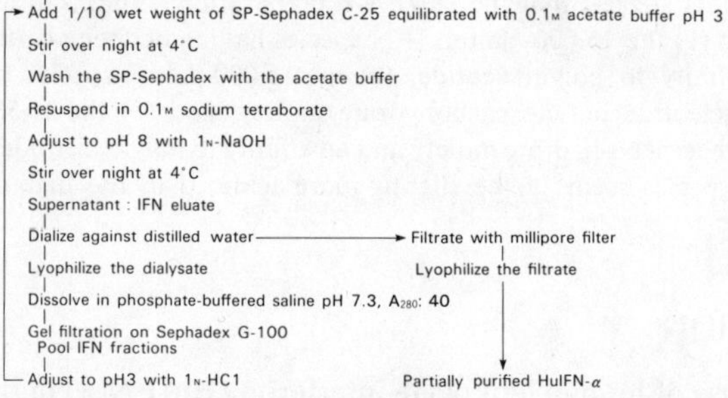

Human leukocyte suspension, 1×10^7 cell/ml in Eagles MEM plus Plasmanate(5%)
IFN priming, 100 IU/ml for 2hr at 37°C
Inoculate purified Sendai virus, 100 HA/ml
Incubate for 20hr at 37°C
Supernatant : crude IFN
Adjust to pH 2 with 10$_N$-HCL
Preserve for 2 days at 4°C : inactivation of Sendai virus
Supernatant
Adjust to pH 3 with 5$_N$-NaOH
Add 1/10 wet weight of SP-Sephadex C-25 equilibrated with 0.1$_M$ acetate buffer pH 3
Stir over night at 4°C
Wash the SP-Sephadex with the acetate buffer
Resuspend in 0.1$_M$ sodium tetraborate
Adjust to pH 8 with 1$_N$-NaOH
Stir over night at 4°C
Supernatant : IFN eluate
Dialize against distilled water ⟶ Filtrate with millipore filter
Lyophilize the dialysate   Lyophilize the filtrate
Dissolve in phosphate-buffered saline pH 7.3, A$_{280}$: 40
Gel filtration on Sephadex G-100
  Pool IFN fractions
Adjust to pH3 with 1$_N$-HC1   Partially purified HuIFN-α

Fig. 1.   Preparation of human leukocyte interferon for clinical use.

feron. SP-Sephadex is a good adsorbent of HuIFN-α as well as of Namalwa interferon.

SDS-polyacrylamide Gel Electrophoresis

Molecular weights were determined under nonreducing conditions to maintain full interferon activity. Dried samples and markers were dissolved in 25% glycerol-1% SDS-0.02 M phosphate buffer, pH 7.2, and kept overnight at room temperature; 0.1% SDS-10% polyacylamide gel was prepared in glass tubes of 0.5 cm in diameter. SDS-treated 20-μl aliquots were placed on the gel; 0.1% SDS-0.1 M phosphate buffer, pH 7.2, was used as the tray buffer. Electrophoresis was carried out for 5 hours at a constant current (8 mA/gel) and temperature. Gel slices of 2-mm thickness were extracted by shaking with 0.5 ml of 0.1% SDS-phosphate buffered saline (PBS), pH 7.2, to measure interferon activity. The marker's gel was stained overnight with a 0.25% Coomassie Brilliant Blue solution ($H_2O:CH_3COOH:MeOH = 5:1:5$) and destained in 7% acetic acid -5% methanol.

Isoelectric Focusing

Isoelectric focusing was performed in an LKB-8100 Ampholine column consisting of a sucrose density gradient from 0 to 50%, and 1% carrier ampholyte ranging from pH 3.5 to 10. A dried sample was dissolved in 2.6 ml of a solution equivalent to the center of the gradient and charged to the center of the column. A current of 300 V was applied for 48 hours at 2°C. Fractions of 3 ml were collected and their A_{280} and pH values were measured. A 1-ml portion of each fraction was added to the same volume of 5% human albumin in PBS and the mixtures were dialyzed against PBS for interferon assay.

Interferon Assay

HuIFN-α was assayed from reduced CPE on the FL cell-VSV system on microtest plates. All titers were expressed in relation to the titer of the international reference preparation 69/19.

Cell-growth Inhibition by the Three Fractions Separated by ConA-Sepharose Chromatography

The SP-Sephadex eluate was chromatographed under the conditions shown in Fig. 5. The ConA-binding and nonbinding fractions and the SP-Sephadex eluate were tested for growth inhibition of Raji cells. Each sample was diluted so as to contain 2,000 IU interferon activity/ml in RPMI 1640 containing 10% fetal bovine serum. The suspension of Raji cells adjusted to 2×10^5 cells/ml with the medium was dispensed in 50-μl quantities into the wells of the semimicroplate (FB-16-24TC, Linbro, Inc.), and 50 μl of a diluted sample was added to duplicate wells. After incubation in a humidified 5% CO$_2$ atmosphere at 37°C, the viable cells were counted at specified intervals.

RESULTS AND DISCUSSIONS

In the purification of HuIFN-α by the procedure shown in Fig. 1, crude HuIFN-α was purified about 5-fold with a recovery of 70% by batch-wise SP-Sephadex C-25 chromatography. Concentration of HuIFN-α with SP-Sephadex C-25 appears to be very useful for preventing loss of the activity on subsequent gel filtration. Gel filtration of the concentrated SP-Sephadex eluate on Sephadex G-100 increased the specific activity 60-fold or more, and most of the activity applied was recovered. Thus, HuIFN-α was purified by these two step by 250-fold or more with a maximum recovery of 50%.

Figure 2 shows the molecular weight distribution of partially purified HuIFN-α in 0.1% SDS-10% polyacrylamide gel electrophoresis under non-reducing conditions. As Stewart and Desmyter.[8] reported, interferon activity were separated into two molecular populations with peaks at molecular weights of about 21,500 and 15,000 daltons. There was much more activity in the 15,000-dalton fraction than in the 21,500-dalton one.

Figure 3 is the pattern of isoelectric focusing of the HuIFN-α preparation. The

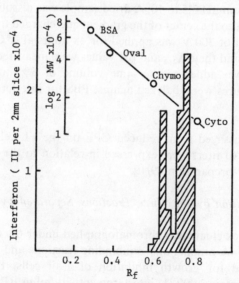

Fig. 2. SDS-polyacrylamide gel electrophoresis of partially purified HuIFN-α without reduction. Input, 85,000 IU; recovery, 93%. Electrophoresis time, 5 h, 8 mA/gel, at room temperature. O——O: molecular weight markers; BSA: bovine serum albumin; Oval: ovalbumin; Chymo: chymotrypsinogen; Cyto: cytochrome c; ▨▨▨: interferon.

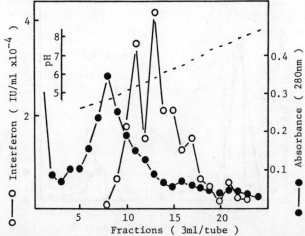

Fig. 3. Isoelectric focusing of partially purified HuIFN-α. Input: 1,735,000 IU; recovery: 35.5%; ●——● : A_{280}; ○——○ : interferon; – – – – : pH.

interferon activity migrated in a broad band ranging from pH 5.0 to pH 7.0, and two activity peaks were detected at pI 5.41 and pI 5.84.

Recently DeMaeyer-Guignard et al.[17] reported that mouse interferon had a high affinity for some polynucleotides, especially poly I and poly U. They purified mouse interferon to about 2×10^9 reference units of specific activity by sequential affinity chromatography on poly U-Sepharose and antibody-agarose columns.[18] We also tried affinity chromatography on poly U-Sepharose for the further purification of HuIFN-α. As shown in Fig. 4, most of the interferon activity (70%) passed through the poly U-Sepharose column under the same conditions as those for mouse interferon, and only 30% was retained.

Moreover, the interferon moved together with the protein contaminant. Accordingly, we could not purify HuIFN-α any further, in contrast to the situation with mouse interferon. However, we found that HuIFN-α was resolved into at least two components by poly U-Sepharose chromatography. The mechanism by which interferon to polynucleotide is not clear, but we speculated that the affinity of interferon is bound to polynucleotide might differ depending upon the carbohydrate moiety of the interferon molecule.

We next attempted the chromatograph of partially purified HuIFN-α on Con-A-Sepharose. Jankowski et al.[13] and Davey et al.[14] reported that HuIFN-α did not bind to ConA-Sepharose, but we found that 20% of the applied interferon activity was bound to ConA-Sepharose under different conditions,[19] and all the activity was recovered with α-methyl-D-glucoside (Fig. 5). It is apparent, therefore, that HuIFN-α can also be resolved into two components by ConA-

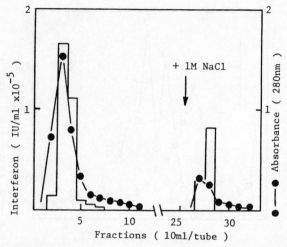

Fig. 4. Affinity chromatography of partially purified HuIFN-α on poly U-Sepharose 4B. Column, 1 × 19 cm, equilibrated with 0.01 M Tris-HCl buffer, pH 7.5, plus 0.02% NaN₃, flow rate, 6 ml/hr, at room temperature. Input, 4,249,000 IU; recovery, 104%; ●——● : A₂₈₀; □ : interferon.

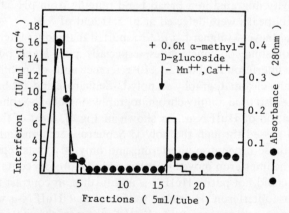

Fig. 5. Affinity chromatography of partially purified HuIFN-α on Con A-Sepharose. Column, 0.9 × 10 cm, equilibrated with 0.02 M Tris-HCl. buffer, pH 6.8 containing 1M NaCl, 10 mM MnCl₂, 10 mM CaCl₂, 0.02% NaN₃, flow rate, 6 ml/hr, at room temperature. Input, 1,908,000 IU; recovery, 110%, ●——● : A₂₈₀; □ : interferon.

Sepharose chromatography, and it is likely that the binding of HuIFN-α to ConA-Sepharose is attributable to the sugar moiety.

In the next experiment, we tried to determine whether the binding property of HuIFN-α to poly U-Sepharose was correlated with that to ConA-Sepharose. Table 1 summarizes the molecular weights and pI of the two components separated by poly U and ConA-Sepharose chromatography. Figures 6 and 7

Table 1. Properties of the components of partially purified HuIFN-α in affinity to poly U and ConA.

Component	Ratio	Molecular weights	pI (range)
Partially purified	70	15,000	5.4, 5.8 (5.0–7.0)
HuIFN-α	30	21,500	
poly U-nonbinding	70	14,500	5.5 (5.0–6.4)
poly U-binding	24, 6	21,000, 15,000	5.9 (5.4–7.0)
ConA-nonbinding	80	13,000	—
ConA-binding	20	21,000	—

show the chromatography of poly U-nonbinding and -binding components on ConA-Sepharose. The poly U-nonbinding component of HuIFN-α bound very title to ConA-Sepharose, but the poly U-binding component was further separated into two components by ConA-Sepharose chromatography.

These data suggest that HuIFN-α preparations contain at least three molecular species, two low molecular species of HuIFN-α having no carbohydrate moiety with and without affinity for polynucleotide, and one high molecular species having a carbohydrate moiety and affinity for polynucleotide. The low molecular species seem to be slightly more acidic than the high molecular species. The binding property of HuIFN-α to polynucleotide may not be due to its carbohydrate moiety.

To differentiate these components of HuIFN-α according to their biological activities, we performed a preliminary experiment on growth inhibition with the ConA-binding and -nonbinding components of HuIFN-α on Raji cell cultures

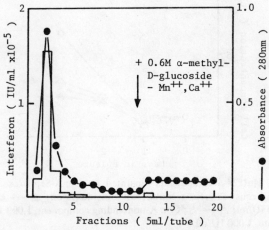

Fig. 6. ConA-Sepharose chromatography of poly U nonbinding component in partially purified HuIFN-α. Column, 0.9 × 10 cm, equilibrated with 0.02 M Tris-HCl buffer, pH 6.8, containing 1 M NaCl, 10 mM MnCl$_2$, 10 mM CaCl$_2$, 0.02 % NaN$_3$, flow rate, 6 ml/hr, at room temperature. Input, 1,902,900 IU; recovery, 55.4%. ●——●: A$_{280}$; ☐: interferon.

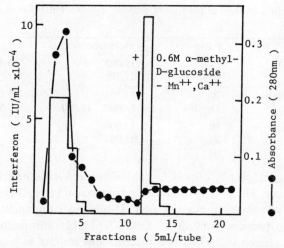

Fig. 7. ConA-Sepharose chromatography of poly U-binding component of partially purified HuIFN-α. Column, 0.9 × 10 cm, equilibrated with 0.02 M Tris-HCl buffer, pH 6.8, containing 1 M NaCl, 10 mM MnCl₂, 10 mM CaCl₂, 0.02% NaN₃, flow rate, 6 ml/hr, at room temperature. Input, 1,779,600 IU; recovery, 82%, ●——●: A₂₈₀; ▢: interferon.

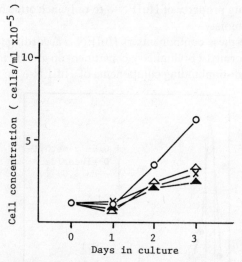

Fig. 8. Effect of HuIFN-α components separated by ConA-Sepharose chromatography on growth of Raji cells. ○——○: control without interferon; ▲——▲: ConA-binding component, 1,000 IU/ml; △——△: Con A-nonbinding component, 1,000 IU/ml; ×——×: SP-Sephadex eluate, 1,000 IU/ml.

(Fig. 8). There was no significant difference in the inhibition of the cell growth among the fractions separated by ConA-Sepharose chromatography.

REFERENCES

1. Kishida, T., Sotomatsu, S., Uyeda, K., Matsuo, A., Negoro, Y., Imanishi, J., and Ito, H.: Human leukocyte interferon and its evaluation. *Proc. Symposium on Clinical Use of Interferon.* Yug. Acad. Sci. Arts, Zagreb, 1 & 2 October 1975, pp. 159–167.

2. Stancek, D., Gressnerova, M., and Paucker, K.: Isoelectric components of mouse, human and rabbit interferons. *Virology*, **41**: 740–750, 1970.

3. Anfinsen, C. B., Bose, S., Corley, L., and Gurari-Rotman, A.: Partial purification of human interferon by affinity chromatography. *Proc. Natl. Acad. Sci. USA.*, **71**: 3139–3142, 1974.

4. Matsuo, A., Hayashi, S., and Kishida, T.: Production and purification of human leukocyte interferon. *Japan J. Microbiol.*, **18**: 21–27, 1974.

5. Borecky, L., Fuchsberger, N., and Hajnicka, V.: Electrophoretic profiles and activities of human interferon in heterologous cells. *Intervirology*, **3**: 369–377, 1974.

6. Berg, K., Ogburn, C. A., Paucker, K., Mogensen, K. E., and Cantell, K.: Affinity chromatography of human leukocyte and diploid cell interferons on sepharose-bound antibodies. *J. Immunol.*, **114**: 640–644, 1975.

7. Havell, E. A., Berman, B., Ogburn, C. A., Berg, K., Paucker, K., and Vilček, J.: Two antigenically distinct species of human interferon. *Proc. Natl. Acad. Sci. USA.*, **72**: 2185–2190, 1975.

8. Stewart, W. E., II and Desmyter, J.: Molecular heterogeneity of human leukocyte interferon: Two populations differing in molecular weights, requirements and cross-species antiviral activity. *Virology*, **67**: 68–78, 1975.

9. Torma, E. T. and Paucker, K.: Purification and characterization of human leukocyte interferon components. *J. Biol. Chem.*, **251**: 4810–4820, 1976.

10. Chen, J. K., Jankowski, W. J., O'Mally, J. A., Sulkowski, E., and Carter, W. A.: Nature of the molecular heterogeneity of human leukocyte interferon. *J. Virol.*, **19**: 425–434, 1976.

11. Mogensen, K. E., Pyhala, L., Torma, E., and Cantell, K.: No evidence for a carbohydrate moiety affecting the clearance of circulating human leukocyte interferon in rabbits. *Acta Path. Microbiol. Scand,* **82**: 305–310, 1974.

12. Besancon, F. and Bourgeade, M. F.: Affinity of murine and human interferon for concanavalin A. *J. Immunol.*, **113**: 1061–1063, 1974.

13. Jankowski, W. J., Davey, M. W., O'Malley, J., Sulkowski, E., and Carter, W. A.: Molecular structure of human fibroblast and leukocyte interferons: Probe by lectin and hydrophobic chromatography. *J. Virol.*, **16**: 1124–1130, 1975.

14. Davey, M. W., Sulkowski, E., and Carter, W. A.: Binding of human fibroblast interferon to concanavalin A-agarose. Involvement of carbohydrate recognition and hydrophobic interaction. *Biochemistry*, **15**: 704–710, 1976.

15. Stewart, W. E., II, Lin, L. S., Wiranowska-Stewart, M., and Cantell, K.: Elimination of size and charge heterogeneities of human leukocyte interferon by chemical cleavage. *Proc. Natl. Acad. Sci. USA.*, **74**: 4200–4204, 1977.

16. Bodo, G.: Production and purification of human lymphoblastoid interferon. *Proc. Symposium on Preparation, Standardization and Clinical Use of Interferon.* Yug. Acad. Sci. Arts, Zagreb, June 1977, pp. 49–57.

17. DeMaeyer-Guignard, J., Thang, M. N., and DeMaeyer, E.: Binding of mouse interferon to polynucleotides. *Proc. Natl. Acad. Sci. USA.*, **74**: 3787–3790, 1977.

18. DeMaeyer-Guignard, J., Tovey, M. G., Gresser, I., and DeMaeyer, E.: Purification of mouse interferon by sequential affinity chromatography on poly (U)-and antibody-agarose columns. *Nature*, **271**: 622–625, 1978.

19. Yang, C. and Srivastava, P. N.: Purification of bull serum hyaluronidase by concanavalin-A affinity chromatography. *Biochim. Biophys. Acta*, **391**: 382–387, 1975.

Discussion

Dr. MACHIDA: I would like to ask you a question concerning antigenic differences among the three types of interferon.

Dr. MATSUO: You mean differences between the high and low molecular weights? Or between the three types—two low and one high molecular weight type?

Dr. MACHIDA: How you ever looked into the antigenic differences of the three types of interferon?

Dr. MATSUO: The answer is no.

Dr. MACHIDA: So is it correct to understand that the only difference between the interferon of 15,000 dalton and the interferon of 21,500 dalton is whether it has the carbohydratechain or not?

Dr. MATSUO: Though the 21,000 molecular weight type has the carbohydrate moiety, I don't think that the carbohydratechain alone accounts for the difference between the two molecular weights of 21,000 and 15,000.

Dr. MAKINO: In the case of leukocyte interferon, purification is conducted in the interest of safety, and I think that the elimination of microorganisms in the sample is one of the major purposes of purification. Weak microorganisms can be inactivated or eliminated in the process of purification. However, highly resistant microorganisms such as hepatitis B type virus or unconventional viruses may not be easily eliminated, possibly remaining in the material. Have you set any conditions for determining which study materials are safe in your purification process? If not, you should consider this point.

Dr. MATSUO: Well, this is a very difficult question. Currently, we are using a blood sample which has been approved by the HB test. However, it is quite difficult to conduct tests for unknown factors, so we are not carrying out such tests at present.

Production and Purification of Human Leukocyte Interferon

I. Béládi, M. Tóth, I. Mécs, S. Tóth, B. Taródi, R. Pusztai, and
M. Koltai

*Institutes of Microbiology and Pharmacology, University Medical Sohool, Szeged, Dóm tér
10, H-6720 Hungary*

SUMMARY

The production and purification procedures adopted by us are composed mainly
of steps already known. Having studied the experimental conditions and possible
modifications we have succeeded in establishing a simple, reliable, and economical
procedure which is suitable to meet the quickly growing demand for human IFN.
Some of the highlights of our current procedures are the following. A double-
assay system consisting of HA and AIE tests permits the selection of appropriate
inducer virus preparations and controls their interferonogenic activity. A simple and
inexpensive balanced salt solution is used as a substitute for Eagle's medium. At the
phase of IFN formation, excess virus and egg proteins are removed and a medium
with a reduced amount of serum is added to the cells. This modification resulted in a
10-fold increase in the specific activity. Finally, the semi-crude material obtained
from this procedure does not need to be purified extensively. By a simplified ion-
exchange chromatographic step it can be purified to a specific activity suitable for
clinical studies.

INTRODUCTION

Production and purification of human leukocyte interferon (HuIFN-α) have
been investigated in our laboratory with the goal of applying the results to
clinical studies. Human trials on a large scale have been hampered by practical and financial problems encountered in the production and purification of
large amounts of IFN. Since the present production facilities and, in particular,
the amount of fresh leukocytes available are limiting factors, improvement in
the recovery and quality of clinical IFN is of prime importance. To this end,
and in an effort to reduce the costs of production, attempts have been made to
modify and to combine methods already available. As a result of 4 years of

31

experience, a routine procedure for the production and purification of HuIFN-α has been established, and in this paper we summarize the results of our work.

METHODS

Production and Assay of Sendai Virus

As an inducer we use the Sendai strain of parainfluenza 1 virus (kindly provided by Dr. K. Cantell) which is grown in 10–11-day-old embryonated eggs. The inoculated eggs are incubated at 37°C for 48 hours, then kept at 4°C overnight. Allantoic fluids are collected and tested for hemagglutinating (HA) activity. For this purpose we have developed a simple microassay, which is carried out in microtiter plates. A standard virus preparation is always included in the assay, the titer of which is determined by Cantell's method.[1] All hemagglutination units (HAU) are expressed with reference to this standard.

For economical mass production of IFN a controled inducer virus with a standard, high IFN-inducing capacity is a strict prerequisite. It has not yet been definitely determined whether the interferonogenic capacity of different virus preparations parallels their hemagglutinating activity. In an effort to elaborate a reliable method to control our inducer virus, we took advantage of the observation that Sendai virus has an anti-inflammatory effect (AIE) in mice,[2] i.e., the acute inflammatory response induced by a subplantar injection of 300 μg of carrageenan is inhibited by a previous intravenous inoculation of Sendai virus. This simple test can easily be performed within 5 hours using Levy's technique.[3] AIE in the virus-treated animals is expressed in percent compared to the group injected with control allantoic fluid. To ascertain whether this phenomenon could be used for testing the quality of inducer virus, a large number of eggs were inoculated with Sendai virus and the allantoic fluids of the same HA titers were pooled, and their interferonogenic activity in human leukocytes was determined. Similarly, all the samples were tested for AIE in CFLP mice. We found a close correlation between interferonogenic activity and HA or AIE (Figs. 1 and 2). Therefore, the Sendai virus preparations produced in our laboratory are always tested for HA and AI activity, since this double assay system seems to be much safer for selecting appropriate inducers. Pools of allantoic fluids obtained from 5–50 infected eggs with HA titer no less than 4,000 HAU/ml and AIE higher than 30% are used for IFN production in human leukocytes.

For economical inducer virus production, the dose of inoculating Sendai virus also seems to be critical. The appropriate quantity of inoculum is 3,000–30,000 egg infective dose$_{50}$/EID$_{50}$/ per egg (Fig. 3). In routine procedure, 5,000 EID$_{50}$ per egg is used as the inoculum. The inducer virus is stored at −70°C without any additives, and it maintains its IFN-inducing activity for more than 6 months.

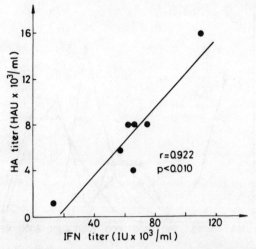

Fig. 1. Relationship of IFN-inducing capacity to HA activity of different Sendai virus preparation. Seven virus preparations were tested. The IFN-inducing capacity of virus preparations were tested in 3 different experiments.

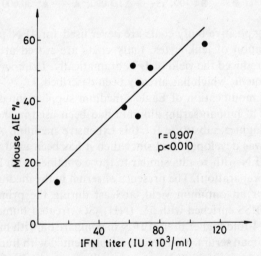

Fig. 2. Correlation between interferonogenic and anti-inflammatory activity of different Sendai virus pools. Seven virus preparations were tested. Each AIE value is an average obtained from the results of the treatment of 15 mice.

Production of Human Leukocyte Interferon
1. Production of crude interferon

The blood is collected from healthy volunteers and buffy coats are pooled. Each donor is tested for HB_sAg by an indirect hemagglutination test, and

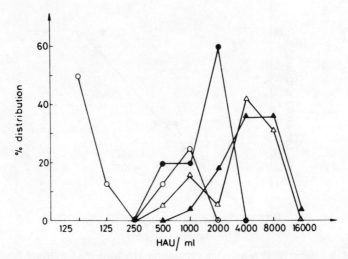

Fig. 3. Effect of the amount of inoculated Sendai virus on the virus yield in infected eggs. The distribution of the HA activity of individual allantoic fluids from eggs infected with the same inoculum is plotted. Groups of 25 eggs were inoculated with the following amounts of virus: ○——○ :1; ●——● : 100; △——△ : 3,000; ▲——▲ : 30,000 EID_{50}/egg.

pools containing positive buffy coats are never used for IFN production. Before the purification of leukocytes, buffy coats are stored at 4°C overnight. Longer storage reduced the yield of IFN dramatically. Leukocytes are purified by NH_4Cl treatment, which has already been described.[4]

The Glasgow modification of Eagle's medium supplemented with 25 μg/ml neomycin and 5% human serum albumin had been used in the cultivation of cells, but we sought a substitute for this expensive medium. A balanced salt solution (BSS) was developed, and since then it has been used routinely in the production of IFN with results similar to those obtained with Eagle's medium (manuscript in preparation). The presence of serum in the medium proved to be indispensable for an optimum yield, at least during the priming period. In our experience, BSS enriched with 5% $(NH_4)_2SO_4$-treated human ("agamma") serum yielded a 4-fold higher titer of IFN in comparison with medium containing untreated human serum. With media supplemented with human "agamma" or normal bovine serum about the same results were obtained.

In the routine procedure, the cell concentration is adjusted to 10^7 cells/ml, and in 2,000 ml round flasks, 500 to 1,000 ml of cell suspensions are incubated at 37°C and agitated slowly on a magnetic stirrer. At the start of incubation, 200 international units (IU) per ml of interferon are added to the cell suspension to prime the cultures. For this purpose high titered crude IFN without acid treatment is used, aliquots of which are stored at −20°C. Two hours later a one-twentieth volume of Sendai virus preparation is added to the cell cultures.

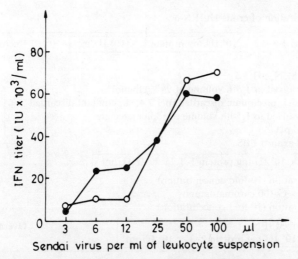

Fig. 4. Effect of dosage of inducer on the yield of IFN in primed leukocytes. HA activity of Sendai virus pools: ○——○ : 4,000; ●——● : 6,000 HAU/ml.

Usually these virus preparations have a titer of 4–6×10^3 HAU/ml, and as Fig. 4 shows, 50 μl of virus inducer is sufficient per ml of leukocyte suspension to attain to the optimum IFN yield. The incubation is continued for about 20 hours. After centrifugation of the cultures the supernatant obtained is a crude IFN with a titer of 5–10×10^4 IU/ml, the specific activity of which is 2–4×10^4 IU/mg protein.

2. Production of semi-crude IFN

A modification has been introduced into the procedure for the production of IFN by which the excess virus and egg proteins are removed, and thus a considerable increase in specific activity is achieved. The production of semi-crude IFN is similar to that of crude IFN, except that 3 hours after infection with Sendai virus the medium is removed by centrifugation and the cells are resuspended in BSS supplemented with 0.5% human serum albumin. As a result, the IFN-producing capacity of the leukocytes is still 60–90% of the unchanged control but a 10-fold increase is gained in specific activity.

Concentration and Purification Procedures

1. Purification of crude HuIFN

The crude IFN is purified by the method of Cantell and Hirvonen[5] with some modifications (Table 1). The IFN is precipitated by acidic KSCN and the precipitate is dissolved in cold ethanol. The pH of this solution is raised by the stepwise addition of small amounts of 0.1 N NaOH. The pH is monitored continuously and a titrations curve is constructed. Precipitates are collected at pH values corresponding to inflexion parts on the titration curve (usually at pH

Table 1.   Purification of crude HuIFN-α.

Crude IFN-α: 1.5–2.5 × 10⁴ IU/mg protein 6 × 10⁴ IU/ml	Recovery range per step (%)
↓ 0.5 M KSCN, pH 3.5	
Sediment dissolved in 1/5th volume of 96% ethanol	
↓ pH 5.2–5.3, precipitate discarded, pH 7.4, supernatant discarded	40–50
Sediment dissolved in 1/50th volume of sodium acetate	
(0.05 M), pH 3.5	
↓ Dialysis against PBS	
IFN-α: 2–4 × 10⁵ IU/mg protein 1–1.25 × 10⁶ IU/ml	
Ultrafiltration (10-fold concentration)	100–120
Sephadex G-100 chromatography	80–100
↓ Ultrafiltration (10-fold concentration)	100–120
Partially purified IFN-α:	Overall recovery
5–10 × 10⁶ IU/mg protein 2–3 × 10⁶ IU/ml	40–50

5.2–5.3 and 5.7–5.8). With a further increase of pH the IFN is precipitated. After centrifugation the pellet is dissolved in 0.05 M sodium acetate, pH 3.5, and dialyzed against phosphate-buffered saline (PBS).

Instead of the second acid-KSCN precipitation used by Cantell, additional concentration of the crude IFN is carried out by ultrafiltration. An Amicon system is used with an ultrafilter having a nominal molecular weight limit of 10⁴. To prevent IFN adsorption it is presoaked in a 1% human serum albumin-containing solution. This material is then subjected to gel filtration performed on a Sephadex G-100 column. IFN is eluted as a fairly symmetrical peak, and the appropriate fractions are collected in siliconized tubes and pooled. Since the gel filtration dilutes the IFN about 10-fold a final ultrafiltration is needed.

This procedure was found to be highly reliable; the recoveries varied from 80 to 100%. The specific activity of the gel filtered IFN appears to be higher than that of the purified IFN obtained by KSCN precipitation, while the overall recovery is only slightly lower (40–50%) than described by Cantell and his coworkers.

2. Concentration and purification of semi-crude IFN

The semi-crude IFN, the result of the modified preparation procedure, is usually acid treated at pH 2 for 24 hours to inactivate residual virus (Table 2). It is then either concentrated by precipitation with 1M KSCN at pH 3.5 in the presence of 1 M NaCl or purified by ion-exchange chromatography. By using SP-Sephadex C-25 batchwise we can partially purify IFN activity direct-ly from the semi-crude material; 5 gm of ion exchanger is sufficient for the total adsorption of activity in one liter of starting material. After stirring overnight at 4°C, gel is poured into a chromatographic column and washed with 0.05 M

Table 2.   Concentration and purification of semi-crude HuIFN-α.

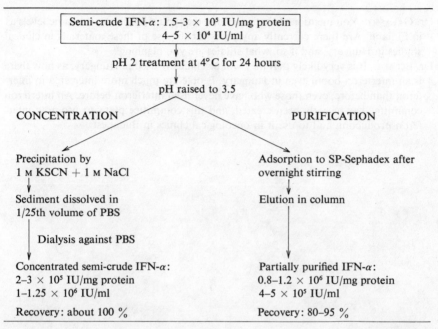

Semi-crude IFN-α: 1.5–3 $\times$ 10^5 IU/mg protein
4–5 $\times$ 10^4 IU/ml

pH 2 treatment at 4°C for 24 hours

pH raised to 3.5

CONCENTRATION

PURIFICATION

Precipitation by
1 M KSCN + 1 M NaCl

Adsorption to SP-Sephadex after
overnight stirring

Sediment dissolved in
1/25th volume of PBS

Elution in column

Dialysis against PBS

Concentrated semi-crude IFN-α:
2–3 $\times$ 10^5 IU/mg protein
1–1.25 $\times$ 10^6 IU/ml

Partially purified IFN-α:
0.8–1.2 $\times$ 10^6 IU/mg protein
4–5 $\times$ 10^5 IU/ml

Recovery: about 100 %

Pecovery: 80–95 %

sodium acetate at pH 3.5. IFN is eluted by 0.1 M sodium phosphate, pH 8, containing 1 M NaCl. The eluate is monitored for its extinction at 280 nm and protein-containing fractions are pooled. The semi-crude IFN is partially purified to a specific activity of about 10^6 IU/mg protein by this simple method, and the recovery in total yields ranges around 80%.

REFERENCES

1. Cantell, K., Hirvonen, S., Nogensen, K. E., and Pyhälä, L.: Human leukocyte interferon: Production, purification, stability, and animal experiments. In: C. Waymouth (ed.), *In Vitro*, The Tissue Culture Association, Rockville, Md., 1974, p. 35.
2. Koltai, M., Mécs, I., and Kásler, M.: On the anti-inflammatory effect of Sendai virus inoculation. *Arch. Virol.* (in press).
3. Levy, L.: Carrageenan paw oedema in the mouse. *Life Sci.*, **8**: 601–606, 1969.
4. Mécs, I. and Béládi, I.: Factors influencing interferon production by human leukocytes. In *Proc. Symp. Preparation, Standardization and Clinical Use of Interferon*. Yugoslav Academy of Sciences and Arts, Zagreb, 1977, pp. 23–26.
5. Cantell, K. and Hirvonen, S.: Large-scale production of human leukocyte interferon containing 10^8 units per ml. *J. Gen. Virol.*, **39**: 541–543, 1978.

Discussion

Dr. GALASSO: You mentioned that you hope that you will achieve the same levels as in Finland. Are there currently any plans for the use of these materials in clinical studies in Hungary, and if so, what studies are you planning?

Dr. BÉLÁDI: It is very likely that they will be clinically used in Hungary, as now there is an interferon boom even in Hungary. People are much more interested in interferon than before, even those who have never used interferon before. An interferon committee has recently been created, and this committee plans to promote interferon production and to use it in oncological clinics in Budapest.

Production of Interferon for Clinical Use from Human Lymphoblastoid Cells

N. B. FINTER, K. H. FANTES, G. D. BALL, and M. D. JOHNSTON

Wellcome Research Laboratories, Langley Court, Beckenham, Kent, England

SUMMARY

We have established a manufacturing system which could be scaled up without apparent limit. The cost of production decreases with the scale, and on a much larger scale, the marginal cost of making the IFN should be quite small. As with other biologicals, the major cost will be for quality control procedures, staff costs, packaging, and so forth. For clinical purposes, the choice between Namalwa cell IFN and IFN derived from *E. coli* cultures by genetic engineering techniques will depend on their relative performance in clinical use. It remain to be seen whether single component materials prepared from bacterial cultures will match the performance of the natural mixture of IFNs prepared from primary or transformed human B-lymphocytes. If the advantage proves to be with the Namalwa cell-derived material, the necessary very large amounts could certainly be prepared.

The important work of Cantell and Hirvonen[1] has established that leukocytes from donated blood (buffy coat cells) can be the source of significant amounts of human interferon (HuIFN-α). Buffy coat cells have been the source of almost all the IFN used in clinical studies to date, but unfortunately they are only available in limited amounts. We therefore decided in 1974 to investigate a potential source of limitless amounts of human IFN, namely transformed human cells grown in suspension. We of course knew that the idea of using such cells as the source of a medicinal product ran contrary to the opinions of most microbiologists. Nevertheless, there are good precedents for the use of less than ideal starting materials in the manufacture of other drugs, and, for example, insulin is made from pancreases collected from abattoirs; the

39

final product is acceptable because the insulin is rigorously purified during manufacture to remove undesirable contaminants. We felt that the same reasoning could be applied to the manufacture of IFN from transformed cells.

Shortly after starting our studies, a paper appeared[2] in which a number of human lymphoblastoid cell lines were induced to form IFN by treatment with Sendai virus. One line, termed Namalwa, gave particularly good yields. Following this lead, we screened a large number of human lymphoblastoid cell lines derived both from normal individuals and from patients suffering from various diseases. Out of the 140 different lines which we tested, 5 gave rise to relatively large amounts of IFN, and among these was the line Namalwa.[3] We chose to carry out further work with Namalwa cells because not only do they produce large amounts of IFN when suitably stimulated, but they also grow well in suspension. We learned to handle them in cultures of increasing volume from 500 ml to 3,000 liters. We use medium RPMI 1640 supplemented with 7% irradiated bovine serum. We find it best to screen serum batches in order to exclude a small number which are unsuitable for use. However, it is unnecessary (and impractical) to use fetal calf serum in large tank cultures.

In our earlier studies, we found a considerable variation in the yields of IFN obtained from one occasion to another. We gained the impression that IFN yields were highest when cells were cultured under conditions such that they grew relatively slowly. We therefore explored the effects on IFN yields of various inhibitors of cell growth, and this led us to study the effects of sodium butyrate. We found that if Namalwa cell suspensions are incubated for 36–48 hours in the presence of sodium butyrate at 1–5 mM, and are then induced to form IFN by addition of Sendai virus, consistent high yields of IFN are obtained.[4,5] The titers are not higher than can sometimes be obtained in the absence of butyrate treatment, but the average titer is much higher. It is necessary to add butyrate before the cells are induced, and preferably it should be removed during the period of IFN formation as large amounts of butyrate present at this time depress IFN yields.

Our preliminary studies were carried out with Namalwa cells grown in fermenters of 50 or 100 liter capacity. Based on the experience gained, we decided in 1977 to build a pilot plant to make IFN for clinical purposes. In this, cell culture medium is made in 300 or 600 liter batches from pretested ingredients and is sterilized by filtration. It is supplied to the cell culture vessels, including one of 1,000 liter capacity, in which the Namalwa cells are maintained in suspension culture for periods of several months at a time. Eventually they are lost as a result of bacterial contamination, mechanical failures, or human error. As required, quantities of up to 500 liters of cell suspension are transferred from this tank to an IFN production tank, where they are treated with sodium butyrate for about 48 hours. Sendai virus (Hemagglutinating Virus of Japan), grown in fertile hen's eggs, is added to induce formation of IFN. After overnight incubation, the crude IFN is separated from the cell suspension and transferred to a holding tank. The crude IFN then passes through a multistage in-line purification procedure. This concentrates the IFN up to 50,000 times and purifies it up to about 10,000 times. All the culture vessels and the purification plant are linked by stainless steel or pyrex glass pipes, which can be sterilized by steam under pressure or by chemical means. Thus, medium, cell suspension, and IFN are moved from one part of the plant to another through sterile lines.

Namalwa cells originated from a Ugandan girl who died with a Burkitt tumor, and it is necessary to regard these cells as potentially being contaminated with a human oncogenic agent. All the cells contain Epstein-Barr (EB) virus, and it likely that this is responsible for their stably transformed nature. EB virus is of course a very common infection of man, and in a relatively few individuals leads to infectious mononucleosis. In the majority, EB virus infection is silent, but most adults have antibodies to it. It is thought that a Burkitt tumor results from abnormal processing of EB virus in an individual who is immunosuppressed as a result of a concomitant malarial infection rather than from some peculiarity of the EB virus itself. Nevertheless, it is necessary to consider that the EB virus in Namalwa cells is indeed a human tumor virus. Since the cells contain only part of the virus genome (approximately 50%), no infectious virus is or can be formed. Nevertheless, among the few viral genes expressed in each cell must be the one or more responsible for the transformed nature of the cells. We therefore looked for the presence in our crude IFN of DNA derived from EB virus that might be oncogenic, but none could be detected in hybridization studies (carried out by Dr. J. Pagano at the University of North Carolina). Indeed, there was only a small amount of DNA derived from the Namalwa cells themselves.

We felt that it was likely that any DNA would be eliminated during our purification process. To prove this, we deliberately added markers, namely heavily radio-labeled preparations of EB virus DNA (385,000 counts per minute) and human cellular DNA (7,095,500 counts per minute) (both provided by Dr. Pagano), to crude IFN which was processed by the routine procedure. No radioactivity above background was detected in the final IFN fraction. Thus, to the limit of detection, all the EB virus and cellular DNA were eliminated during processing.

We similarly added other markers to crude IFN which was then processed. In every case, none of the agent concerned could be found in the final preparation. Among the markers were virus representatives of many different classes, including large and small viruses, viruses containing RNA and DNA, and mammalian, avian and bacterial viruses. Thus, if Namalwa cells are contaminated with some as yet undiscovered tumor virus, the overwhelming likelihood is that this would also be eliminated by our purification procedure. In collaboration with Dr. Hunter, Agricultural Research Council Laboratories, Compton, England, we also worked with scrapie agent, a representative of the class of very stable "slow" viruses. This agent added to crude IFN was also eliminated by our purification procedure.

Such marker studies cannot prove that every single molecule of the agent concerned is eliminated during purification. They do, however, indicate that the degree of contamination is likely to be very small indeed. Absolute safety cannot be guaranteed for any medicinal product, but in view of our data, we believe that our lymphoblastoid IFN is probably safer than any other biological agent so far used in human medicine. It should be noted that our material has been approved for clinical trials in the United Kingdom and the United States by the control authorities in these countries.

Our procedures not only render the product safe, but also result in a very high degree of purity. Conventionally, the purity of an IFN preparation is measured in terms of its specific activity, that is to say the ratio between the biological activity (expressed in international units of activity) and the protein content. Unfortunately, as the purity of a preparation becomes greater, so the amount of protein available for measurement becomes smaller and smaller, and so measurements of specific activity become less reliable. Fantes and Allen,[6] from our laboratories have developed a chromatographic procedure for analyzing the purity of IFN preparations. Briefly, purified IFNs are chromatographed on Sephadex G-75 and eluate fractions are collected. Their protein content is assessed from the optical absorption at 206 nm, and the IFN activity is measured by bioassay. A representative chromatograph is shown in Fig. 1. There is a characteristic double peak in which all the IFN activity is found (we term this region the "interferon peaks"), unless preparations are tested at a very high concentration, when there may be some dimerization and a consequent change in the characteristic curve. When SDS-polyacrylamide gel electrophoresis is carried out on fractions from the IFN peak region, at least 8 different protein bands are seen, and all of these have IFN activity. No other proteins are found in this region. Thus, from the ratio of the area under the IFN peaks to the total area under the protein trace, an assessment of the purity of the IFN preparation can be obtained. Also, by calibrating the chromatography column, an estimate of the amount of protein in the IFN peaks region can be made. (Control studies have shown that it is valid to use the optical density at 206 nm for measuring amounts of protein which differ very considerably in their optical absorbance at, for example, E_{280}.) Data thus obtained for the purity of 7 successive large batches of IFN used for clinical purposes are shown in Table 1, together with their specific activities

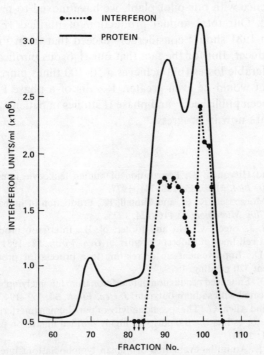

Fig. 1. Sephadex G-75 chromatography of a routinely prepared and purified batch of lymphoblastoid IFN. From the elution profile, the purity of this preparation is calculated to be 87%.

Table 1. Chromatographic estimation of purity and specific activity for 7 successive batches of IFN prepared for clinical use.

Clinical batch no.	Purity (%)	Specific activity (IU × 10⁶/mg total protein)[a]
3	77	42.7
4	97	96.3
5	ND	ND
6	88, 80[b]	62.5, 88.9[b]
7	88	70.7
8	92	133
9	85	112
10	78	133

a) Protein estimated from column elution profile.
b) Duplicate estimations.
ND: not done by this method.

based on protein values calculated by chromatographic estimation. As can be seen, the minimum purity recorded was 77%.

After experience with our pilot plant, we have moved to production on an industrial scale. Our total annual production of purified IFN is now substantial, and in 1981 should considerably exceed that from Finland, hitherto the largest producer. But for the fact that our rigorous purification procedure involves considerable losses (but achieves a 50–100 times more pure product), our total output would be even greater. Results of a phase I study with our material have been published,[7] and phase II studies in patients with melanoma and myeloma are now in progress.

REFERENCES

1. Cantell, K. and Hirvonen, S.: Preparation of human leukocyte interferon for clinical use. *Texas Rpts. Biol. Med.*, **35**: 138–141, 1977.
2. Strander, H., Morgensen, K. E., and Cantell, K.: Production of human lymphoblastoid interferon. *J. Clin. Microbiol.*, **1**: 116–124, 1975.
3. Christofinis, G. J., Steel., C. M., and Finter, N. B.: Interferon production by human lymphoblastoid cell lines of different origins. *J. Gen. Virol.*, **52**: 1981 (in press).
4. Johnston, M. D.: Improvements in or relating to a process for producing interferon. European Patent 520 pending. 1979.
5. Johnston, M. D.: Enhanced production of interferon from human lymphoblastoid (Namalwa) cells pre-treated with sodium butyrate. *J. Gen. Virol.*, **50**: 191–194, 1980.
6. Fantes, K. H. and Allen, G.: The specific activity of pure human interferons and a non-biological method for estimating the purity of highly purified interferon preparations. *J. Interferon Res.*, **1**: 1981.
7. Priestman, T. J.: An initial evaluation of human lymphoblastoid interferon in patients with advanced malignant disease. *Lancet*: July 19, 1980.

Purification of Human Lymphoblastoid Interferon by Highly Specific Anti-Interferon Antibody and Competitive Radioimmunoassay for Human Interferon-α

Shin YONEHARA

Tokyo Metropolitan Institute of Medical Science, Honkomagome, Bunkyo-ku, Tokyo 113, Japan

SUMMARY

Human Namalwa cell interferon (IFN), induced by Sendai virus and composed of a single species with molecular weight 17 K, was purified to 4.5×10^8 international reference units (IU)/mg protein by a combination of salt precipitation, ion-exchange chromatography, metal chelate chromatography, hydrophobic chromatography, and polyacrylamide gel electrophoresis in the presence of sodium dodecyl sulfate. By immunization of a rabbit with this purified IFN and extensive absorption with Namalwa cells and an impurity column, highly specific antibody was obtained.

Namalwa cells, treated with 5-bromo-2′-deoxyuridine (BrdU), produced 10-fold more IFN upon induction by Sendai virus. IFN in this case was composed of heterogeneous species with molecular weights ranging from 15 K to 24 K. These heterogeneous IFN molecules were purified to 7.6×10^8 IU/mg protein by successive chromatography using immobilized anti-IFN antibody, Blue Sepharose, and immobilized antirabbit IgG antibody. The overall recovery of IFN was 72%, and the purity was ascertained by polyacrylamide gel electrophoresis in the presence of sodium dodecyl sulfate.

Namalwa cell IFN, treated with BrdU and induced by Sendai virus, was labeled with (^{3}H)-leucine added to the culture fluid during active synthesis and precipitated quantitatively from the culture fluid using anti-IFN antibody and formalin-fixed *Staphylococcus aureus*, strain Cowan I. The material recovered from the precipitate was shown, upon polyacrylamide gel electrophoresis in the presence of sodium dodecyl sulfate, to be essentially pure in radioactivity.

By using this purified radioactive IFN and anti-IFN antibody, at least 100 IU of HuIFN-α could be measured by radioimmunoassay.

INTRODUCTION

Much progress has been mabe in the purification of IFN, some mouse and human IFNs having been obtained in an essentially pure state.[1-9] Fairly rapid methods of purification with good rates of recovery were reported for some human and mouse IFNs of fibroblast origins,[2,5,8] but in the case of human leukocyte interferon[6,9] and human lymphoblastoid cell interferon,[7] the methods developed to date have usually been complex and time-consuming, and the recovery rate has often been low.

In this study, highly specific antibody against Namalwa cell IFN was prepared in a rabbit. This antibody was found to be highly effective for the purification of lymphoblastoid cell IFN when coupled to Sepharose and, when precipitated with IFN labeled with radioactive amino acid.

EXPERIMENTAL PROCEDURES

Initial Purification Procedures
1. Preparation of crude IFN

Namalwa cells in phosphate buffer saline (PBS) containing Ca^{2+} and Mg^{2+} at $2–5 \times 10^7$ cells/ml were infected with Sendai virus (50 hemagglutinating units/10^6 cells). After standing for 26–36 hours at a concentration of 0.5–1.0 $\times 10^7$ cells/ml in RPMI 1640 containing 15 mM Hepes, the culture fluid was harvested and concentrated by zinc acetate precipitation.[10]

2. SP-Sephadex column chromatography

The concentrated IFN was dialyzed against Buffer A (McIlvein's citrate/phosphate buffer, pH 4.0, containing 20% glycerin) and charged onto a SP-Sephadex C-25 column (200 ml bed volume) equilibrated with Buffer A. The IFN active materials were eluted by a NaCl gradient to 1.0 M NaCl in Buffer A. The eluate was concentrated by 80% ammonium sulfate precipitation. The precipitate was dissolved in Buffer B (20 mM sodium phosphate buffer, pH 7.1, containing 0.2 M NaCl and 20% glycerin).

3. Cu chelate column chromatography

$CuSO_4$ solution was applied to an imidodiacetic acid-conjugated Sepharose CL-6B (30 ml bed volume) until the color of the whole bed turned blue. Then, ammonium sulfate precipitate was applied to the column, equilibrated with Buffer B, and IFN was eluted by a pH gradient formed by mixing Buffer B and 20 mM sodium citrate buffer, pH 2.0, containing 0.2 M NaCl and 20% glycerin.

4. Octyl-Sepharose column chromatography

The eluate from the Cu chelate column was applied to an octyl-Sepharose column (1.5 ml bed volume), equilibrated with Buffer B containing 0.1 mM EDTA. IFN was eluted by the same buffer containing 2% sodium dodecyl sulfate (SDS) at room temperature.

Preparation of Anti-IFN Serum

Antiserum against highly purified Namalwa cell IFN was prepared in a rabbit. The details are described elsewhere.[11] In brief, a total of approximately 4×10^7 IU of highly purified IFN (the eluate from the SDS-polyacrylamide gel in the initial purification, 4.5×10^8 IU/mg protein), together with Freund's complete adjuvant, was injected into a rabbit subcutaneously at about 10 day intervals. The resulting antiserum was absorbed by Sendai virus-infected Namalwa cells and an impurity column as described elsewhere.[11]

Purification of IFN by Affinity Chromatography

1. Preparation of crude IFN

Namalwa cells treated with 5-bromo-2'-deoxyuridine (BrdU) were infected by Sendai virus and the induced IFN was used for the subsequent purification.

2. Anti-IFN column chromatography

The original culture fluid was directly applied to an anti-IFN column (1.4 gm IgG of anti-IFN serum was conjugated to 27 gm of CNBr-activated Sepharose 4B) equilibrated with 0.2 M sodium acetate, pH 7.3, containing 0.5 M NaCl, 0.1 mM EDTA, and 20% glycerin. IFN was eluted by 0.2 M acetic acid, pH 3.0, containing 0.5 M NaCl, 0.1 mM EDTA, and 20% glycerin.

3. Blue Sepharose column chromatography

The antibody column eluate was diluted 1.7-fold with 0.02 N NaOH, and then applied to a Blue Sepharose column (1 ml bed volume) equilibrated with 0.1 M sodium acetate buffer, pH 3.5, containing 0.3 M NaCl, 0.1 mM EDTA, and 20% glycerin. The column was washed by Buffer C (20 mM Sodium phosphate buffer, pH 7.1, containing 0.1 mM EDTA and 20% glycerin) containing 0.1 M NaCl. IFN was eluted by Buffer C containing 0.5 M NaCl

4. Antirabbit IgG Sepharose column chromatography

Twenty-three mg IgG of goat anti-rabbit IgG serum (1 ml; Fujizoki Pharmaceutical Company, Tokyo), purified by Protein A Sepharose, was conjugated to 1 gm of CNBr-activated Sepharose. The Blue Sepharose column eluate was diluted 1.7-fold by Buffer C and was applied to a column (2 ml bed volume) equilibrated with Buffer C containing 0.3 M NaCl. IFN was not adsorbed.

Induction of Radioactive IFN

BrdU-treated and Sendai virus-infected Namalwa cells were washed with Earle's balanced salt solution (EBS) and suspended at 5×10^6 cells/ml in EBS containing 15 mM Hepes, 500 μg/ml glutamine, and 90 μCi/ml ^{3}H-leucine (1.8 Ci/mM). After standing for 17.5 hours at 33°C, the culture fluid was harvested, and viruses were inactivated by 0.5% Triton X-100.

In order to obtain highly radioactive IFN, Sendai virus-infected Namalwa cells were cultured without ^{3}H-leucine at 33°C for 4.5 hours, and at 4.5 hours after infection, 100 μCi/ml of ^{3}H-leucine (160 Ci/mM) was added. After further incubation for 4 hours at 33°C, the culture fluid was harvested.

Immune Precipitation of Radioactive IFN

One ml of the original culture fluid was adsorbed with 0.15 ml of PAA (protein A adsorbent; 10% solution of formalin-fixed *Staphylococcus aureus*, strain Cowan I), and the unadsorbed fraction was incubated with 25 μl of anti-IFN serum at 37°C for 30 min and then 4°C overnight. Next, 0.15 ml of PAA was added and the precipitate, formed after 15 min at 37°C, was collected by centrifugation. After washing the precipitate with Buffer C containing 0.5 M NaCl and 1% Triton X-100 4 times, and with 1 ml of Buffer C containing 0.2 M NaCl 4 times, IFN was dissolved in 0.16 ml of Buffer C containing 0.2 M NaCl and 5% SDS. After incubation at 50°C for 15 min, PAA was removed by centrifugation and the supernatant was heated at 100°C for 1 min.

Radioimmunoassay for HuIFN-α

RIA Buffer, used in the radioimmunoassay, is Buffer C, containing 0.2 M NaCl, 5 mg/ml bovine serum albumin, 1% Triton X-100, and 0.02% NaN$_3$. In the assay, 0.2 ml of IFN sample and 0.1 ml of RIA Buffer containing 0.2 μl anti-IFN serum were incubated at 40°C for 15 min; then 0.2 ml/sample of radioactive IFN (65 IU/600 cpm) was added and the sample was incubated at 40°C for 45 min. Next, a 20 μl/sample of PAA was added and the sample was incubated at 40°C for 15 min. The precipitate, collected by centrifugation, was washed by PBS once and IFN was dissolved in a 0.2 ml/sample PBS containing 2% SDS. After incubation at 50°C for 5 min, PAA was removed by centrifugation, and the radioactivity of the supernatant was measured.

RESULTS

Initial Purification of IFN

Namalwa cell IFN with molecular weight 17 K, induced by Sendai virus, was first purified for use as an immunogen to obtain anti-IFN serum of high specificity.

1. Preparation of crude IFN

IFN from about 1×10^{10} Namalwa cells was usually harvested at one time. In total, 1.65×10^8 IU in 18 liter (2.4×10^4 IU/mg protein) of the original culture fluid were used for the present purification. The material concentrated by zinc acetate precipitation was frozen until all the fractions were pooled (1.4×10^8 IU in 2.9 liters, 2.0×10^5 IU/mg protein).

2. Column chromatography

The zinc acetate precipitate was applied to a SP-Sephadex column and IFN was eluted by a NaCl gradient (8.6×10^7 IU in 570 ml, 7.1×10^5 IU/mg protein). The eluate, concentrated by 80% ammonium sulfate precipitation (8.2 × 10^7 IU in 40 ml, 1.1 × 10^6 IU/mg protein), was applied to a Cu chelate column, and IFN was eluted by pH gradient (3.8 × 10^7 IU in 88 ml, 4.9 × 10^7 IU/mg protein). The effluent was purified by an octyl-Sepharose column (3.0 × 10^7 IU in 3.6 ml, 1.2 × 10^7 IU/mg protein).

3. SDS polyacrylamide gel electrophoresis

The octyl-Sepharose eluate was electrophoresed in 12.5% polyacrylamide gel in the presence of SDS. A protein band associated with IFN activity was observed. This protein represented 2.4% of all the protein in the densitometer tracing of the stained gel, and 90% of IFN applied to the gel was recovered from the band. Therefore, the specific activity of IFN recovered from the gel band was estimated to be 4.5 × 10^8 IU/mg protein.

Purification of IFN by Affinity Chromatography

IFN induced from BrdU-treated Namalwa cells by Sendai virus, was composed of electrophoretically heterogeneous species with molecular weights ranging from 15 K to 24 K. These heterogeneous IFN molecules were purified by a 3-step procedure.

1. Preparation of crude IFN

Initially, 1.7 × 10^{10} Namalwa cells treated with BrdU (20 liter culture) were infected with Sendai virus, and the culture fluid containing 1.47 × 10^8 IU in 1,700 ml (5.9 × 10^5 IU/mg protein) was used for purification.

2. Antibody column chromatography

The original culture fluid was directly applied to the anti-IFN column. IFN was eluted by pH 3 solution (1.1 × 10^8 IU in 75 ml, 8.6 × 10^7 IU/mg protein). The major protein components of the eluate, revealed by protein staining of the SDS-polyacrylamide gel, were two proteins with molecular weights of more than 100 K and a broad protein band. This broad band lay in the range of molecular weights from 15 K to 24 K and coincided closely with IFN activity (Fig. 1A). In contrast, SDS-polyacrylamide gel electrophoresis of BrdU-untreated Namalwa cell IFN, purified by antibody column, revealed a comparatively sharp protein band, comigrating together with IFN activity, with a molecular weight of 17K (Fig. 1B).

3. Blue Sepharose and antirabbit IgG Sepharose column chromatography

The main proteins with molecular weights of more than 100 K in the eluate from the anti-IFN column were removed by a Blue Sepharose column followed by an antirabbit IgG Sepharose column. The anti-IFN column eluate was applied to a Blue Sepharose column, and IFN was eluted by 0.5 M NaCl (1.1 × 10^8 IU in 10 ml, 3.5 × 10^8 IU/mg protein). The effluent was passed through an antirabbit IgG column (1.1 × 10^8 IU in 18 ml, 7.6 × 10^8 IU/mg protein). Of the IFN activity in the original culture fluid, 72% was recovered. The purified IFN was analyzed by SDS-polyacrylamide gel electrophoresis. An

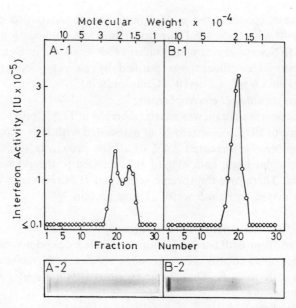

Fig. 1. SDS-polyacrylamide gel electrophoresis of IFN from (A) BrdU-treated Namalwa cells and (B) BrdU-untreated Namalwa cells purified by anti-IFN columns. (A) Concentrated antibody column eluate of BrdU-treated Namalwa cell IFN, containing 2.3×10^6 IU/34 µg protein, was applied and the recovery of IFN activity was 40%. (B) BrdU-untreated Namalwa cell IFN (1.5×10^7 IU in 800 ml, 5.3×10^4 IU/mg protein) was purified by antibody column (1.3×10^7 IU in 75 ml, 7.8×10^7 IU/mg protein), followed by octyl-Sepharose column (1.3×10^7 IU in 2.2 ml, 1.0×10^8 IU/mg protein). Purified IFN, containing 1.6×10^6 IU/16 µg protein, was electrophoresed and the recovery of IFN activity was 73%. (A-1) and (B-1) indicate the distribution of interferon activity (O——O). Another gel run in parallel was stained for protein and the photograph of the stained gel is inserted in (A-2) and (B-2).

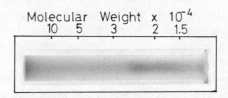

Fig. 2. Photograph of protein stained gel. IFN was electrophoresed after antirabbit IgG Sepharose column chromatography (3.5×10^6 IU/5 µg protein).

IFN peak with a molecular weight ranging from 15 K to 24 K comigrated with a broad protein band, and no conspicuous impurities were detectable other than minor ones, indicating that the final preparation was essentially pure. A photograph of the stained gel is shown in Fig. 2.

Purification of Radioactive IFN by Immune Precipitation
1. Preparation of Crude Radioactive IFN

BrdU-treated and Sendai virus-infected Namalwa cells produced IFN from at least 2 to 17.5 hours after infection with the virus (Fig. 3). The times of addition of ^{3}H-leucine (O hr) and of harvest (17.5 hr) were thus determined. When using 1.8 Ci/mM and 90 μCi/ml of ^{3}H-leucine, ^{3}H-incorporation into the total acid-insoluble material proceeded nearly linearly with time during the period of IFN production (Fig. 3), indicating that the quantity of added leucine was not limiting.

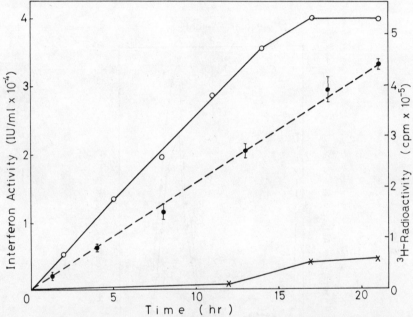

Fig. 3. Time course of IFN production and ^{3}H-leucine incorporation after Sendai virus-infection. BrdU-treated and Sendai virus-infected Namalwa cells at 5×10^6 cells/ml in 6 mm wells of a microtiter plate (Linbro) were fed with 50 μl of medium containing ^{3}H-leucine (90 μCi/ml, 1.8 Ci/mM). At the time indicated, 50 μl of 10% trichloroacetic acid was added and the precipitated radioactivity was measured (●----●). From another well, the fluid was withdrawn and assayed for IFN (O——O). IFN from BrdU-untreated and Sendai virus-infected Namalwa cells is also indicated (×——×).

2. Immune precipitation of radioactive IFN

IFN was purified from the ^{3}H-leucine-labeled fluid by the use of rabbit anti-IFN serum and PAA. The original culture fluid contained 2.3×10^4 IU and 3.1×10^5 cpm in 1 ml, and the immune precipitate contained 2.3×10^4 IU and 5.7×10^4 cpm. The precipitated material was electrophoresed in polyacrylamide gel in the presence of SDS (Fig. 4). Only one broad radioactive band was observed in the electropherogram, and it coincided closely with IFN activity. The radioactivity associated with IFN activity (2.2×10^4 IU) was 3.0×10^4 cpm, 9.7% that of the original culture fluid and 0.43% that of the total incorporation (6.6×10^6 cpm of cells and debris and 3.1×10^5 cpm of the culture fluid). The radioactive peaks, which comigrated with IFN activity, were specific for anti-IFN serum and IFN-induced culture fluid because normal rabbit serum did not precipitate the radioactive peak associated with IFN and the radioactive peak was not precipitated by anti-IFN serum from Sendai virus-uninfected culture fluid (data not shown).

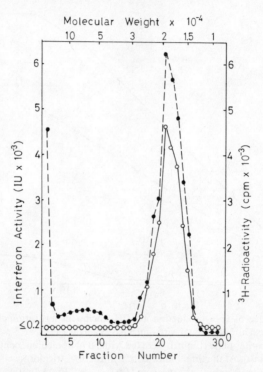

Fig. 4. SDS-polyacrylamide gel electrophoresis of immune-precipitated IFN. O——O: IFN activity; ●----●: radioactivity. The material precipitated with anti-IFN antibody, containing 2.2×10^4 IU and 5.6×10^4 cpm, was electrophoresed. The recovery was 78% and 96%, respectively.

In order to obtain highly radioactive IFN, Sendai virus–infected Namalwa cells were pulse-labeled with ³H-leucine of high specific activity. This highly radioactive IFN purified by immune precipitation and SDS-polyacrylamide gel electrophoresis contained 9.2 cpm/IU and was used for the radioimmunoassay.

Radioimmunoassay for HuIFN-α

A competitive radioimmunoassay for HuIFN-α was established by the use of highly radioactive IFN, anti-IFN serum, and PAA. Figure 5 shows the results of the radioimmunoassay. Two hundred IU of HuIFN-α (Namalwa cell IFN and leukocyte IFN) inhibited 50% of the immune precipitation between radioactive IFN and antibody, and about 100 IU of IFN-α could be measured by the radioimmunoassay (Fig. 5). However, more than 10^4 IU of HuIFN-β, mouse IFN-α, and mouse IFN-β did not inhibit the formation of an immune precipitate (Fig. 5).

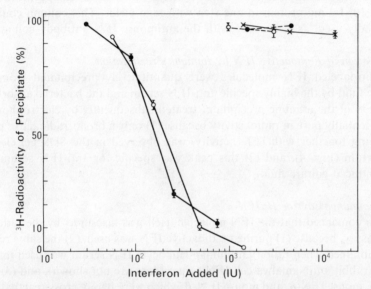

Fig. 5. Radioimmunoassay for IFN. Percent inhibition of immune precipitation between labeled IFN and antibody, measured by radioactivity, is plotted against the quantity of added IFN. The titer of added IFN, indicated in the figure, was measured by biological assay. One hundred percent of the radioactivity corresponded to 295 cpm. ●——●: Namalwa cell IFN purified by anti-IFN column (about 1×10^7 IU/mg protein); ○——○: HuIFN-α (Le) (about 1×10^5 IU/mg protein); ×——×: HuIFN-β ($>1 \times 10^7$ IU/mg protein), kindly supplied Dr. K. Kobayashi (Basic Research Laboratory, Toray Industries, Inc.); ○——○: mouse IFN-α (about 1×10^7 IU/mg protein); ○----○: mouse IFN-β (about 1×10^7 IU/mg protein). Mouse IFNs were kindly supplied by Dr. Y. Kawade (Institute for Virus Research, Kyoto University).

DISCUSSION

Purification of IFN by Affinity Chromatography

IFN produced by BrdU-treated and Sendai virus-infected Namalwa cells was purified in high yields to 7.6×10^8 IU/mg protein by a simple procedure consisting of 3 chromatographic procedures. The final preparation was judged essentially pure, because (1) only a broad protein band which coincided closely with IFN activity was observed in the SDS-polyacrylamide gel electropherogram of the final preparation (Fig. 2), 2) this broad protein band was not observed with the purified homogeneous interferon protein obtained from BrdU-untreated Namalwa cells (Fig. 1B), and (3) the specific activity is comparable to the value of purified human leukocyte IFN reported by Berg and Heron[9] and is higher than that reported by Zoon et al. for Namalwa cell IFN.[7]

The essential feature of our purification is the introduction of a highly specific antibody affinity column as the first step, which allows the purification of nearly 10^8 IU/mg protein in one step with high yields. This column could be repeatedly used, as is the case with the antimouse IFN antibody column.[2,3]

Purification of Radioactive IFN by Immune Precipitation

Radio-labeled IFN molecules were quantitatively precipitated from the culture fluid by the highly specific anti-IFN serum and the bacterial adsorbent. The IFN of the immune precipitate, treated subsequently by electrophoresis, was essentially pure in radioactivity because (1) only a broad radioactive peak, migrating together with IFN activity, was observed in the SDS gel electropherogram (Fig. 4), and (2) this peak was specific for anti-IFN serum and IFN-induced culture fluid.

Radioimmunoassay for HuIFN-α

I am convinced that the IFN molecule itself was measured by the radioimmunoassay, because (1) purified radioactive IFN was used, (2) the same results were obtained when rabbit antihuman leukocyte IFN serum was used instead of the rabbit antiNamalwa cell IFN serum (data are not shown), and (3) HuIFN-β, mouse IFN-α, and mouse IFN-β, which were barely cross-reactive with HuIFN-α in antigenicity, did not inhibit the formation of an immune precipitate between anti-IFN antibody and radioactive IFN (Fig. 5).

At least two days are needed to measure IFN activity with a biological assay, but the quantity of IFN protein can be measured within one day with this radioimmunoassay. Radioimmunoassays will be effective for measuring the quantity of IFN in serum for clinical applications because viral inhibitors in serum often obstruct biological assays of IFN.

Acknowledgments

I would like to thank Ms. Y. Yanase (Tokyo Metropolitan Institute of Medical Science), Mr. M. Imai (Immunology Division, Jichi Medical School), Dr. S. Nakasawa (Department of Pediatrics, School of Medicine, Keio University), and Dr. H. Mori (Yokohama City Institute of Health) for Namalwa cell cultures and Sendai virus preparations. I am also grateful to Dr. K.

Nishioka (Tokyo Metropolitan Institute of Medical Science) and Dr. Y. Kawade (Institute for Virus Research, Kyoto University) for useful discussions.

REFERENCES

1. Kawakita, M., Carber, B., Taira, H., Rebello, M., Slattery, E., Weideli, H., and Lengyel, P.: Purification of interferon from mouse Ehrlich ascites tumor cell. *J. Biol. Chem.*, **253**: 598–602, 1978.
2. De Maeyer-Guignard, J., Tovey, M. G., Gresser, I., and De Maeyer, E.: Purification of mouse interferon by sequential affinity chromatography on poly (U)- and antibody-agarose column. *Nature*, **271**: 622–625, 1978.
3. Iwakura, Y., Yonehara, S., and Kawade, Y.: Purification of mouse L cell interferon: Essentially pure preparation with associated cell growth inhibitory activity. *J. Biol. Chem.*, **253**: 5074–5079, 1978.
4. Tan, T. H., Barakato, F., Berthold, W., Smith-Johansen, H., and Tan, C.: The isolation and amino acid/sugar composition of human fibroblast interferon. *J. Biol. Chem.*, **254**: 8067–8073, 1979.
5. Knight, E., Jr., Hunkapiller, M. W., Korat, B. D., Hardy, R. W. F., and Hood, L. E.: Human fibroblast interferon: Amino acid analysis and amino terminal amino acid sequence. *Science*, **207**: 525–526, 1980.
6. Rubinstein, M., Rubinstein, S., Familletti, P. C., Miller, R. S., Waldman, A. A., and Pestka, S. : Human leukocyte interferon: Production, purification to homogeneity, and initial characterization. *Proc. Natl. Acad. Sci. USA*, **76**: 640–644, 1979.
7. Zoon, K. C., Smith, M. E., Bridgen, P. J., Nedden, D., and Anfinsen, C. E.: Purification and partial characterization of human lymphoblastoid interferon. *Proc. Natl. Acad. Sci. USA*, **76**: 5601–5605, 1979.
8. Yonehara, S., Iwakura, Y., and Kawade, Y.: Rapid purification of mouse L cell interferon labeled with radioactive amino acid by immune precipitation. *Virology*, **100**: 125–129, 1980.
9. Berg, K. and Heron, L. : The complete purification of human leucocyte interferon. *Scand. J. Immunol.*, **11**: 489–502, 1980.
10. Yamamoto, Y., Tsukui, K., Ohwaki, M., and Kawade, Y.: Electrophoretic characterization of purified mouse L cell interferon of high specific activity. *J. Gen. Virol.*, **23**: 23–32, 1974.
11. Yonehara, S., Yanase, Y., Sano, T., Imai, M., Nakasawa, S., and Mori, H.: Purification of human lymphoblastoid interferon by a simple procedure with high yields. *J. Biol. Chem.*, **256**: 3770–3775, 1981.

Discussion

Dr. TAIRA: I have two questions. First, a very diffused band is observed after the antibody column purification. However, we see one peak after tritium leucine labeling in SDS-PAGE. Why is there such a peak? Second, is it possible to conduct radioimmunoassay by ^{125}I-labeled interferon? Have you ever tried it?

Dr. YONEHARA: As for the first question, I apologize that my figure was not clear. There is a broad protein band even in SDS-PAGE of labeled IFN. We don't see any sharp interferon band. Regarding the second question, we believe iodine-labeled interferon is very valuable for radioimmunoassay. However, the interferon receptor analysis that I am planning for the future may not be possible using iodine-labeled interferon due to the possible inactivation of interferon.

Dr. KOBAYASHI: Have you ever applied Namalwa cell interferon clinically to patients and measured it by radioimmunoassay?

Dr. YONEHARA: You mean in the serum?

Dr. KOBAYASHI: Yes.

Dr. YONEHARA: No, we have not tried it in patients' sera. I think that we have to improve this method before we can measure interferon in human sera by RIA and that the sensitivity of the method is not sufficient yet for clinical application.

Dr. OHTSUKI: Is the specitic activity of heterogeneous IFN protein in radioactivity heterogeneous or homogeneous?

Dr. YONEHARA: It is rather homogeneous.

Dr. OHTSUKI: In other words, the synthesis of heterogeneous IFN protein is homogeneous.

Dr. YONEHARA: Well, I have not looked at the time course, whether each IFN is in the early production or later production. But in any case, I believe it is homogeneous.

Preparation of Human Fibroblast Interferon for Clinical Trials

Sigeyasu KOBAYASHI,* Masahiko IIZUKA,* Michio HARA,* Hitoshi OZAWA,* Takashi NAGASHIMA,* and Jiro SUZUKI[2]*

* Basic Research Laboratories, Toray Industries, Inc., Kamakura, Japan 248, [2]* Tokyo Metropolitan Institute of Medical Science, Honkomagome, Bunkyo-ku, Tokyo 113, Japan

SUMMARY

Several strains of human diploid fibroblasts were identified as good producers of human fibroblast interferon (HuIFN-β), among which the DIP-2 cell was one of the best. A new multi-tray culture apparatus was developed for mass culture of anchorage-dependent cells and large-scale production of HuIFN-β. Using this culture system, over 10^{10} international reference units (IU) of crude HuIFN-β per month were produced from DIP-2 cells. Large amounts of crude Hu IFN-β were routinely purified to more than 10^7 IU/mg protein of specific activity by a relatively simple procedure. The purified and lyophilized HuIFN-β was assayed for its safety for clinical use under the regulation of the National Institute of Health of Japan. The clinical evaluation of this HuIFN-β is now in progress.

INTRODUCTION

Human interferons (HuIFNs) are being prepared on a large scale for clinical evaluation.[1] So far, at least three types of human tissue-derived cells have been used for preparing large amounts of HuIFNs. These are buffy coat leukocytes,[2] diploid fibroblast strains,[3] and lymphoblastoid cell lines.[4] The leukocyte IFN (HuIFN-α) was the only type available in sufficient amounts for some clinical trials.[1] However, greater quantities of HuIFN must be produced for proper evaluation in extended clinical trials.

A large supply of fresh human leukocytes is difficult to obtain in common laboratories. On the other hand, the human diploid fibroblast strains can be readily prepared from neonatal foreskins and embryonic tissues, among other sources.[5] Furthermore, these appear to be suitable substrates for preparing safe HuIFN for clinical trials.[6] However, large-scale production systems for HuIFN-β using the diploid fibroblast strains have seldom been reported.[3,7] One major reason is that these anchorage-dependent cells can grow only in monolayer culture conditions and their growth rates are slow in comparison with those of other estiablished cell lines.

To date, laboratories have employed either roller bottles or large flasks both for the mass culture of these cells and for IFN production on a large scale. Several new types of culture apparatus for large-scale monolayer culture have been reported,[8,9] but these techniques may prove to be impractical. We have also developed an apparatus for mass culture and for large-scale HuIFN-β production in our laboratory. This multi-tray culture apparatus[10] is similar to the "NUNC Multitray Unit System."[8] We have accomplished routine pilot plant preparation, purification, and safety testing of HuIFN-β for clinical trials.

MATERIALS AND METHODS

Cell Cultures

Several hundred strains of human fibroblasts have been derived from various kinds of tissue such as neonatal foreskin, embryonic tissues, and amnion in our laboratory. Some cell strains have been selected as good sources for HuIFN-β production in accord with our criteria for cell selection (see Table 1). Stocks of the cells at the 6th population doubling level (PDL), 14th PDL, and 22nd PDL were kept frozen in ampoules in liquid nitrogen (2×10^6 cells/ampoule). The growth medium for both stock cultures and mass cultures was Eagle's minimum essential medium (MEM; Nissui Seiyaku Co., Japan) supplemented

Table 1.   Criteria for selection of human diploid cell strains.

Characteristics		Ranking				
		A	B	C	D	E
1. Growth rate[a]	Days	1–3	4–5	6–7	8–9	>10
2. Density	10^4 cell/cm^2	>7	3–7	0.7–3	0.07–0.7	<0.07
3. Split ratio	Dilution	×32	×16	×8	×4	×2
4. Life span	PDL	>50	40–50	30–40	20–10	<20
5. IFN production	IU/ml	>5,000	3–5,000	1–3,000	0.2–1,000	<200
6. Serum requirement	%	<5	5–10	10–15	15–20	>20
7. Durability	Days	>14	10–14	6–9	3–5	<3
8. Stability in liquid N$_2$[c]	Days	<3	4–7	8–14	15–20	>21
9. Diploidy	%	>90	80–90	70–80	60–70	<60

a) Time required for cells inoculated at 1:4 dilution to form confluency.
b) After confluency.
c) Time required ampouled cells to form confluency in Roux bottle.

mainly with 5% precolostrum newborn calf serum (PNCS; Mitsubishi Kasei Institute for Life Science, Japan).

An ampoule of the cells at the 22nd PDL is routinely used to supply the starting cells for large-scale IFN production. As shown in Fig. 1, the starting cells are grown to about the 42nd PDL by using over a hundred units of the multi-tray culture apparatus. At this stage, sufficient numbers of the cells (over 5×10^{10} cells) can be obtained to produce IFN.

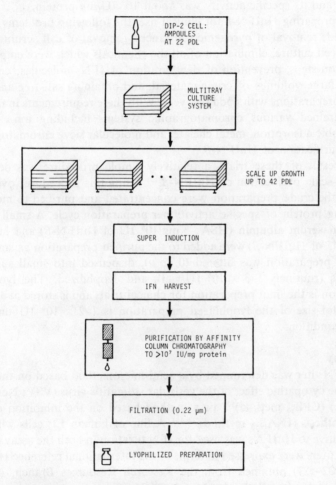

Fig. 1.   Mass production system of HuIFN-β.

IFN Production and Purification

Confluent monolayer cultures in the multi-tray culture apparatus were first primed by the addition of a low dose of HuIFN-β prior to IFN induction.[11]

HuIFN-β was superinduced by treating the primed cells with poly I:poly C (Yamasa Shoyu Co., Japan), cycloheximide (CH; Sigma Co., U.S.A.), and actinomycin D (Act-D; Mackor Co., Israel). The superinduction procedure used was very similar to the methods reported by Havell and Vilček,[5] Billiau et al,[7] and Horoszewicz et al.,[3] except for the use of serum-free medium in the whole process of IFN production. The average yield of crude HuIFN-β was approximately 10,000 international reference units (IU)/ml of harvest medium, and its specific activity was about 10^5 IU/mg protein.

When preparing HuIFN-β for clinical use, the following problems must be considered: removal of pyrogenic substances, removal of calf serum proteins used for cell culture, elimination of all the chemicals which were employed in preparation steps, prevention of denaturation of IFN molecules, easy handling of large volumes of crude material, and obtaining salt-free and highly purified preparations with good recovery. With these requirements in mind, we have examined various chromatographic systems including ion-exchange, hydrophobic adsorption, metal chelate, and molecular sieve chromatographies for the purification of HuIFN-β.

As a result of these trials, a relatively simple procedure was developed for large-scale purification of HuIFN-β.[12] Using this procedure, over 1,000 liters of the crude preparation were concentrated and purified to more than 10^7 IU/mg protein of specific activity per preparation cycle. A small amount of human serum albumin (HSA; 3 mg/10^6 IU of HuIFN-β) and lactose (1 mg/10^6 IU of HuIFN-β) were added to the purified preparation as stabilizers. Then the preparation was filtered (0.22 μ), dispensed into small siliconized glass-vials (routinely 1–3 × 10^6 IU/vial), and lyophilized. The lyophilized preparation is the final preparation for clinical trials and is stored at 4° C until used. A lot-size of the lyophilized preparation is 1–2 × 10^9 IU under the present conditions.

IFN Assay

The IFN titer was determined by a semi-micromethod based on the inhibition of the cytopathic effect of the vesicular stomatitis virus (VSV; New Jersey sero type) (CPE_{50} method)[13] or a method based on the inhibition of VSV-RNA synthesis ($INAS_{50}$ method).[14,15] A line of human FL cells which was very sensitive to HuIFNs was used for IFN titration in both the assay systems. The IFN titers were expressed in terms of the international reference HuIFN-β (G-023–902–527) obtained from the Research Resources Branch, National Institutes of Health, Bethesda, Maryland, U.S.A.

Other Tests

The Cell number was counted in a hemocytometer, in most cases directly, or after staining with 0.17% trypan blue for exact viability count. Karyotypic analyis of the cells was carried out according to the method of Furuyama and Chiyo.[16] Protein concentration was mainly determined by the Coomasie Brilliant Blue G-250 method of Sedmak and Grossberg,[17] using bovine serum albumin (BSA), fraction five, (Seikagaku Kogyo Co., Japan) as a standard. In some cases, the concentration was also calculated from the results of amino acid analysis by a Hitachi model 835 analyzer. Electrophoresis on 15% polyacrylamide slab gels in the presence of sodium dodecyl sulfate (SDS-PAGE) was performed using the method of De Maeyer-Guignard et al.[18]

RESULTS

Selection of Cell Stains for Production of HuIFN-β

Table 1 shows 9 characteristics used for the selection of cell strains as good producers of HuIFN-β. Five rankings were set up to evaluate the response of the cells. It has been difficult to find cell strains which achieve a high ranking for all the items, although a few hundred cell strains have been derived from human tissues, as described in Materials and Methods. However, several cell strains demonstrated A abilities in most items and B abilities in a few. These cell strains were selected as candidates for the production of HuIFN-β. Ampoule stocks of the candidate cells at the 6th PDL were kept in liquid nitrogen as the primary cell stocks.

Table 2 indicates the properties of DIP-2 cells, derived from neonatal foreskin and one of the best candidate cell strains for HuIFN-β production. The cell strain has abilities which rank A in 7 items and rank B in 2.

Table 2.   Characteristics of Dip-2 cells.

Characteristics	Ranking
Growth rate	A
Density	A
Split ratio	A
Life span	A
IFN producibility	A
Serum requirement	A
Durability	B
Stability in liquid N_2	B
Karyology (diploidy)	A

DIP-2 cells have typical fibroblast morphology and grow well to form a uniform monolayer. The *in vitro* life span was approximately 60 PDL. As shown in Fig. 2, karyotypic analysis indicated that over 90% of the cells have the normal diploid chromosomes for the human male karyotype (46, XY) and maintain this diploidy even in older generations (i.e., 47 PDL).

Table 3 shows that DIP-2 cells exhibit no tumorigenicity in nude mice. When

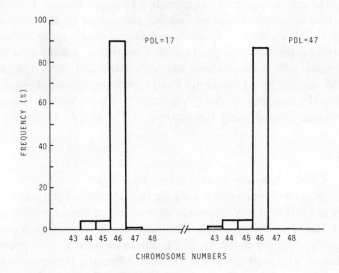

Fig. 2. Karyotypic analysis of DIP-2 cells.

Table 3. Tumorigenicity of DIP-2 cells in nude mice.[a]

Cells	Cells/mouse	Tumor animals/tested animals
Hela	10^6	5/5[b]
DIP-2 (32nd PDL)	10^7	0/5[c]

a) Mice used are 12-week-old males (nu/nu).
b) At 24 days after *SC* inoculation of the cells, tumors with the size of about $2 \times 1 \times 0.5$ cm^3 occurred in all mice tested.
c) Observation was carried out for 50 days after the inoculation.

10^6 HeLa cells were inoculated into each of 5 nude mice, tumor formation was clearly observed in all mice tested. But even the injection of 10^7 DIP-2 cells per mouse did not cause tumor formation. DIP-2 cells were free of detectable adventitious agents such as viruses, mycoplasma, bacteria, and fungi. We therefore decided to use this cell strain as the primary source for large-scale preparation of HuIFN-β for clinical use.

Properties of HuIFN-β Preparation

Mass production of HuIFN-β from DIP-2 cells and purification of large amounts of the crude preparation are described in Materials and Methods. As shown in Fig. 3, SDS-PAGE analysis of the purified HuIFN-β revealed antiviral activity associated with a single band, which had a molecular weight (MW) of about 25,000 daltons. The activity at a MW of 25,000 was not consistent with that at the MW of 21,000 reported by Knight,[19] but it was the same as the value estimated by Otto *et al.*[20] and Vilček *et al.* (personal communication). The difference in these values may be attributed to a dissimilarity of carbohydrate components.

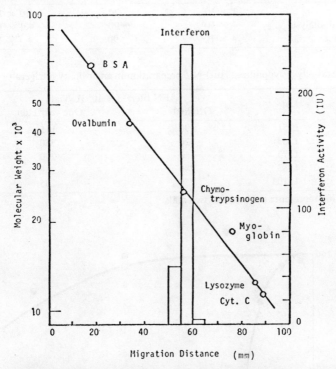

Fig. 3. Molecular weight of HuIFN-β by SDS-PAGE analysis. About 12% of charged IFN activity was recovered at the band with a molecular weight of 25,000.

The specific activity of the purified HuIFN-β preparation was determined by 3 methods: high speed liquid partition chromatography (HLPC), amino acid analysis, and dye binding (Bio-Rad reagent).[17] Table 4 shows that the specific activity of purified HuIFN-β is over 10^7 IU/mg protein in all cases.

The lyophilized HuIFN-β preparation was stable in an ordinary refrigerator (4–7°C) for over a year. Table 5 presents an example of stability tests for the preparations preserved in the refrigerator. As shown in the table, all the lyophilized preparations tested retained their original antiviral activities without any loss for a year.

For clinical trials the lyophilized preparation is reconstituted in physiological saline and has been used for subcutaneous, intramuscular, intravenous, and intrathecal injection. The stability of the reconstituted preparation was also investigated. Figure 4 indicates the stability of three lots at 4°C and 25°C for

Table 4. Specific activity of purified HuIFN-β.

Method of protein analysis	IFN activity (IU/ml)	Protein content (μg/ml)	Specific activity (IU/mg protein)
HPLC	2×10^6	20	10×10^7
Amino acid analysis	4×10^6	90	4.4×10^7
Dye-binding	4×10^6	90	4.4×10^7

Table 5. Stability of lyophilized HuIFN-β preparation in an ordinary refrigerator (4–7°C).

Lot	IFN titer[a] ($\times 10^4$ IU/vial)	
	Original	One year later
L-51	90	115
L-53	320	360
L-73	280	290
L-83	280	235
L-103	250	235

a) Each value represents the mean of two vials.

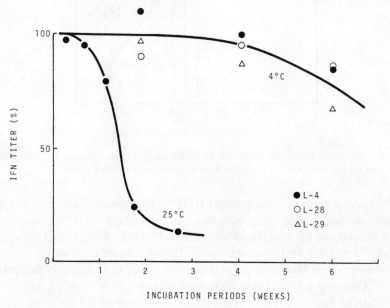

Fig. 4. Stability of lyophilized HuIFN-β preparation reconstituted in physiological saline. L-4, L-28, and L-29 are lot numbers of the lyophilized preparations.

several weeks. The injection was fairly stable at 4°C for over a month, although a significant loss of activity occurred at 25°C incubation within a couple of weeks.

Quality Control and Safety of HuIFN-β for Clinical Trials

The final HuIFN-β preparation was evaluated according to the tentative guidelines of the National Institute of Health (NIH) of Japan on general safety, pyrogenicity, sterility, potency, contaminants, and other factors. These guidelines are very similar to those issued by the Food and Drug Administration (FDA) of the U.S.A. in 1981. Table 6 shows the results of negative tests for various contaminants (such as poly I:poly C, Act-D, CH, or BSA), potency (IFN titer), moisture content, and isotonicity (in one ml of the saline) in the final container. As shown in Table 7, the final preparation also easily passed the tests for general safety, pyrogenicity, and sterility. These quality control and safety tests have been routinely performed for each lot in the final container in both our laboratory and the NIH of Japan.

Table 6. Safety tests for final container (I).

Test	Method	Results
Potency	IFN titration	$1-3 \times 10$ IU/vial
Contaminants		
Poly I:poly C	Cytopathic effect[a]	<0.5 μg/vial
Act-D	Inhibition of RNA synthesis[b]	$<10^{-3}$ μg/vial
CH	Inhibition of protein synthesis[b]	$<10^{-2}$ μg/vial
BSA	Hemagglutination-inhibition of SRBC[c]	<0.1 μg/10^6 IU
Moisture content	Weight measuring	$<3\%$
Osmosis	Osmo-meter	Isotonic

a) Using mouse L cells.
b) Using human FL cells.
c) SRBC: sheep red blood cells.

Table 7. Safety tests for final container (II).

Test	Method	Results
Sterility		
Bacteria	National guidelines	Negative
Fungi	for	Negative
Mycoplasma	biological products	Negative
Tuberculosis		Negative
General safety		
Guinea pig	I. P., 2.5×10^6 IU/animal	Negative[a]
Mouse	I. P., 1.5×10^6 IU/animal	Negative[b]
Pyrogenicity		
Limulus	Endotoxin detection (3×10^6Iu/ml)	Negative
Rabbit	I. V., 10^6 IU/kg	Negative[c]

a) Seven days' observation using 5 animals.
b) Seven days' observation using 5 animals.
c) Three hours' observation using 3 rabbits.

DISCUSSION

We have developed a new type of mass culture system, the multi-tray culture apparatus, for anchorage-dependent cells such as human fibroblasts. The apparatus can also be applied, with careful handling, to the production of HuIFN-β from the above fibroblast cell strains.

Mass production of HuIFN-β for clinical investigation using the above system was initiated in our laboratory early in 1977. In one set of the apparatus, $0.5-1 \times 10^9$ cells can be routinely grown (2–3 liters of culture medium per set). It is, therefore, not difficult to prepare several hundred liters of crude HuIFN-β (over 10^9 IU of IFN titer) from the fibroblast cell strains at one time by employing more than a hundred sets. In fact, we are now producing over 10^{10} IU of the crude HuIFN-β per month and preparing highly purified and safety-tested HuIFN-β for clinical trials on a large scale, as described in Materials and Methods. However, these amounts of HuIFN-β are not enough for a proper clinical evaluation in a wide variety of diseases. So we are also studying an improved microcarrier culture system for larger scale production of HuIFN-β, as reported by Giard and Fleischaker.[9] The development of this system may enable us to prepare enough HuIFN-β for an adequate clinical evaluation in the near future.

Each lot of our final HuIFN-β preparation for clinical use ($1-2 \times 10^9$ IU/ lot) has passed the quality control and safety tests under the regulations of the NIH of Japan for use by the IFN research groups for clinical trials organized by the Ministry of Health and Welfare of Japan. That is, we have completed all the quality control and safety tests of HuIFN-β from the cell culture through the production and purification of IFN with the support of the Japanese government. Since mid-1979, these IFN research groups have started phase I or phase II studies using our HuIFN-β preparations with various viral and neoplastic diseases such as viral warts, herpetic keratitis, chronic active hepatitis, melanoma, medulloblastoma, glioblastoma, lymphoma, and leukemia. The results are presented elsewhere in this volume.

Acknowledgments

This work was supported, in part, by a research grant for important technology from the Ministry of International Trade and Industry of Japan.

We thank Dr. K. Okada, Dr. R. E. Gills, and Mrs. S. Ruskey for supplying tissue sources of human fibroblasts. We are indebted to Dr. Y. Kiuchi for his help in nude mouse experiments. The advice of Dr. C. W. Walter in the preparation of the manuscript is gratefully acknowledged. Our thanks are also due to all the members of the Interferon Labs at the Basic Research Laboratories of Toray Industries, Inc., and the Tokyo Metropolitan Institute of Medical Science for their technical assistance.

REFERENCES

1. Stewart, W. E., II: *The Interferon System*. Springer-Verlag, Vienna and New York, 1979.
2. Mogesen, K. E. and Cantell, K.: Production and preparation of human leucocyte interferon. *Pharmacol. Ther. C.*, **1**: 369–381, 1977.
3. Horoszewicz, J. S., Leong, S. S., Ito, M., Dibernardine, L. A., and Carter, W. A.: Aging *in vitro* and large-scale interferon production by 15 new strains of human diploid fibroblasts. *Infect. Immun.*, **19**: 720–726, 1978.
4. Adams, A., Lindin, B., Strander, H., and Cantell, K.: Spontaneous interferon production and Epstein-Barr virus antigen expression in human lymphoid cell lines. *J. Gen. Vitrol.*, **28**: 219–223, 1975.
5. Havell, E. A. and Vilček, J.: Production of high titered interferon in cultures of human diploid cells. *Antimicrob. Agents Chemother.*, **2**: 476–484, 1972.
6. Hayflick, L.: The choice of a cell substrate for preparation of human interferon. In: C. Waymouth (ed.), The Production and Use of Interferon for the Treatment and Prevention of Human Virus Infections. Tissue Culture Association, Rockville, Md., 1973, pp. 4–11.
7. Billiau, A., Joniau, M., and De Somer, P.: Mass production of human interferon in diploid cells stimulated by poly I: poly C. *J. Gen. Virol.*, **19**: 1–8, 1973.
8. Skoda, R., Pakos, V., Hormann, A., Spath, O., and Johansson, A.: Communicating vessel system for mass cell culture of anchorage dependent cells. *Develop. Biol. Standard.*, 121–126, 1979.
9. Giard, D. J. and Fleischaker, R. J.: Examination of parameters affecting human interferon production with microcarrier-grown fibroblast cells. *Antimicrob. Agents Chemother.*, **18**: 130–136, 1980.
10. Iizuka, M.: Cell culture propagation apparatus. U.S. Patent, 4, 228, 243, Oct. 14, 1980.
11. Ito, F. and Kobayashi, S.: Enhancing effect of interferon pretreatment on interferon production. *Japan. J. Microbiol.*, **18**: 223–228, 1974.
12. Hosoi, K. and Ozawa, H.: Purification method of human fibroblast interferon. Japanese Patient Applications, Japan Kokai 55–62902 (May, 1980), 55–64799 (May, 1980), and others in application.
13. Armstrong, J. A.: Semi-micro dye-binding assay for rabbit interferon. *Appl. Microbiol.*, **21**: 723–725, 1971.
14. Suzuki, J., Akaboshi, T., and Kobayashi, S.: A rapid and simple method for assaying interferon. *Japan. J. Microbiol.*, **18**: 449–456, 1974.
15. Suzuki, J., Iizuka, M., and Kobayashi, S.: Assay of interferon by reduction of viral RNA synthesis: A convenient assay for tracer experiments with monolayer cultures. In: S. Pestka (ed.), Methods in Enzymology. **78A**, Academic Press, New York, 1981 (in press).
16. Furuyama, J. and Chiyo, T.: The methods for chromosome analysis. *Clinical Laboratory*, **7**: 281–288, 1977 (in Japanese).
17. Sedmak, J. J. and Grossberg, S. E.: A rapid, sensitive and versatile assay for protein using coomassie brilliant blue G250. *Anal. Biochem.*, **79**: 544–552, 1977.
18. De Maeyer-Guignard, J., Tovey, M. G., Gresser, I., and De Maeyer, E.: Purification of mouse interferon by sequential affinity chromatography on poly (U)- and antibody-agarose columns. *Nature*, **271**: 622–625, 1978.
19. Knight, E., Jr.: Interferon: Purification and initial characterization from human diploid cells. *Proc. Natl. Acad. Sci. USA*, **73**: 520–523, 1976.
20. Otto, M. J., Sedmak, J. J., and Grossberg, S. E.: Enzymatic modifications of human fibroblast and leukocyte infections. *J. Virol.*, **35**: 390–399, 1980.

Discussion

Dr. MACHIDA: What do you mean by the stability of the cells in liquid nitrogen?

Dr. KOBAYASHI: Some cells deteriorate while being stored. The question is how fast living cells are recovered in case of transfer from liquid nitrogen.

Dr. MACHIDA: You mentioned durability in your presentation. Does this refer to the number of days that cells are alive?

Dr. KOBAYASHI: That is correct. In the production of interferon, we have to consider the aging factor and other enhancing factors. At the same time, it is true that when a cell is confluent and can be maintained for a long time, it is easier to make a schedule.

Dr. MACHIDA: Do you use priming for interferon induction?

Dr. KOBAYASHI: Yes, we do. It is like insurance.

Dr. NOBUHARA: You mentioned that if 2×10^5 u/kg i.v. rabbit is negative, it is considered to be pyrogen-free. However, in the case of humans, for example in Japanese, their average weight is 50 kg, so that is 10 million u per body. Wouldn't your preparations cause a pyrogenic reaction in humans?

Dr. KOBAYASHI: In fact, it does cause pyrogenic reactions. I think many doctors will refer to this point in tomorrow's sessions. Our interferon is mostly administered intravenously. The i.v. administration of interferon generates a temporary pyrogenic reaction. It is reported that in some patients it produces severe reactions. However, in cases of subcutaneous or local administration no pyrogenicity is observed.

Human Fibroblast Interferon: Subpopulations with Different Pharmacokinetic Behavior

J.W. HEINE, A. BILLIAU, J. Van DAMME, and P. De SOMER

Rega Institute for Medical Research, University of Leuven, B-3000 Leuven, Belgium

SUMMARY

Human fibroblast interferon, prepared from diploid cells or from an osteosarcoma cell line, was chromatographically separated into two distinct fractions. Upon intramuscular injection in rabbits, one of these yielded concentrations of antiviral activity in the serum comparable to those obtained with leukocyte interferon. The interferon contained in the other fraction yielded only very low blood concentrations.

Human interferon exists in at least three molecular types for which a recently proposed nomenclature is HuIFN-α, HuIFN-β, and HuIFN-γ.[1] Preparations containing mainly HuIFN-α (leukocyte interferon preparations) and HuIFN-β (fibroblast interferon preparations) are increasingly being used for systemic administration in clinical trials on patients with virus infections or malignancies.[2]

A comparison of blood titers obtained in patients injected with these IFNs revealed that intramuscular injection of 3×10^6 units of leukocyte IFN resulted in maximal blood titers of up to 500 units/ml.[3,4] In contrast, similar doses of fibroblast IFN yielded blood titers of less than 30 units/ml,[4] suggesting that it may be less effective clinically. This difference in pharmacokinetic behavior between the two IFN types was unexpected in view of earlier studies in rabbits where intramuscular injections of either IFN had yielded comparable blood curves of antiviral activity.[5] Subsequent re-examination of the pharmacokinetics in rabbits then did reveal a considerable difference between leukocyte and fibroblast IFN in one study[6] and a minor difference in another.[7]

We here present data which may clarify this confusion in that they reveal the heterogeneity of current fibroblast IFN preparations, with different variants

69

possessing different pharmacokinetic behavior. In particular, it was found that fibroblast IFN eluted from zinc chelate columns as two apparent subpopulations.[8,9] As the pH of the eluant buffer was lowered, a first peak eluted at pH 5.9, together with about 5% of the contaminating proteins, and a second peak at pH 5.2 without fluorimetrically detectable proteins. Since the zinc chelate method had preparative capacity, it was possible to obtain each subpopulation in sufficient quantity to perform comparative pharmacokinetic experiments in rabbits.

The results of these experiments are illustrated in Fig. 1. The injection of leukocyte IFN (panel a) resulted in a maximum serum level of about 600 units/ml, a value comparable to that described in the literature.[5,13] With fibroblast IFN the serum levels differed depending on the cellular origin of the IFN and on the method of fractionation. Fibroblast IFN from MG-63 cells, eluting from zinc columns at pH 5.9, yielded blood titers (panel b) comparable to those obtained with leukocyte IFN. The fraction eluting at pH 5.2, on the contrary, gave very low blood values (panel d). Similar low values were obtained with a preparation of fibroblast IFN from diploid cells (E_1SM strain) that had not undergone fractionation by zinc chelate chromatography (panel c). This was concordant, however, with the observation that this IFN represented more than 90% of the subpopulation which eluted at pH 5.2.[8]

It thus appears that the two variants of fibroblast IFN which are separable from each other by zinc chelate chromatography have different pharmacokinetic behavior. All pharmacokinetic experiments done in the past[5-7] have used unfractionated fibroblast IFN preparations. The discrepancy between the results obtained in these studies may have resulted from differences in the relative amounts of the two variants contained in the IFNs used by various investigators. Thus, fibroblast IFN prepared from the osteosarcoma cell line MG-63 invariably contained the two components in a 50/50 proportion.[8] Fibroblast IFN from most of the diploid cells tested in our laboratory contained only 5 to 10% of the pH 5.9 variety.[8,9] Some diploid cell strains produced a larger fraction of this IFN when reaching a high passage level.[8]

The molecular basis for the observed difference in pharmacokinetics is still unclear. The two variants of fibroblast IFN might differ in glycosylation or they may also have different amino acid sequences. They might also simply differ in that one of them is bound to a carrier protein. Another unresolved question is the significance of the pharmacokinetic difference for clinical effectiveness. What happens with the IFN population that does not appear in the circulation? Is it retained and degraded at the injection site? Or is it quickly removed from the circulation by certain organ systems? The fact that intramuscular injection of fibroblast IFN in patients causes activation of NK cell activity without achieving high serum levels favors the second possibility.[11]

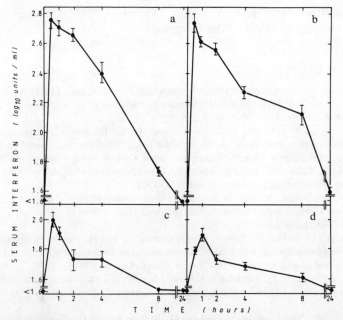

Fig. 1. Levels of IFN in the serum of rabbits injected intramuscularly with different IFN preparations.

Rabbits ($\sim$ 1.5kg) were injected intramuscularly with 10^6 units of the IFN preparations. Blood samples were taken from the ear vein, before and at indicated times after the injection. IFN assays were done on the serum samples using a CPE-inhibition method on diploid human skin fibroblasts with VSV as a challenge virus and neutral red as a dye to measure cell viability.[10] IFN concentrations are expressed in international units. Aliquots of the injected material were diluted in pre-bleeding serum or in saline, and these mixtures were included in the assays in order to monitor the destruction of the IFN activity by the serum. No such inactivation was seen. Each curve represents an average from data on 6 rabbits. Human leukocyte IFN was a fift from Dr. K. Cantell (State Serum Institute, Helsinki, Finland). Fibroblast IFN was prepared in our laboratory by superinduction of either diploid human skin fibroblasts or of the osteosarcoma cell line MG-63, as described.[11,12] This material underwent purification and concentration by adsorption to controlled pore glass. When indicated it was also fractioned on zinc chelate columns.

Panel a: Leukocyte IFN.

Panel b: Fibroblast IFN from MG-63 cells purified by controlled pore glass adsorption plus zinc chelate chromatography; fraction eluting at pH 5.9.

Panel c: Fibroblast IFN from diploid cell strain E_1SM, purified by controlled pore glass adsorption only.

Panel d: As in c; fraction eluting at pH 5.2.

Acknowledgment

This study was supported by the Cancer Research Foundation of the Belgian General Savings and Retirement Fund (ALSK/CGER) and by Research Contract No. 76/81-IV of the "Geconcerteerde Onderzoeksacties" (Belgian Ministry of Science Administration).

REFERENCES

1. International Committee: Interferon Nomenclature. *Nature*, **286**: 110, 1980.
2. Scott, G. M. and Tyrrell, D. A. J.: Interferon, therapeutic fact or fiction for the '80s? *Brit. Med. J.*, **280**: 1558–1562, 1980.
3. Greenberg, S. B., Harmon, M. W., and Couch, R. C.: Exogenous interferon: Stability and pharmacokinetics. In:D. A. Stringfellow (ed.), Interferon and Interferon Inducers, Clinical Applications. Marcel Dekker Inc., New York & Basel, 1980, pp. 57–87.
4. Edy, V. G., Billiau, A., and De Somer, P.: Non-appearance of injected fibroblast interferon in the circulation. *Lancet*, **1**: 451–452, 1978.
5. Edy, V. G., Billiau, A., and De Somer, P.: Comparison of rate of clearance of human fibroblast and leukocyte interferon from the circulatory system of rabbits. *J. Infect. Dis.*, **133**: A18–A21, 1976.
6. Billiau, A., De Somer, P., Edy, V. G., De Clercq, E., and Heremans, H.: Human fibroblast interferon for clinical trials: Pharmacokinetics and tolerability in experimental animals and humans. *Antimicrob. Agents Chemother.*, **16**: 56–63, 1979.
7. Vilček, J., Sulea, L. T., Zerebeckyi, I. L., and Yip, Y. K.: Pharmacokinetic properties of human fibroblast and leukocyte interferons in rabbits. *J. Clin. Microbiol.*, **11**: 102–105, 1980.
8. Heine, J. W., Van Damme, J., De Ley, M., Billiau, A., and De Somer, P.: Purification of human fibroblast interferon by zinc chelate chromatography. *J. Gen. Virol.*, **54**: 47–56, 1981.
9. Heine, J. W., De Ley, M., Van Damme, J., Billiau, A., and De Somer, P.: Human fibroblast interferon purified to homogeneity by a two-step procedure. *Ann. N. Y. Acad. Sci.*, **350**: 364–373.
10. Finter, N. B.: Dye uptake methods for assessing viral cytopathogenicity and their application to interferon assays. *J. Gen. Virol.*, **5**: 419–427, 1969.
11. Billiau, A., Van Damme, J., Van Leuven, F., Edy, V. G., De Ley, M., Cassiman, J. J., Van den Berghe, H., and De Somer, P.: Human fibroblast interferon for clinical trials: Production, partial purification, and characterization. *Antimicrob. Agents Chemother.*, **16**: 49–55, 1979.
12. Billiau, A., Edy, V. G., Heremans, H., Van Damme, J., Desmyter, J., Georgiades, J. A., and De Somer, P.: Human interferon: Mass production in a newly established cell line, MG-63. *Antimicrob. Agents Chemother.*, **12**: 11–15, 1977.
13. Cantell, K., Pyhälä, L., and Strander, H.: Circulating human interferon after intramuscular injection into animals and man. *J. Gen. Virol.*, **22**: 453–455, 1974.

Discussion

Dr. Hosoi: What was the molecular weight of interferon obtained at pH 5.2 from zinc chelate column?

Dr. Billiau: The 5.2 material was put on a SDS gell and the molecular weight was around 22,000. The 5.9 material, as you have noticed on the profile, is impure. It comes out with most of the protein of the zinc chelate. So we could not label it, and we have not examined its molecular weight as yet. We are now in the process of purifying this material on an antibody column; since the technique works very nicely, we will label it and put it on a gel. Unfortunately, the amount of 5.9 material produced by the cells varies. And although we had much of it in the beginning, our cells are failing to produce very much of it right now. This is what happens in the laboratory. When you want it to happen, it doesn't.

Dr. VILČEK: I wonder whether you have examined the stability of the pH 5.9 fraction in SDS.

Dr. BILLIAU: No, we haven't done it yet. We have to do it.

Dr. VILČEK: The reason I am asking is to see whether this is perhaps the elusive β-2 subspecies. One of the reasons why perhaps this does not show up in the usual type of test on SDS gels—it is apparently homogeneous in terms of molecular weight— is that this subspecies might be perhaps more labile on SDS treatment. That is only a speculation at this point.

Dr. BILLIAU: It's a very good hypothesis. It may be the elusive β-2 type. There are some experiments under way in the sense that we are trying to isolate two messengers from the MG63 cells. If this can be done, it will more or less settle the question.

Dr. BORDEN: I missed whether that was intramuscular or intravenous injection of the rabbits.

Dr. BILLIAU: It was the intramuscular injection.

Dr. BORDEN: Have you looked at any other biological activities of the 5.9 material? For example, does it have heterospecies activity in terms of antiviral effects on other cells?

Dr. BILLIAU: As far as we can see, the host range is the same. We looked at bovine cells, Vero cells; that I can remember now. It was not done very extensively, but the hot spots were examined, and it looked similar.

Dr. YAMAZAKI: I am very interested in the pH 5.9 material. As Dr. Vilček's question pointed out, you did not use SDS. But what about the hydrophobicity?

Dr. BILLIAU: We have not done that yet. It's a good suggestion.

Dr. YAMAZAKI: I think that Sepharose column would be a good way to look at hydrophobicity. Many researchers who experienced the purification of fibroblast interferon have observed that some fractions will attach but others will not. There is the possibility of overlooking the existence of such fractions. The glycoprotein or sugar moiety may have some connection with the pH difference; what do you think about this possibility?

Dr. BILLIAU: Actually, there are several possibilities. One is that it is a different primary structure, and so a β-2 type interferon. The other possibility is that it is differently glycosylated. Jochen Heine tried to show in some experiments that tunicamycin treatment affected the production of the two components in a different way. Actually, it did not. It depressed both the 5.2 and 5.9 materials to the same extent. But what we first want to do is to get it more pure than we have it now by passing it through the antibody column, and then we will characterize it in different ways, including, among others, looking at hydrophobicity.

Dr. REVEL: In line with what has been suggested, maybe you could try to see if your

material binds to SH sepharose column, because the only indication we have about the β-2 interferon —this is the product of heavy messenger RNA— is that it binds to SH Sepharose column while the product of the light messenger RNA— β-1— does not bind. So it will be interesting to know if your 5.9 binds to SH Sepharose.
Dr. Billiau: Thank you for your suggestion.

Interferon Induced in Human Leukocytes by Mitogens: Production, Partial Purification, and Characterization

Marc De Ley,* Joseph Van Damme,* Hendrik Claeys,[2]* Hans Weening,* Jochen W. Heine,* Alfons Billiau,* Carl Vermylen,[2]* and Piet De Somer*

*Rega Institute, Division of Microbiology, Department of Human Biology, University of Leuven, Belgium, [2]*Belgian Red Cross Blood Transfusion Center, Leuven Belgium

INTRODUCTION

Human α- and β-type interferons (HuIFN-α and -β) have been prepared and purified in sufficiently large quantities to allow the study of their molecular structure and their application in clinical trials. Their mRNAs have been isolated and their cDNA has been built into bacteria. The production by bacteria of still larger amounts of these IFNs is expected for the near future.

Little is known, however, about the molecular structure of γ-type IFNs. Their production and purification on a large scale have recently been initiated,[1] but they are not yet available for human application. Based on experiments in mice, however, one can predict a more pronounced activity against tumors. It has indeed been shown that lymphokine preparations, rich in γ-type IFN, were 100-fold more active as antitumor agents than preparations of classical α- or β-type IFN of comparable antiviral potency.[2]

Therefore, it seemed of particular interest to investigate the conditions for optimal production and purification of human γ-type IFN.

Elaboration of Optimal Conditions for the Production of HuIFN-γ from Blood Leukocytes

Several T-cell mitogens and cell culture conditions have been compared for the production of immune interferon by fresh human buffy clat leukocytes. After treatment with ammonium chloride to remove the erythrocytes,[3] blood leukocytes were suspended in medium RPMI 1640, with added proteins, and stimulated by the addition of either SEA (0.02 μg/ml), PHA-P (1/1,000), or ConA (10 μg/ml). Incubation of the cell cultures was continued at 37°C either in half-gallon roller bottles (rotating at 2 rpm) or in spinner vessels. After 24 hours of incubation, the supernatant fluids were clarified by centrifugation (3,000 rpm, 20 min) and stored at —70°C. IFN titrations were carried out by the CPE-inhibition method on diploid human embryonic skin and muscle cells with vesicular stomatitis virus as a challenge and reduction of neutral red uptake as a measure of CPE.[4]

Internal laboratory standard preparations (preserved at —70°C) allowed the expression of antiviral activity of fibroblast and leukocyte IFNs in international units. An internal laboratory standard of controlled pore glass (CPG) and gel filtration-purified immune IFN was assigned an arbitrary value which corresponded to the reciprocal of the average titration endpoint by the above-mentioned method. Table 1 shows the IFN yields, expressed per 10^6 cells.

Table 1.　Comparison of different protocols for the induction of HuIFN-γ.

Inducer	Cell density (cells/ml ÷ 10^6)	Protein additive	IFN yield ($\log_{10}$ units/10^6 cells)
SEA	5	10% agamma plasma	2.5
PHA-P	1	10　agamma plasma	2.8
ConA	2	2　agamma plasma	2.8
	2	2　HPPF	3.2

It can be seen that the highest IFN yields were obtained after stimulation with ConA in the presence of human plasma protein fraction (HPPF) as a protein additive. This reaction was therefore studied in more detail. From the time course of the IFN production (data not shown) it was seen that antiviral activity was detected as soon as 5 hours after stimulation with ConA. A maximum level of production was reached after 8 to 12 hours. From these experiments an optimal induction scheme for the routine production was deduced: fresh buffy coat leukocytes at a cell density of 5×10^6 cells/ml suspended in EMEM were stimulated with ConA (10 μg/ml) in the presence of 1 mg/ml HPPF and incubated in spinner vessels at 37°C for 20 hours. The average IFN yield amounted to $10^{3.2}$ units per 10^6 cells and was found to be remarkably constant throughout multiple production runs. This method has the particular advantages that no fractionation of leukocytes is required and that ConA is the only non-human protein in the production medium. Bovine serum and SEA used in other systems may be harmful in clinical trials if not removed completely.

Initial Purification of ConA-induced IFN

The supernatant fluids were immediately processed for initial purifications. After clarification at 3,000 rpm for 20 min, the fluids were subjected to CPG adsorption and desorption by ethylene glycol (EG) containing buffers as described by Langford *et al.*[1] with slight modifications. Briefly, clarified culture

Table 2. Partial purification and concentration of immune IFN on CPG.

Fraction	Volume (ml)	IFN titer (log₁₀ units/ml)	Protein concentration (mg/ml)	Specific activity (log₁₀ units/mg protein)	Total IFN content		Purification factor
					$\log_{10}$ units	percent of input	
Crude IFN harvest (clarified culture supernatant)	4,470	3.7	7.20	2.84	7.35	100	1
Unadsorbed fraction	4,470	2.7	7.23	1.84	6.35	10	—
Wash no. 1 (PBS)	200	<1.7	1.97	—	<4.00	—	—
Wash no. 2 (1.5 M NaCl)	200	<1.5	0.32	—	<3.80	—	—
Wash no. 3 (1.5 M NaCl)	200	<2.2	0.32	—	<4.50	—	—
Eluate no. 1 (50 % ethylene glycol)[a]	4.5	6.7	23.4	5.33	7.35	100	309
Eluate no. 2 (50 % ethylene glycol)[a]	4.5	5.7	10.9	4.66	6.35	10	66

a) Concentrated 40-fold by dialysis against polyethylene glycol.

supernatants were gently stirred for 3 hours at 4°C with CPG beads (5 mg/ml). The beads were allowed to settle, the unadsorbed material was decanted, and the beads were washed once with Dulbecco's phosphate-buffered saline and twice with 1.5 M NaCl, 8 mM phosphate, pH 7.4. The immune IFN was then eluted with 1/20 of the starting volume 1.5 M NaCl, 8 mM phosphate, pH 7.4, containing 50% (v/v) ethylene glycol. The eluted IFN was further concentrated by dialysis against polyethylene glycol 20,000. The data in Table 2 from a typical experiment show that with this method a 300-fold purification could be achieved with 100% recovery of the antiviral activity at a specific activity of $10^{5.3}$ units/mg. A second elution yielded minor amounts of immune IFN at lower specific activities. It was observed that the overall recovery in several purification runs varied widely and often exceeded 100%. This may be an indication of the presence in our preparations of components with either synergistic or antagonistic effects which are eliminated during the purification to different degrees. Most of the characterization experiments described below were carried out on this CPG-purified material.

Characterization of CPG/ethylene-glycol-purified Immune IFN
Physicochemical properties

In order to achieve a further purification, and as an initial characterization, the CPG-purified material was subjected to gel filtration on Ultrogel AcA44 or Sephacryl S-200. Under the conditions used, more than 90% of the antiviral activity eluted as a single peak corresponding to a molecular weight of 45,000 daltons. On average, 65% of the applied antiviral activity could be recovered at a specific activity of $10^{6.5}$ units/mg. In several gel filtration runs, a distinct trace of antiviral activity was found which eluted at a position corresponding to a molecular weight of 22,000 daltons. The biological activity of this material was relatively more pronounced when titrated on embryonic skin and muscle cells, as compared to HEp-2 cells.

The CPG-EG-purified, ConA-induced IFN was found to be inactivated by heat (10 min, 56°C), by dialysis against an acid buffer (pH 2), and by incubation with trypsin.

Serologic properties

The serologic characterization of our CPG/EG-purified immune IFN was carried out by titration in the presence of potent antisera against fibroblast and leukocyte IFN. Triplicate dilution series of leukocyte, fibroblast, and immune IFN samples were made, and suitable amounts of antisera were added. After incubation the dilutions were used for a regular IFN titration. Neutralization could thus be shown by a shift in the IFN titration endpoint. The specificity of the antisera was verified by including fibroblast and leukocyte IFNs as controls. As shown by the data in Table 3, the antiserum against fibroblast IFN was highly specific, while that raised against leukocyte IFN showed some cross-reactivity with fibroblast IFN. The activity of the immune IFN preparations was slighty but definitely inhibited by the antiserum against fibroblast IFN and minimally by the antiserum against leukocyte IFN.

Table 3. Serological characterization of CPG/EG-purified, ConA-induced IFN.

Antibody added in titration	Titration endpoints obtained with sample of		
	Fibroblast IFN	Leukocyte IFN	Immune IFN
None	2.65	2.90	3.45
Antifibroblast IFN	<0.90	2.90	2.80
Antileukocyte IFN	1.40	<0.90	3.25

Biological properties

(1) *Heterologous activity.* The host range of both crude and CPG-EG-purified immune IFN was examined by titration on cell cultures of different animal species. Leukocyte and fibroblast IFNs were included for comparison. From the data summarized in Table 4 it can be seen that, in contrast to leukocyte and fibroblast IFNs, no activity of immune IFN could be detected in any

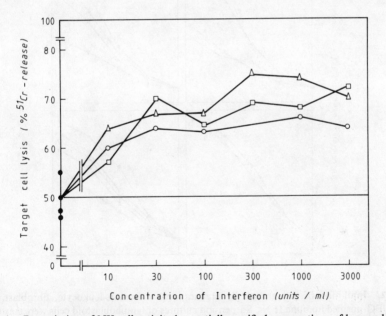

Fig. 1. Potentiation of NK cell activity by partially purified preparations of human leukocyte, fibroblast, and CPG/EG-purified immune IFNs. Lymphocytes were exposed to IFN for 16 hours and incubated for 4 with labeled target cells at a ratio of 12/1. (●: base level; ○: leukocyte-IFN; □: fibroblast IFN; △: ConA-induced, CPG/EG-purified IFN).

heterologous system tested so far. As a result of this, protection experiments with mitogen-induced IFN in monkeys, as predictive models for clinical trials in man, seem to be precluded.

Table 4. Titration endpoints of human leukocyte, fibroblast, and immune IFNs on heterologous cells.

Cell type	Leukocyte IFN	Fibroblast IFN	ConA-induced IFN	
			Crude	CPG-purified
Human embryonic skin and muscle	3.5	4.7	3.9	5.5
Rabbit kidney	<1.5	1.5	<1.5	<1.5
Feline lung	3.8	1.6	<1.5	<1.5
Fetal calf kidney	4.5	2.5	<0.5	<0.5
Cynomolgus kidney	2.5	2.9	<1.5	<1.5
VERO	1.7	3.1	<1.5	<1.5
Mouse embryo fibroblast	1.7	2.3	<1.5	<1.5

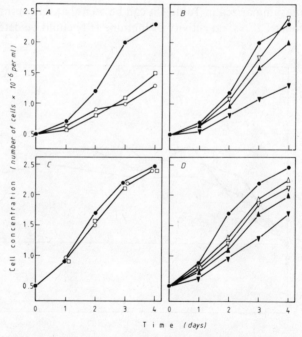

Fig. 2. Inhibition of cell growth by preparations of human leukocyte, fibroblast, and CPG/EG-purified immune IFNs. Suspension cultures of lymphoblastoid cells were started at 0.5×10^6 cells/ml in the presence of IFNs. Panels A and B: Daudi cells; panels C and D: Molt-4 cells. ●: no IFN added; ○: leukocyte IFN (10 units/ml); □: fibroblast IFN (100 units/ml); △: ConA-induced IFN (30 units/ml); ▽: idem (100 units/ml); ▲: idem (300 units/ml); ▼: idem (1,000 units/ml).

(2) *Natural killer activity.* The stimulation of NK cell activity of fresh lymphocytes from healthy donors by semipurified immune IFN was tested on K-562 cells as target in a ^{51}Cr release assay.[5] Leukocyte and fibroblast IFNs were included for comparison. From the dose-response curves shown in Fig. 1 it is clear that, on the basis of antiviral activity, immune IFN was not significantly more active in stimulating NK cell activity than leukocyte or fibroblast IFN.

(3) *Cell growth inhibition.* The cell growth inhibitory action of CPG-EG-purified immune IFN was investigated using several lymphoblastoid cell lines. The results obtained with Daudi cells, as an example of a B-cell line, and of Molt-4 cells, as an example of a T-cell line, are shown in Fig. 2. As expected, the growth of Daudi cells was inhibited by as little as 10 U/ml of leukocyte IFN or 100 U/ml of fibroblast IFN. A comparable result was only obtained with 1,000 U/ml of immune IFN. Molt-4 cells were markedly less sensitive to leukocyte and fibroblast IFNs. They showed, however, definite inhibition of cell growth by immune IFN at concentration of $\geqslant$ 30 U/ml.

REFERENCES

1. Langford, M. P., Georgiades, J. A., Stanton, G. J., Dianzani, F., and Johnson, H. M.: Large-scale production and physicochemical characterization of human immune interferon. *Infect. Immun.*, **26**: 36, 1979.
2. Crane, J. L., Jr., Glasgow, L. A., Kern, E. R., and Younger, J. S.: Inhibition of murine osteogenic sarcomas by treatment with type I or type II interferon. *J. Nat. Cancer Inst.*, **61**: 871, 1978.
3. Cantell, K., Hirvonen, S., Mogensen, K. E., and Pyhälä, L.: Human leukocyte interferon: production, purification, stability and animal experiments. In: In Vitro, Monograph Vol. 3, In: C. Waymouth (ed.), The Tissue Culture Association, Rockville, Md., 1974, p. 35.
4. Finter, N. B.: Dye uptake methods for assessing viral cytopathogenicity and their application to interferon assays. *J. Gen. Virol.*, **5**: 419, 1969.
5. Bolhuis, R. L. H., Schuit, H. R. E., Nooyen, A. M., and Ronteltap, C. P. M.: Characterization of natural killer (NK) cells and killer (K) cells in human blood: discrimination between NK and K cell activities. *Eur. J. Immunol.*, **8**, 731, 1978.

Discussion

Dr. VILČEK: Concerning the question whether you have or don't have β interferon present in the preparation, you said you made an antibody that has a very high neutralizing titer of 1 to 100,000. Is that neutralization specific for γ interferon or is it not specific?

Dr. BILLIAU: It is specific for γ interferon although one would expect it to act also against fibroblast interferon, because the antigen contains some of the fibroblast component. It is not acting against our fibroblast interferon. But that may be the lack of immunization of the animal.

Dr. VILČEK: Well, I wonder whether, with your antiserum against fibroblast interferon in the first place, you may perhaps be seeing some antigenic cross-reaction. I say this because, on some occasions, with certain batches of either anti-α or anti-β serum, we did see partial neutralization of what we are pretty sure is γ interferon. I describe that although I have no absolute proof of an antigenetic cross-reaction. The second point I'd like to make is that we consider pH 2 stability or lability a very bad criterion. And we also had some batches of material that were rather stable. We could not destroy the activity at pH 2, at least not all of it. I just wonder whether you are not mistakenly assuming that you have had some β interferon when indeed it is, at least the bulk of it, γ interferon.

Dr. BILLIAU: Of course we have thought of this possibility, because we see cross-reactivity with the most pure immune interferon that we have. We also find some cross-reactivity using that specific antibody. But the strange thing is that if you take the crude immune interferon, or the one that has already undergone the CPG purification, and you dialyze that at pH 2, you lose some activity, not very much perhaps. But what remains then is completely wiped out by the anti-β. So it is not a little bit of cross-reactivity that you see at that time; you just wipe it out.

Dr. VILČEK: Well could you perhaps by pH 2 dialysis unfold the molecule so that it then becomes more easily neutralizable by the serum? If you really have a specific antiserum to γ interferon, then you can further analyze this question and get the final answer.

Dr. BILLIAU: Of course, that's what we will do.

Dr. BORDEN: Could you tell us what was the target cell for your NK cell assays?

Dr. BILLIAU: Yes. It was the classical K562.

Dr. BORDEN: Have you looked at other targets to see whether the range of relative activity of the three interferons that you reported differs for different targets?

Dr. BILLIAU: Not yet.

Dr. KAWADE: I have some experience with murine γ interferon induced by con-A. And I found some acid-stable component which needs anti-γ in addition to anti-α and -β to completely neutralize. So that seems to be a subcomponent of mouse γ.

Dr. BILLIAU: This is interesting. Dr. Falcoff from the Institut Curie in Paris, I think, has similar findings that he may not have published yet, but he also finds an acid-resistant fraction. I am not quite sure what the neutralization pattern of that interferon is.

Dr. KOBAYASHI: Thank you, Dr. Billiau.

Floor Discussion

Dr. KAWADE: I'd like to ask Dr. Billiau a question. I have found some inhibitor of γ interferon in various rabbit sera, either normal or anti-α and anti-β. This is in the case of mouse interferon. I wonder if you have similar experience in sera of rabbits or other animals—non-specific inhibitor of gamma interferon which is not active on α or β.

Dr. BILLIAU: I don't think we tested for this. I am aware of your studies. I don't think we tested for such inhibitors.

Dr. KAWADE: So some anti-α and -β antisera look as if they show cross-reaction with γ. Some of your results might be related to this inhibitor.

Dr. BILLIAU: Yes. What we did to control this is that the goat that was used to make the anti-β antibody was extensively bled before the immunization procedure. So we have a pre-serum, and this has no activity whatsoever on the immune interferon preparations. I think that was the best control that we could get to control non-specific neutralization.

Dr. BEKTIMIROV: I have a question to Dr. Kobayashi. In your presentation, you talked about the preliminary study on the microcarrier system. Can you give some details about the microcarrier systems? What kind of microcarrier do you use? What is the density of the cells? What is the yield of interferon? Because you said it worked very well.

Dr. KOBAYASHI: I didn't say it worked very well. I said that it is under way and it works "fairly well," but I did not say "very well." It's very difficult to explain. I cannot give you detailed information now, but mainly we are using very similar conditions to those of the MIT group. But we have had many troubles in growing cells. Because our cells are very different from their cells, we need optimal conditions for our cells in the microcarrier system. The conditions are not so different from those of the MIT group.

Dr. ISHIDA: Is there anyone here who can comment on the *in vitro* tumor cell static activity of three types of interferon in connection with their site of action—which is higher and which is lower?

Dr. BILLIAU: I have no data from our laboratory on this question. But somebody else might have some data. I think it is too premature to discuss it. Maybe next year we will know the answer. As far as the microcarrier is concerned, we have limited experience in our laboratory using diploid cells. And we use a commercial microcarrier that we buy from the Flow Company. This is not an advertisement, but that's where we buy it. And we have worked for months with small-scale setups and we have seen the yields improve with two variables. The first variable was the batch of microcarrier that we received. As new batches kept coming in, they improved. And the second variable is the kitchenery of it—the amount of serum that you put into, the speed of stirring it, the split ratio and all sorts of other things. But if you have all these things optimized, then you get—and this is on 10 or 20 runs, that order of magnitude—the same amount of interferon unit per cell that you have in the system at the time of induction. So you can optimize it. Then we discontinued work with this, because we calculated that the microcarrier at this time was still more expensive than the ordinary roller bottle. So this is a matter of development. They have to work on the manufacture of the beads until they get to the point where it is less expensive than the ordinary roller bottle. But it works if you have all the variables right and works reproducibly. The MG63 cell, the tumor cell line, which has the added advantage of producing about 3 to 4 times more interferon per cell, doesn't like the beads; it doesn't stick on them. Cells come off the beads, so you cannot use the MG63 cells in the system.

Dr. KOBAYASHI: Thank you very much, Dr. Billiau, for giving us very valuable information.

Dr. YAMANE: I'd like to ask you, Dr. Vilček, a question concerning the isoelectric point of your immune interferon preparation. You mentioned that pH is 8.6. Do you have some chemical explanation for this isoelectric point? Because the immune interferon is a kind of glycoprotein and most glycoproteins should contain some sialic acid, most of such glycoprotein should be acidic in the isoelectric point. So could you give us some chemical explanation for this isoelectric point?

Dr. VILČEK: I don't have a chemical explanation; I am sorry. But in my defense, I can say that our data are not very different from those obtained by the Galveston group. The one exception is that the material that we use appears to be more homogeneous. We have really only one major peak while the Texas group has reported three peaks with most of the activity around 8.6. So I don't have the chemical explanation that you ask for, but we are quite sure that this is the isoelectric point. If you remember, we showed the isoelectric profile of α interferon which was analyzed on the gel run concurrently, and the values that we obtained there agree with the values found by other people.

Dr. YAMANE: Thank you.

Dr. ISHIDA (Asahi Kasei): I'd like to ask a question to Dr. Vilček. How much blood do you need to get 1 mg of γ interferon with the present technique?

Dr. VILČEK: I would need a Japanese calculator to give you the answer, and I don't have it right now. But clearly you would need a lot of blood. And we would be quite happy if you could make a few microgram of pure γ interferon.

Dr. ISHIDA: Then how many years will it take to elucidate the amino acid sequence?

Dr. VILČEK: Well, if you have the methods that the people at the California Institute of Technology have—they apparently can do sequencing with as little as one microgram of protein—we hope to be able to produce that much.

Dr. REVEL: I'd like to ask a question to Dr. Billiau about the 45,000 molecular weight of β-like interferon that you mentioned. Is it possible that you have a dimer like what Dr. Knight reported a year ago? Do you have a dimer of fibroblast interferon? Or could you comment on the dimer?

Dr. BILLIAU: The 45,000 material is only minimally cross-reacting with fibroblast. It is probably the other one that we can separate. But it is cross-reacting, and the most fancy hypothesis we could dream up was that there would be two β molecules which are linked up, so that they hide most of the antigenic sites and therefore they are only minimally cross-reactive. If they open up by the pH 2 treatment, then they are completely neutralized. So we have thought of the dimer hypothesis. But it is a little bit far-fetched at this moment. One can only dream it at night.

Dr. KUMAGAI: I'd like to ask a question concerning the interferon-producing cells to Dr. Vilček or any of the other speakers. Is it correct to understand that α interferon is produced by NK or B cells and γ interferon by T cells? I'd like to ask another question to Dr. Billiau. If leukocytes produce β interferon, then what about T cells and macrophages?

Dr. VILČEK: We don't have definitive results about the source of γ interferon in our system. But we have done some experiments in our own laboratory and some in collaboration with others. And the preliminary evidence seems to be that, indeed, you need only T cells or a T cell-enriched fraction, and that the macrophages do not appear to be necessary for the production of this interferon. That answers I think, my part of the question.

Dr. BILLIAU: We haven't done any experiment to find out which cells are responsible.

Dr. KOBAYASHI: I think this question can be answered by Dr. Samuel Baron.

Dr. BARON: There have been a number of groups who have examined the cell of origin of the α interferon. Dr. Roberts of Rochester points out that in his system with virus induction, the macrophage is the primary producer. With B cell mitogens, one can get α interferon, and with deletion of the B cells, indicating that the B cells can be a producer. Then finally there is very good evidence that reaction to foreign cells by the NK cells can give rise to it. The German group in, I guess, Heidelberg, has produced that information. So it looks like there are at least three types of cells within the leukocyte cells which can produce the α interferon, perhaps depending on the stimulus, perhaps on the culture conditions.

Dr. FINTER: I wonder if we get too concerned about a particular cell producing any one sort of interferon. I think Lois Epstein, some years ago, showed interferon of the immune type formed by both B and T lymphocytes depending on the time. With our lymphoblastoid cells, we know that they produce both the α and β types of interferon. The product that we prepared is extremely stable and persists for a long time on storage at pH 2. But we quite consistently see a small initial drop in the activity when the material is first prepared. And although I've never looked at this, I wonder whether there is in fact some γ type interferon produced by these cells also. The genes to make all these different interferons are presumably present in all human cells, and under some conditions may be activated. It could be that with the appropriate stimulus, one could use many cells to produce almost any type of interferon. But probably, normally and preferentially, they produce one or the other type.

Dr. BILLIAU: Of course, the people who ask these questions are interested in knowing which cells produce it, so they can then enrich the population. I think it was from the practical point of view that they raised this question.

Spontaneous and Potential Interferon Producing Cell Lines Transformed from Human Cord Blood Lymphocytes and Grown in Serum-free Medium

Isao YAMANE,* Takeshi SATO,* Yoshiki MINAMOTO,* Toshio KUDO,²* and Takehiko TACHIBANA²*

*Department of Microbiology and ²*Immunology, Res. Inst. for TB & Cancer, Tohoku University, Sendai, Japan

SUMMARY

Lymphoblastoid cell lines were established by transforming human adult peripheral and cord blood lymphocytes, by infection with Epstein Barr virus. The majority of cell lines obtained from cord blood lymphocytes were found to be spontaneous producer of interferon (IFN), while lymphoblastoid cell lines derived form the peripheral blood lymphocytes were not. These spontaneous producers grew well in a newly developed serum-free culture medium based on Dulbecco's modified Eagle's medium supplemented with nonessential amino acid, vitamins, nucleotides, trace metals, human transferrin, insulin and bovine or human serum albumin (Cohn Fr. V). In the serum-free medium, the cells spontaneously produce IFN as well as in the serum-containing conventional medium (RPMI-1640). About 10,000U/ml of IFN could be harvested every day, by collecting the serum-free culture fluid and refeeding the cells with fresh medium to give the saturation cell density (10^7 cells/ml). The IFN was shown to be HuIFN-α by its physicochemical and serologic characteristics.

INTRODUCTION

Several workers have described the spontaneous production of IFN by lymphoblastoid cell lines.[1-7] Although they produces high titer of IFN upon viral induction,[8,9] only a very small amount of IFN is found in their culture media without the induction.[1-7,9] Therefore it is almost impossible to prepare large amount of IFN without the viral induction. Fetal bovine or calf serum is usually added to the culture medium of animal cells. A tested and approved batch of serum is a very expensive ingredient which may represent 80 to 90% of the total cost of the culture medium. Moreover, it is very difficult to remove all traces of bovine serum proteins completely in the purification of IFN. The mass production of human IFN has been impeded by this problem. Although serum -free media or media containing a low level of serum can be used in the preparation of IFN from human lymphocytes[10,11] or Namalwa cells,[12,13] such cultures are viable only for short periods as the media can not support cell growth.

In this report we examin the possibility of establishing new cell lines which spontaneoulsy produce IFN in high titer. Among a number of lymphoblastoid cell lines which had been obtained by transformation of adult peripheral blood lymphocytes (PBL) and umbilical cord blood lymphocytes (CBL) by EBV, several established lines were found to produce IFN without further stimulation. We have also attempted to cultivate the cells in a novel serum-free medium in order to facilitate the large scale purification of IFN.

MATERIALS AND METHODS

Preparation of Lymphocytes

Lymphocyte preparations were obtained from fresh heparinized adult peripheral blood (PBL) of 8 volunteers, and from fresh heparinized umbilical cord blood (CBL) of 13 newborn infants. PBL and CBL were isolated with Ficoll Isopaque density gradient as described by Böyum.[14] They were cultured with RPMI-1640 medium in the presence of 10% fetal bovine serum (FBS) at 37°C in an atmosphere of 5% CO_2.

Transformation of Lymphocytes

Epstein Barr virus (EBV) strain B95-8 was used to transform these lymphocytes. Permanent lines of PBL (Tr-PBL) were established after about 3 weeks and lines of CBL (Tr-CBL) in 1 week.

Other Lymphoblastoid Cell Lines

The RITC-1000 cell line was established in our laboratory by Dr. M. Uno from normal peripheral blood lymphocytes without treatment with EBV. HL-60 was established from a case of promyelocytic leukemia by Collins[15] *et al.* RPMI-1788[16] cell line was obtained from Flow laboratories (McLEAN, Virginia 22102 U.S.A.). NC-37, Daudi and Namalwa cell lines were kindly supplied from Dr. G. Klein's laboratory.[17-19]

Determination of EBV-specific Antigen

EBV-specific virus capsid antigen (VCA) was determined by the method of Henle.[20] EBV nuclear antigen (EBNA) was determined by the method of Readman and Klein.[21]

Preparation of Serum-free Culture Medium

Powdered RPMI-1640 and Dulbecco's modified Eagle's medium (DEM) were supplied by Nissui Pharmaceutical Co., Ltd. Amino acids and nucleic acid precursors were obtained from Kyowa Hakko Kogyo Co., Ltd. Vitamins, metalsalts and organic chemicals were purchased from Wako Pure Chemicals Co., Ltd. Bovine or human albumin (fraction V), human transferrin, bovine insulin, and sodium β-glycerophosphate were purchased from Sigma Chemical Co. Other bovine serum fraction were the products of Miles Co.

Table 1.   Composition of the RITC 55–9 medium.

Composition of medium RITC 55–9	
DEM[a]	(mg/l) 9,800
Amino acids	
L-alanine	20
L-asparagine·H_2O	56
L-aspartic acid	20
L-cysteine·HCl·H_2O	40
L-glutamic acid	20
L-proline	20
Vitamins	
Ascorbic acid	10
Biotin	0.2
Folinic acid	0.01
Vitamin B_{12}	0.1
Organic compounds	
Glucose	1,000
Glutathione	1.0
Putrescine·2HCl	0.1
Hypoxanthine	4
Thymidine	0.7
Deoxycytidine	0.03
Deoxyadenosine	1.0
6,8-dihydroxypurine	0.3
Inorganic compounds	
$FeSO_4$·$7H_2O$	0.8
$ZnSO_4$·$7H_2O$	0.02
Na_2SeO_3	0.004
$CaCl_2$	100
Buffer	
β-glycerophosphate·2Na	1,500
$NaHCO_3$	1,300
Hormones	
Insulin	10
Transferrin (Human)	5

a) Powdered Dulbecco's modified Eagle medium (DEM) was dissolved at a slightly lower concentration in order to adjust the osmotic pressure of the medium (285 ± 5 mOsm/Kg).

The composition of our chemically defined medium, RITC 55-9, is presented in Table 1. After the powdered culture medium, DME, and buffer salts had been dissolved in distilled water, a mixed solution of other supplements prepared as a 100 fold concentrate, was added. When it was necessary to add lyophilized serum fractions, pH of the medium was adjusted to 7.3–7.4 under 5% CO_2 with N-NaOH or N-HCl. The medium was sterilized by membrane filtration (TM-3, Toyo Roshi Co., Ltd.) and stored in tightly stoppered bottles at 4°C until use.

Cell Count

The number of cells was counted by the trypan blue dye exclusion method.

IFN Production and Assay

(a) *Virus induced IFN*: Transformed PBL, CBL and other lymphoblastoid cell lines were cultured at a concentration of 1×10^6 cells/ml for 2 days in 10% FBS RPMI-1640 medium containing 100HAu/ml of Sendai virus at 37°C under 5% CO_2. The culture fluid was collected by centrifugation and kept until the IFN assay. (b) Spontaneous IFN (Sp-IFN) production: Transformed lymphocytes and other cell lines were cultured for 4 to 5 days with an initial concentration of 2 to 5×10^5 cells/ml in 10% FBS RPMI-1640 or RITC 55-9 medium. The culture fluid was collected and kept until the IFN assay.

These culture fluids were dialyzed against Tris-HCL buffer, pH 2 at 4°C for 2 days, and the pH was adjusted to 7.2 by the addition of phosphate buffered slaine (PBS). The IFN content were assayed with a semimicroassay method based on the inhibition of the cytopathic effect (CPE) of vesicular stomatitis virus (VSV) on FL cells.[22]

Characterization of Spontaneous IFN

(a) *Partial purification of IFN*: A total of 1,200 ml of the culture fluid was applied to a Matrex gel blue A (Amicon Corp.) in 1.6×20 cm column at a flow rate of 25 ml/hr/cm.[2] The column was washed with 300 ml of 0.01M phosphate buffer pH 7.5 (E_0), and IFN was eluted by $E_0 + 0.5$M NaCl (E_1), $E_0 + 1$M NaCl(E_2), and $E_2 + 30$% ethyleneglycol(E_3).[23] The IFN partially purified by the affinity chromatography was further purified by gel-permeation chromatography using Toyopearl HW-55 superfine (Toyo Soda Mfg. Co., Ltd.) with 3.2×90 cm column in E_2 buffer.

The molecular weight of the partially purified IFN was determined by gel-permination chromatography on Toyopeare HW-55 superfine (column size 1.6×90 cm). The following internal markers were used; Cytochrome-C (12,500), Chymotrypsinogen (25,000), Ovalbumin (45,000), Bovine serum albumin (75,000), Bovine γ-globuline (150,000) and Blue dextran.

(b) *Acid-inactivation test*: The samples were dialysed against pH 2 Tris-HCl buffer at 4° C for 24 hr.

(c) *Heat-inactivation*: The samples in PBS were heated in a water bath at 56° C for 1 hr.

(d) *Sedimentability*: Samples were centrifuged at 100,000 × g at 4° C in the RPS-65 rotor of a Hitachi ultracentrifuge.

(e) *Trypsinization*: Equal volume each of a 0.2% solution of 3 times crystallized trypsin in PBS and the IFN preparation were mixed and incubated for 1 hr at 37° C. The hydrolysis was then stopped by addition of soybean trypsin inhibitor.

(f) *Neutralization by antiserum*: An anti-human leukocyte IFN serum[24] which could neutralize 32,000 units of IFN-α was the kind gift of Dr. Kishida (Department of Microbiology, Kyoto Prefectural University). An equal volume of the anti-serum was added to the IFN preparation in PBS, and the sample was incubated for 3 hours at room temperature.

RESULTS

Spontaneous and Virus-induced Production of IFN by Lymphoblastoid Cells

Table 2 summarized the spontaneous and virus-induced IFN production by newly established Tr-CBL, Tr-PBL and other lymphoblastoid cell lines. All of the cell lines except the one derived from promyelocytic leukemia were EBNA positive. Of the Tr-PBLs, 8 lines did not produce IFN spontaneously. Only RITC-1000 and RPMI 1788 cell lines were found to produce IFN spontaneoulsy in low titer. Namalwa cells produced IFN spontaneoulsy to some extent, as reported previously.[9,10] Surprisingly, all strains of Tr-CBLs were found to produce 200 to 6,000 U/ml of IFN spontaneously. They were named "UMCL cells." Almost all of the tested cell lines produced fairly large amounts of IFN when induced by Sendai virus.

All of UMCL cells were EBNA-positive, but VCA and infectious EBV were not detectable. Moreover, the culture fluids and the extracts of UMCL cells did not induce IFN synthesis in mouse spleen or L-929 cells.

Growth and Spontaneous IFN Production of the Cells in Serum-free Medium

Growth and spontaneous production of IFN by UMCL cells was monitored in various test media which contained no serum. Since DEM was superior to RPMI-1640 as the basal medium, the former was further strengthened by supplementation with various effective components, shown in Table 1. The final serum-free medium (RITC 55-9) consisted of DEM supplemented with non-essential amino acids, vitamins, nucleic acid derivatives, trace metals and hormones. However this medium supported very limited growth of UMCL

Table 2. Spontaneous and virus-induced IFN production by newly established lymphoblastoid cells and other lymphoblastoid cell lines.

Origin	Cell line	IFN (10^{-3} units/ml)[a]		EBNA
		Spontaneous[b] (4 day)	Sendai virus[c] (2 day)	
Normal adult	FU–01	<0.05	2.2	+
peripheral	KU–01	<0.05	0.3	+
lymphocyte	SA–02	<0.05	1.5	+
	KN–01	<0.05	3.3	+
	MI–01	<0.05	NT[d]	+
	SU–01	<0.05	NT	+
	UE–01	<0.05	NT	+
	RITC–1000	0.14	0.45	+
	RPMI–1788	0.36	0.37	+
	NC–37	<0.05	<0.05	+
Cord blood	CB–1007	6.6	11.2	+
lymphocyte	CB–1205	1.2	3.6	+
	CB–2205	0.17	1.3	+
	CB–1428	1.0	0.9	+
	CB–2510	1.4	0.8	+
	CB–3512	2.9	NT	+
	CB–4514	0.13	1.0	+
	CB–5516	1.4	NT	+
	CB–6516	0.28	NT	+
	CB–7516	5.8	NT	+
	CB–8516	0.35	NT	+
	CB–9520	2.9	1.6	+
	CB–0524	1.1	0.9	+
	CB–11714	2.9	NT	+
Promyelocytic leukemia	HL–60	<0.05	<0.05	–
Burkitt's lymphoma	Daudi	<0.05	1.0	+
	Namalwa[e]	0.03	0.36	+

a) Interferon titers determined in triplicate experiments are expressed in reference units per ml.
b) Spontaneous IFN production was determined after 4 days of culture with an inoculum size of 5×10^5 cells/ml.
c) Virus-induced IFN production was determined 2 days after infection with 100 HAu/ml of Sendai virus at cell density of 1×10^6 cells/ml.
d) Interferon production were not tested.
e) Namalwa cells were cultured with an inoculum size of 3×10^6 cells/ml.

cells as compared with REMI-1640 medium supplemented with 10% FBS. We therefore determined which serum proteins were necessary as supplements for the synthetic medium. As shown in Fig. 1, Chon Fr. V, i.e., the albumin fraction, showed the expected effect; the optimal concentration of bovine serum albumine (BSA) or human serum albumin (HSA) was found to be 0.5% in RITC 55–9 medium.

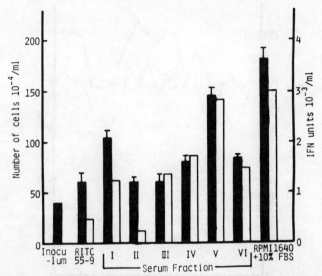

Fig. 1. Effect of bovine serum fractions on cell growth and spontaneous IFN production by UMCL cells. Cohn fraction of bovine serum was added to RITC 55-9 medium at a concentration to 0.5 mg/ml. Cells were suspended at 4×10^4 cells/ml and incubated at $37°C$ in $5\% CO_2$ for 4 days. Solid bars, cell number; blank bars, interferon production in the cultured medium.

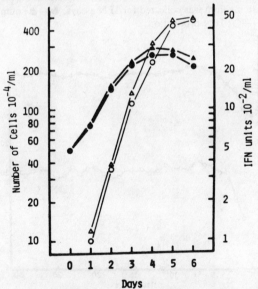

Fig. 2. Kinetics of cell growth and spontaneous production of IFN by UMCL cells. ●—● : cell number; ○—○ : IFN production in RITC 55-9 medium supplemented with 0.5% human serum albumin. ▲—▲ : number of cells; △—△ : IFN production in RPMI-1640 medium supplemented with 10% fetal bovine serum.

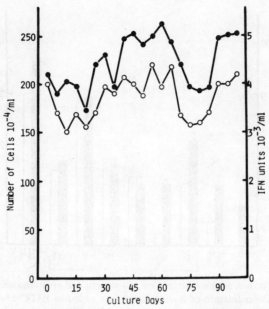

Fig. 3. Growth and spontaneous IFN production by UMCL cells in serial passages in serum-free medium. Cells were inoculated at 5×10^4 cells/ml in RITC 55–9 medium supplemented with 0.5% bovine serum albumin. On the day 5 of cultivation the cells were subcultured and the culture medium was collected for IFN assays. ●—● : number of cells on the day 5 of culture; ○—○ : IFN production

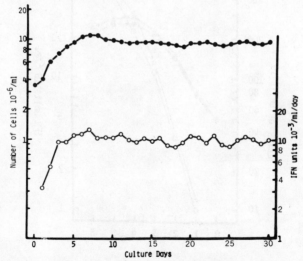

Fig. 4. Spontaneous IFN production by UMCL cells maintalned at their saturation cell density in a serum-free medium. Cells were suspended at 3.5×10^6 cells/ml in RITC 55–9 medium supplemented with 0.5% bovine serum albumin and the medium was changed every day. ●—● : number of cells; ○—○ : IFN production in the cultured medium.

The kinetics of cell growth and Sp-IFN production in RITC 55–9 medium supplemented with 0.5% HSA and in 10% FBS RPMI-1640 medium are shown in Fig. 2. Every 24 hours aliquots were removed from the cultures for interferon assays and cell counts. In RITC 55–9 supplemented with human serum albumin, UMCL cells proliferated and spontaneously produced IFN at about the same rate as in the conventional serum-containing medium. The cell number exceeded 2×10^6 cell/ml on day 6 of the culture, and the spontaneously produced IFN exceeded 4×10^3 U/ml. Moreover, as shown in Fig. 3, the RITC 55–9 + 0.5% BSA supported proliferation and serial passages of UMCL cells. The amount of Sp-IFN on day 5 of the culture did not change throughout the serial passage (more than 3 months). In order to determine the maximum amount of IFN obtainable with this method, a high density culture was attempted in the serum-free medium. As shown in Fig. 4, whene the saturation density of cells (10^7 cells/ml) was maintained by changing the medium every day, we were able to obtain about 10,000 U/ml of IFN in each daily harvest for up to 30 days. This corresponded to a production of 3×10^7 U of IFN by a culture of only 100 ml. These results suggest that the high density culture of UMCL cells in the serum-free medium is one of the most promising methods for the mass production of IFN.

Partial Purification and Characterization of Sp-IFN

Sp-IFN was separated and purified from the culture fluid of the UMCL

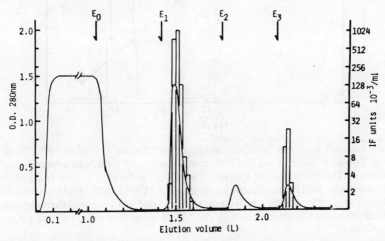

Fig. 5. Chromatography of Sp-IFNs on a Matrex gel blue A column. 1,200 ml of culture fluid, total 3.1×10^6 units of IFN, was applied on a column (1.6×15 cm) at a flow rate of 50 ml/hr. The column was washed with 0.01 M phosphate buffer pH 7.5 (E_0) and then washed in succession with 0.01 M phosphate buffer + 0.5 M NaCl (E_1), E_0 + 1 M (E_2) and E_2 + 30% ethylene glycol buffer (E_3). Concentration of protein: (——); IFN activities: (☐). (Recovery of IFN activity with E_1 was 90%, and with E_3 was 10%.)

cells, CB-3512, by the following methods. The results of chromatography of the IFN on a Matrex gel blue A column are shown in Fig. 5. The IFN completely bound to the column when the culture fluid was applied. About 90% of the IFN activity was eluted by increasing the ionic strength of the E_0 buffer to 0.5 M NaCl (E_1). About 10% of the total IFN was recovered in the 30% ethylene glycol solution (E_3). The specific activity of the fraction eluted by E_1 was 1.5 $\times$ 10^4 U/mg protein, indicating a purification of about 100 times. The E_1 fraction was further purified by gelpermeation chromatography with Toyopearl HW-55 superfine. The IFN activity eluted as a single peak, and the specific activity of this fraction was 6.2 $\times$ 10^5 U/mg protein. The resulting IFN was purified about 1,000 times from the starting material. The partially purified IFN was rechromatographed with Toyopearl HW-55 superfine column to determine its molecular weight. The major peak of IFN activity corresponded to a molecular weight of 23,000 (Fig. 6).

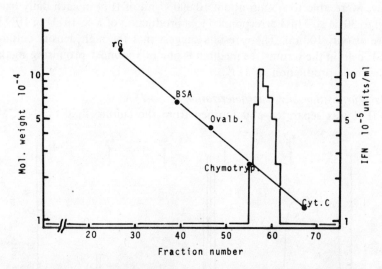

Fig. 6. Estimation of the molecular weight of Sp-IFN on Toyopearl HW-55 superfine column. Two ml of partially purified IFN, containing 5 $\times$ 10^6 units, were applied to a column (1.6 $\times$ 90 cm). The IFN was eluted with 0.01 M phosphate buffer pH 7.5 $+$ 1 M NaCl. Molecular weight standards: (rG) bovine serum gamma globulin, M. W. 15,000; (BSA) bovine serum albumin, M. W. 67,000; (Ovalb.) ovalbumin, M. W. 45,000; (Chymotryp.) chymotrypsinogen, M. W. 25,000; (Cyt-C) cytochrome-c M. W. 12,500. Fractions collected were assayed for IFN activity (□).

Several tests were carried out to determine whether the Sp-IFN had the general properties of IFNs. As shown in Table 3, the antiviral activity of the purified IFN was stable when treated at 56°C for 1 hr and at pH 2 for 24 hr, and it did not sediment at 100,000 g for 2 hrs. The activity disappeared when treated

Table 3.   Characterization of spontaneously produced IFN.

Treatment	Assay cells	Antiviral titer[a] of IFN	
		Spontaneous[b]	Virus-induced[c]
		UMCL	PBL
Non	FL	620	1,200
pH 2, 24 hrs	FL	620	1,160
56°C, 1 hr	FL	620	1,200
100,000 × g, 2 hrs	FL	730	1,200
0.1% Trypsin	FL	< 4	< 4
Anti-IFN serum	FL	< 2	< 2
Non	L-929	10	25

a) Reciprocal of the dilution at the endpoint of CPE.
b) 5,500 U/ml of Sp–IFN.
c) 10,000 U/ml of leucocyte IFN.

with trypsin or with anti-IFN-α serum. The antiviral activity was reduced to about 1% when assayed on mouse L-929 cells. These results show that the Sp-IFN from UMCL cells can be classed as human leukocyte IFN (Hu-IFN-α).

DISCUSSION

The spontaneous production of small amounts of IFN from human lymphoblastoid cell lines has been reported. It was suggested that human IFN might be mass produced if we could succeed in increasing the amount of autogenous IFN produced by either the addition of some drug, or by improvements in the culture technique. Tovey et al.[9] and Klein and Vilček[25] reported that the spontaneous IFN production by Namalwa cells could be enhanced by treatment with 5-bromodeoxyuridine or 5-iododeoxyuridine. However, the titer was only about 300 units/ml. We also confirmed that Namalwa and RPMI-1788 cells autogenously produced low concentrations of IFN.

In contrast, new cell lines established from human umbilical cord blood lymphocytes with EBV (UMCL cells) were shown to produce 100 times more Sp-IFN than Namalwa cells. There was no correlation between Sp-IFN production and the presence of EBV nuclear antigen (EBNA) (Table 2). Therefore, EBV infection dose not seems to be a reason for the spontaneous IFN production of UMCL cells. UMCL cells reacted to de novo IFN induction by Sendai virus in similar fashion as Tr-PBL cells which lack spontaneous productivity. Consequently all newly-established lymphoblastoid cells have a similar capacity to produce IFN on viral induction. These findings suggest that the structural gene(s) of IFN expressed continually in UMCL cells because of unknown anomalies of regulator gene function, but there is no alteration in cellular reactivity toward an external IFN inducing stimulus.

We have designed a new serum-free medium for the culture of lymphoblastoid cell lines. Although a serum-free medium for the culture of mouse spleen lymphocytes has been reported by Iscove and Melchers,[26] a serum-free medium which can continuously support the growth and functions of human lymphoblastoid cells has not previously been elaborated. In the serum-free medium (RITC 55–9) supplemented with bovine or human serum albumin, UMCL cells were found to proliferate and produce Sp-IFN just as they do in a conventional serum-containing medium. This albumin containing serum-free medium can also support the growth of Namalwa cells almost as well as RPMI-1640 medium supplemented with 10 % fetal bovine serum (data not shown).

Among the ingredients of the serum-free medium, serum albumin was a primary contributor to the cell growth. It seems to act as a carrier of lipids, i.e.,[27,28] unsaturated fatty acids, because defatted albumin did not have the same stimulatory effect on cell growth. Trace metal ions and nucleotides were also necessary components for the continued growth of UMCL cells, as has been found with other serum-free media.[29,32] Transferrin and insulin have been reported to stimulate the growth of some cells, such as mouse spleen cells,[30] rat pituitary cells,[31] and hamster and human fibroblasts.[31,32] They also showed a favorable effect on the growth of UMCL cells in the present serum-free medium. Reducing substances such as L-cysteine, glutathione, or ascorbate may lower the oxidation-reduction potential in the same manner as the 2-mercaptoethanol contained in Iscove's medium. Addition of amino acids and vitamins to the present medium was advantageous for the spontaneous production of IFN. This appears to explain why DEM, which contains rich quantities of amino acids and vitamins, is preferable to RPMI-1640 medium for the production of IFN. Since the UMCL cells were cultivated to synthesize IFN in a chemically defined medium supplemented with human serum albumin, we can expect fewer problems in the subsequent purification of IFN.

To produce a large amount of IFN, a high density culture of UMCL cells with daily exchange of medium seems to be the best manipulation. With this procedure, 10^7 U per day of IFN can be harvested from a 1,000 ml culture. Since no inducer virus, bovine or human serum is required for the production of IFN and for the maintainance of continuous cell growth, this method will be of practical use in the mass production of human IFN.

The Sp-IFN in the UMCL cell culture fluid were separated into two fractions by blue sepharose affinity chromatography; about 90 % of the total IFN was eluted into a major fraction by E_1 buffer and the remaining 10 % was eluted as a minor fraction by E_3 buffer. This elution pattern was similar to that of human leukocyte IFN as reported by Jankowski *et al.*[23] The E_1 eluted Sp-IFN seems to belongs to the class of human IFN-α from its physicochemical characterization and antigenicity. This Sp-IFN appeared to have a molecular weight of 23,000 by gel-permeation chromatography.

REFERENCES

1. Deinhardt, F. and Burnside, J.: Spontaneous interferon production in cultures of a cell line from a human myeloblastic leukemia. *J. Nat. Cancer Inst.*, **39**: 681–683, 1967.
2. Northrop, R. L. and Deinhart, F.: Production of interferonlike substances by human bone marrow tissues *in vitro. J. Nat. Cancer Inst.*, **39**: 685–689, 1967.
3. Swart, B. E. and Young, B. G.: Inverse relationship of interferon production and virus content in cell lines from Burkitt's lymphoma and Acute leukemias. *J. Nat. Cancer Inst.*, **42**: 941–944, 1969.
4. Kasel, J. A., Haase, A. T., Glade, P. R., and Chessin, L. N.: Interferon production in cell lines derived from patients with infectious mononucleosis. *Proc. Soc. Ex;. Biol. Med.*, **128**: 351–353, 1968.
5. Zajac, B. A., Henle, W., and Henle, G.: Autogenous and Virusinduced interferons from lines of lymphoblastoid cells. *Cancer research*, **29**: 1467–1475, 1969.
6. Haase, A. T., Johnson, J. S., Kasel, J. A., Margolis, S.,and Levy, H. B.: Induction of interferon in lymphoblastoid cell line. *Proc. Soc. Exp. Biol. Med.*, **133**: 1076–1083, 1970.
7. Adams, A., Lidin, B., Strander, H., and Cantell, K.: Spontaneous interferon production and Epstein-Barr Virus antigen expression in human lymphoid cell lines. *J. gen. Virol.*, **28**: 219–223, 1975.
8. Volckaert-Vervliet, G. and Billiau, A.: Induction of interferon in human lymphoblastoid cells by Sendai and measlesvirus. *J. gen. Virol.*, **37**: 199–203, 1977.
9. Tovey, M. G., Begon-Lours, J., Gresser, I., and Morris, A. G.: Marked enhancement of interferon production in 5-bromodeoxyuridine treated human lymphoblastoid cells. *Nature*, **267**: 455–457, 1977.
10. Strander, H.: Production of interferon in serum-free human leukocyte suspensions. *Appl. Microbiol.*, **18**: 810–815, 1969.
11. Goore, M. Y., Dickson, J. H., Lipkin, S., and DiCuollo, C. J.: The production of human leukocyte interferon in a serumfree medium. *Proc. Soc. Exp. Biol. Med.*, **142**: 46–49, 1973.
12. Brigden, P. J., Anfinsen, C. B., Carley, L., Bose, S., Zoon, K. C., and Rüegg, U. T.: Human lymphoblastoid interferon, Large scale production and partial purification. *J. Biol. Chem.*, **252**: 6585–6587, 1977.
13. Zoon, K. C., Bukler, C. E., Bridgen, P. J., and Gurari-Rotman, D.: Production of human lymphoblastoid interferon by Namalwa Cells. *J. Clin, Microbiol.*, **7**: 44–51, 1978.
14. Böyum, A.: A one stage procedure for isolation of granulocytes and lymphocytes from huham blood. *Scand. J. Clin. Lab Invest.*, **21**: 51–76, 1978.
15. Collins, S. J., Ruscetti, F. W., Callagher, R. E., and Gallo, R. C.: Terminal differentiation of human promyelocytic leukemia cells induced by dimethyl sulfoxide and other polar compounds. *Proc. Natl. Acad. Sc,i. USA*, **57**: 2458–2642, 1978.
16. Huang, C. C. and Moore, G. E.: Chromosomes of 14 hematopoietic cell lines derived from peripheral blood of persons with and without chromosome anomalies. *J. Nat. Cancer. Inst.*, **43**: 1119–1128, 1969.
17. Durr, F. E., Monroe, J. H., Sehmitter, R., Traul, K. A., and Hirshaut, Y.: Studies on the infectivity and cytopathology of Epstein-Barr virus in human lymphoblastoid cells. *Int. J. Cancer*, **6**: 436–449, 1970.
18. Klein, E., Klein, G., Nadkarni, F. S., Nadkarni, J. J., Wigzell, H., and Clifford, P.: Surface IgM-kappa specificity on a Burkitt lymphoma Cell *in vivo* and in drived culture lines. *Cancer research*, **28**: 1300–1310, 1968.
19. Klein, G. and Dombos, L.: Relationship between the sensitivity of EBV-carrying lymphoblastoid lines to super infection and the inducibility of the resident viral genome. *Int. J. Cancer*, **11**: 327–337, 1973.

20. Henle, G. and Henle, W.: Immunofluorescence in cells derived from Burkitt's lymphoma. *J. Bact.*, **91**: 1248–1256, 1966.
21. Reedman, B. M. and Klein, G.: Cellular localization of an Epstein-Barr virus (EBV)-associated comprement-fixing antigen in producer and non-producer lymphoblastoid cell lines. *Int. J. Cancer*, **11**: 499–520, 1973.
22. Gresser, I., Bandu, M. T., Brouty-Boye, D., and Tovey, M.: Pronounced antiviral activity of human interferon on bovine and porcine cells. *Nature*, **251**: 543–545, 1974.
23. Jankowski, W. J., von Muenchhausen, W., Sulkowski, E., and Carter, W. A.: Binding of human interferons to immobilized cibacron blue F3GA: The nature of molecular interaction. *Biochemistry*, **15**: 5182–5187, 1976.
24. Mogensen, K. E., Phyhälä, L., and Cantell, K.: Raising antibodies to human leucocyte interferon. *Acta. path. microbiol. scand. sect. B*, **83**: 443–450, 1975.
25. Klein, G. and Vilček, J.: Attempts to induce interferon production by Id Urd Induction and EBV superinfection in human lymphoma lines and their hybrids. *I. gen, Virol.*, **46**: 111–117, 1980.
26. Iscove, N. N. and Melchers, F.: Complete replacement of serum by Albumin, Transferin and Soybean Lipid in culture of lipopolysaccharide-reactive B lymphocytes. *J. Exp. Med.*, **147**: 923–933, 1978.
27. Yamane, I., Murakami, O., and Kato, M.: Serum-free culture of various mammalian cells and the role of bovine albumin. *Cell struct Funct.*, **1**: 279–284, 1976.
28. Nilausen, K.: Role of fatty accids in growth-promoting effect of serum albumin on hamster cells *in vitro. J. Cell. Physiol.*, **96**: 1–14, 1976.
29. Murakami, O. and Yamane, I.: Effect of basic polymers on growth of tumor cells in suspension cultures with "serum-free" medium. *Cell Struct. Funct.*, **1**: 285–290, 1976.
30. Vogt. A., Mishell, R. I., and Dutlon, R. W.: Stimulation of DNA synthesis in cultures of mouse spleen cell suspensions by bovine transferrin. *Exp. Cell. Res.*, **54**: 195–200, 1969.
31. Hayashi, I. and Sato, G.H .: Replacement of serum by hormones permits growth of cells in a defined medium. *Nature* (London), **259**: 132–134, 1976.
32. Yamane, I., Kan, M., and Hoshi, H.: Hormonal control of cells in culture. In Growth and Growth Factors, (Univ. of Tokyo Press, Tokyo, Japan) pp. 13–25, 1979.

Discussion

Dr. FINTER: Could I ask Dr. Yamane: what strain of EB virus did you use to transform the cord blood lymphocytes in your study?

Dr. YAMANE: I got the strain from Dr. Hinuma, but I do not know the exact name of this virus.

II.

CLINICAL APPLICATIONS

Interferon Therapy in Viral Infections and Malignant Disease

Thomas C. MERIGAN

Division of Infectious Diseases, Stanford University School of Medicine, Stanford, California 94305, U. S. A.

SUMMARY

Interferon (IFN) therapy has been used by our group in several viral infections and in lymphomas in recent years. Our studies in herpes zoster in patients with lymphoma reveal a requirement for not only early initiation of adequate dosage, but the necessity of prolonged therapy for optimum disease response. We are currently attempting to extend these results to both late prophylaxis or early treatment of varicella in children with leukemia. The dosage we find is required for zoster improvement does not appear to influence the varicella-zoster specific humoral or cellular immune responses in the treated patients compared to controls.

Another use which our group has observed for human leukocyte IFN is to supplement the action of adenine arabinoside in producing eradication of Dane particle production in patients with chronic hepatitis B virus infection. Our current open trial results suggest that patients in whom Dane particle eradication is achieved have both better liver function and absence of infectious virus in their serum as assessed by primate infectivity studies. Given these results, we feel it is now necessary to test the ability of our most effective combination antiviral regimen in a randomized placebo controlled trial with double-blind follow-up.

Studies utilizing IFN in malignancy are not as well advanced because of the lack of highly specific markers and variability of disease course in individual patients. At present, we believe human IFN can cause tumor shrinkage in lymphoma patients, but the optimum dose for an enduring response has not been clarified and the mechanism is yet to be understood. Present trials are directed toward determining the optimum dosage and range of malignancy diseases which can be affected. Only after this is known can we initiate the necessary controlled trials to determine whether IFN will add to conventional therapy or produce unique effects which are not observed with other agents.

INTRODUCTION

Although there has been much interest in the clinical application of human

IFN in viral infections, little material has been produced for this purpose over the years. Fortunately, since 1973 our group has been supplied with material by Dr. Kari Cantell of the State Serum Institute in Helsinki, Finland. This paper will summarize our studies in both viral infections and malignancies.

RESULTS AND DISCUSSION

We tested the effect of human leukocyte interferon (HuIFN-α) on early localized herpes zoster infections in three placebo-controlled, randomized double-blind trials involving 90 patients with cancer.[1] There were no significant differences in pretreatment severity of infection or the nature of the underlying disease in the groups. Higher doses of more purified IFN in the second and third trials produced a significant ($p < 0.01$) decrease in cutaneous dissemination. No dissemination occurred in those receiving the highest dosage (5.1×10^5 units (U)/kg/d) ($p < 0.025$). The number of days of new vesicle formation in the primary dermatome decreased (mean, 2.2 days; $p < 0.05$) in this group. Treated patients had a trend toward less acute pain and significantly ($p < 0.05$) diminished severity of postherpetic neuralgia at the two highest dosage levels. Visceral complications were six times less frequent in interferon recipients. High dose IFN thus appeared effective in limiting cutaneous dissemination, visceral complications, and progression within the primary dermatome.

The design of the localized zoster trials involved early administration of HuIFN-α with between 10^5 and 10^6 U/mg/protein for 5 to 7 days or, in other words, the full period during which patients are at risk for visceral complications. In the second and third trials, patients were started on treatment at an average time of 2 days after onset of the rash in the primary dermatome. This strategy took advantage of the fact that the patients were selected from a large lymphoma clinic in which the current combination therapy utilized produced a 30–35% incidence of zoster in the first year after therapy was started. Therefore, patients could be informed about the possiblity of experimental antiviral therapy before they had disease and thus could be brought into therapy regimen when they were still at risk for continuing pathology due to continued virus replication.

More recently, we have analyzed the results of a fourth placebo-controlled, randomized double-blind trial in the same population involving only 48 hours of therapy at the dosage used in the third trial.[2] However, in this trial there was no effect on acute pain or disease progression in the primary dermatome. A modest but significant effect was noted in that distal cutaneous spread was diminished in the treated patients compared to controls, and the treated patients had diminished severity and duration of postherpetic neuralgia. The results of this study indicated that, in addition to a high dosage, a significant duration of treatment with HuIFN-α is required to modify herpes zoster infections in patients with cancer. The effect on distal cutaneous spread seems most likely to be mediated through an effect on viremia. Viremia has been documented in cancer patients during the first 3 days after onset of disease in the primary dermatome,[3] the period in which IFN therapy was being given in this study. Interestingly enough, there also appeared to be an effect on virus replication in the ganglia as manifested by less postherpetic neuralgia in the treated patients compared to controls.

Another parameter which was studied in these trials was the effect of IFN administration on the production of varicella zoster antibodies. There was no evidence for a delay in the production of complement-fixing antibody titers in the treated patients compared to controls.[1] In addition, we observed that virus-specific lymphocyte transformation developed as expected for immunosuppressed patients among the IFN recipients.[2] Although there was fever and a very transient granulocyte depression from the thrid to the fourth day after the start of IFN no significant toxicity was observed.[1,2]

Because of our results in zoster, we have also undertaken to extend this approach to primary infection by the same virus, that is, varicella in children with cancer. Eighteen patients who developed varicella while being treated for a malignancy received HuIFN-α in a small randomized, placebo-controlled trial.[4] These studies were conducted only with the lower two doses used in our initial zoster trial, that is, 4.2×10^4 U/kg or 2.55×10^5 U/kg. The average treatment in this trial was 6.4 days. Complications of varicella occurred in 6 of the 9 placebo recipients but were observed in only 2 of the 9 IFN recipients. In addition, the IFN was tolerated without significant side effects. Because of these results, we have undertaken a randomized double-blind study of HuIFN-α prophylaxis for varicella in immunocompromised children whose exposure to the virus has not been identified until the incubation period, when no benefit from passive antibody prophylaxis is expected. This study is being pursued in a national multicenter format utilizing not only patients treated through Stanford, but those of the Children's Cooperative Cancer Study Group A. Our other trial in varicella which is ongoing is a randomized double-blind study of HuIFN-α for the treatment of early varicella in immunocompromised children with cancer utilizing the same patient population.

We have also attempted to treat chronic viral infections, first focusing on neonates. Although high-dose IFN-α transiently diminished cytomegalovirus viruria in infants, side-effects were recognized.[5] Because of the decreased weight gain and transient liver enzyme elevation, and the transient nature of the antiviral effect, these observations were not pursued further with the IFN preparations then available.

We have recently concluded studies of 3 infants with rubella in whom we could quantitate virus excretion. Although pharyngeal shedding ceased in one of the 3 following treatment, there was no constant effect on virus excretion in the urine or the pharynx of the other individuals.[6] Hence, we conclude that in neonatal infections, although large doses of IFN can be used, the immune deficits which are associated with the infection significantly impair the usefulness of IFN therapy.

On the other hand, we have had more success in utilizing IFN in the treatment of chornic hepatitis B infection.[7] Over the past four and a half years, 32 patients with chronic hepatitis associated with persistent hepatitis B virus (HBV) infection have received 16 courses of HuIFN-α 6 courses of adenine arabinoside, and 21 courses of these two agents used in combination. The aims of this study were to: (1) follow the effects of these agents on HBV markers in serum and liver tissue: (2) evaluate different regimens in order to select one with a reasonable toxicity/efficacy ratio which could be used in a controlled multicenter trial; and (3) attempt to identify patients' clinical and virological characteristics which might influence the outcome of therapy.[8]

IFN was given as subcutaneous or intramuscular injections in dosages varying from 2.5 to 20×10^6 units daily. Adenine arabinoside was given intravenously at dosages of 5 to 15 mg/kg daily. An additive effect of adenine arabinoside was observed on the suppression of viral markers induced by IFN. IFN was shown to maintain viral markers at low or undetectable levels when prior adenine arabinoside therapy was discontinued. Combination course of overlapping cycles of IFN and adenine arabinoside were developed. The mean treatment period ranged from 4 to 6 months.

Twenty patients with chronic active hepatitis (CAH) and 12 patients with chronic persistent hepatitis (CPH) who had been surface antigen (HB$_s$Ag)-positive for at least one year and who had been shown to have stable detectable levels of HBV-associated DNA polymerase (DNAP) activity in their serum were studied. DNAP was used as the most sensitive index of ongoing viral replication. HB$_e$Ag and HB$_s$Ag titers, and their respective antibodies, were followed in all patients. Immunofluorescent staining of liver biopsies for HB$_s$Ag and core antigen (HB$_c$Ag) was also carried out.

Three types of responses were observed in the patients. Within 48 hours of starting IFN or adenine arabinoside there was a predictable fall in DNAP activity in all patients. In the majority of patients treated with a single agent, this effect continued only as long as therapy was maintained (Type III response). With IFN alone, 4 out of 16 patients showed a permanent fall in DNAP activity to undetectable levels and permanent loss of HB$_e$Ag (Type II response). In 2 of these patients, serum HB$_s$Ag also became undetectable (Type I response) and one developed antibody to hepatitis B surface antigen.

In 6 patients treated with adenine arabinoside alone, only one patient became permanently DNAP- and HB$_e$Ag-negative, while HB$_s$Ag remained detectable at low titers. Four of 6 females in the study had permanent responses to a single agent (3 following IFN and one following adenine arabinoside). Only one out of 11 males responded to IFN alone and none of 5 treated with adenine arabinoside alone.

With multiple cycles of combined IFN and adenine arabinoside, 7 out of 16 patients became permanently DNAP- and HB_eAg-negative. One of these patients became HB_sAg-negative (Type I), and there was a marked drop in HB_sAg titers in the remaining 6 (Type II). Anti-HB_e became detectable in 4 and anti-HB_s in 5 of these patients.

In 69 patients who met the criteria for admission to the program, spontaneous falls in DNAP activity without treatment were observed in only 9% over a mean observation period of 10 months. Only one patient became HB_sAg-negative. Treatment with IFN therefore appears to be effective in permanently reducing HBV markers in female patients, whereas combination therapy with adenine arabinoside is superior in male patients.

Patients with chronic active hepatitis and lower initial DNAP levels responded significantly better than other patients. There was a strong association between a successful response to therapy and a rise in serum glutamic oxaloacetic transaminase (SGOT) values during treatment (mean rise, 145 ± 106 IU in Type I and II patients compared to $40 \pm$ IU in Type III patients). The rise was more pronounced in females and in patients with CAH and was associated with a fall in DNAP activity. This rise might indicate host immune responses working in conjunction with the antiviral agents.

In the patients with Type I and II responses there was a marked improvement in symptoms following treatment. SGOT values fell significantly in these patients but there were no changes in the Type III patients. All Type I and II patients had SGOT levels within twice the normal range at a mean period of 16 months following discontinuation of treatment. An improvement in serum total bilirubin, alkaline phosphatase, albumin, and globulin was seen but reached statistical significance only for bilirubin ($p < 0.05$). On blind review of the liver biopsies, there was a significant reduction in inflammatory activity in the Type I and II patients compared to the Type III patients ($p < 0.01$). There was also a change in histologic classification from CAH to CPH in 5 responsive patients and there were no changes in the unresponsive patients. There was also marked loss of infectivity in sera from Type I and Type II patients following treatment, as evidenced by chimpanzee infectivity studies. Inoculation of pretreatment sera from one Type I and six Type II patients studied led to HBV infection in 7 chimpanzees at dilutions varying between 10^{-2} to $10.^{-7}$ Inoculation of undiluted posttreatment sera from these same patients did not lead to infection in 7 other chimpanzees.

Fever, general malaise, and falls in neutrophil and platelet counts were the main observed side-effects resulting from IFN therapy. Gastrointestinal and neurologic side-effects were encountered following adenine arabinoside treatment. These side-effects were found to be dose-related and were also increased by concurrent administration of IFN. This has led to the use of these drugs consecutively rather than concurrently, that is, cycles of adenine arabinoside followed by IFN. It is proposed that these observations be tested in a prospectively controlled, randomized trial.

In addition to these studies in viral infections, we have studied the action of IFN in human maligancies, specifically non-Hodgkin's lymphoma. Initially we failed to show the effect of 4 weeks of daily high dose IFN treatment in rapidly advancing histiocytic lymphoma which had not responded to other therapy. However, we did get significant tumor shirinkage with the same regimen in 3 consecutive patients with nodular, poorly differentiated lymphoma.[9] Therefore, we went on to further expand this group. At present we have observed one complete, 3 partial, and 2 minimal responses in 5 of 7 evaluable patients with nodular non-Hodgkin's lymphoma.[10] The duration of the response appears to be from 6–12 months. Interestingly enough with this one month course of therapy, one patient achieved a second partial response on re-treatment with IFN despite having received chemotherapy between his courses of IFN. Much further work needs to be done to determine the optimal way to use HuIFN-α in these and malignancies. Because of the chronic and recurrent nature of cancer and the other multiple modes of therapy available for such patients, a number of different dosage regimens of IFN alone, and in combination with other therapy, must be explored eventually in controlled trials.

The studies I have described thus represent a significant experience with this material for a single group of investigators. Now that new sources of IFN have appeared, particularly through the use of recombinant DNA, there is a need for new investigators to enter this field. We need their imagination and skills to deal with the significant problems remaining in exploring the clinical utilization of human IFN in disease.

REFERENCES

1. Merigan, T. C., Rand, K. H., Pollard, R. B., Abdallah, P. S., Jordan, G. W., and Fried, R. P.: Human leukocyte interferon for the treatment of herpes zoster in patients with cancer. *New Engl. J. Med.*, **298**: 981–987, 1978.
2. Merigan, T. C., Gallagher, J. G., Pollard, R. B., and Arvin, A. M.: Short course human leucocyte interferon in the treatment of herpes zoster in patients with cancer. *Antimicrob. Agents Chemother.*, 1981 (in press).
3. Feldman, S., Chaudary, S., Ossi, M., and Epp, E.: A viremic phase for herpes zoster in children with cancer. *J. Pediatr.*, **91**: 597–600, 1977.
4. Arvin, A. M., Feldman, S., and Merigan, T. C.: Human leukocyte interferon in the treatment of varicella in children with cancer: A preliminary controlled trial. *Antimicrob. Agents Chemother.*, **13**: 605–607, 1978.
5. Arvin, A., Yeager, A., and Merigan, T. C.: The effect of leukocyte interferon on urinary excretion of cytomegalovirus in infants. *J. Infect. Dis.*, **133** (Suppl.): A205–A210, 1976.

6. Arvin, A. M., Schmidt, N., Cantell, K., and Merigan, T. C.: Interferon administration to infants with congenital rubella. *Antimicrob. Agents Chemother.*, 1982 (in press).
7. Greenberg, H. B., Pollard, R. B., Lutwick, L. I., Gregory, P. B., Robinson, W. S., and Merigan, T. C.: The effect of human leukocyte interferon on hepatitis B virus infection in patients with chronic active hepatitis. *New Engl. J. Med.*, **295**: 517–522, 1976.
8. Scullard, G. H., Pollard, R. B., Smith, J. L., Sacks, S. L., Gregory, P. B., Robinson, W. S., and Merigan, T. C.: Antiviral treatment of chronic hepatitis B virus infection. 1. Changes in viral markers with interferon combined with adenine arabinoside. *J. Infect. Dis.*, **143**: 772–783, 1981.
9. Merigan, T. C., Sikora, K., Breeden, J. H., Levy, R., and Rosenberg, S. A.: Preliminary observations on the effect of human interferon in non-hodgkin's lymphoma. *New Engl. J. Med.*, **288**: 1449–1453, 1978.
10. Louie, A. C., Gallagher, J. G., Sikora, K., Rosenberg, S. A., and Merigan, T. C.: Follow-up observation on the effect of human leukocyte interferon in non-Hodgkin's lymphoma. *Blood*, **58**: 193–195, 1981.

Discussion

Dr. GALASSO: Dr. Merigan, I do not think it was clear from your discussion whether your prospective study is for sequential treatment of the two drugs or in combination. Also you mentioned that when you looked at the drugs in combination, you had neurotoxicity. Have you seen the same kind of neurotoxicity when you have given the drugs sequentially?

Dr. MERIGAN: Thank you for the question. I did not give you the actual regimen we plan in a control trial. We decided to work with adenine arabinoside monophosphate because we can use entirely intramuscular preparations and have the patient take the drug at home and do not have to be in the hospital on I.V.s. In addition, we give the interferon alternately with adenine arabinoside, so that they are not given together. When they are not given simultaneously, we do not have the altered metabolism of adenine arabinoside, and have not seen the toxicity. So by giving the drug sequentially—one month adenine arabinoside AMP and one mouth interferon—we have avoided the toxicity. Hopefully we will maintain the benefit.

Dr. OGAWA: I have a question to Dr. Merigan. You did not touch upon your study concerning non-Hodgkin's lymphoma. Could you kindly tell us the result of your study?

Dr. MERIGAN: I'll be glad to do so. The shortage of time prevented me from discussing it. We have conducted the study supported by the National Cancer Institute. Nine courses of interferon therapy are under way in patients with measurable non-Hodgkin's lymphoma. In 4 of the patients, there has been an objective response. In 3 of them it has been striking. One of the patients, almost two years after stopping the treatment, is still free of disease. The other patients have all relapsed about 6–12 months after stopping therapy. When we re-treated one of them, we got a second response after one month's therapy. It's not as striking as the first response, but it's clear that we can get the second response even after multiple cycles of chemotherapy in that patient. So we think that interferon is not a panacea. It's very important to take Dr. Nagano's suggestion that we proceed cautiously in our claims about our interferon, but we think it has activity against this tumor and other tumors. But we do not yet know the best way to use it, whether alone or in combination, at low dose or high dose. There are many questions as yet unanswered as to how to use it optimally. It's really going to depend upon those questions whether interferon takes a special place in the treatment of any malignancy.

Preliminary Clinical Studies with Poly (ICLC)

Hilton Levy,* Freddie Riley,* Arthur Levine,[2]* Andres Salazar,[3]* W. King Engle,[3]* Brian Durie,[4]* Brigid Leventhal,[5]* John Whiznant,[6]* B. Lampkin[7]* and Susan Krown[8]*

*Laboratory of Viral Diseases, National Institute of Allergy and Infectious Diseases, the [2]*Pediatric Oncology Branch, National Cancer Institute, and the [3]*Medical Neurology Branch, National Institute of Neurological and Communicative Disorders & Stroke, National Institutes of Health, Bethesda, Maryland, U.S.A.; [4]*Department of Oncology, University of Arizona, Tucson, Arizona; [5]*Department of Oncology, Johns Hopkins Hospital, Baltimore, Maryland; [6]*Department of Oncology, University of North Carolina, Chapel Hill, North Carolina;[7]* Children's Hospital Medical Center, Cincinnati, Ohio; and [8]*Sloan Kettering Institute, New York, U.S.A.

INTRODUCTION

Interferon (IFN) was first named in 1957 by Isaacs and Lindemann.[1] At about the same time Nagano and Kojima[2] and Chany[3] were reporting analogous findings. The clinical potential of this broad spectrum antiviral agent was soon realized, but the difficulty of obtaining sufficient quantities of the material has made clinical application slow. Although the situation has improved a good deal, IFN is still very expensive and in very short supply.

Attention turned to finding nonviral inducers that would cause the host to synthesize large quantities of its own IFN, and a number of such materials were found; but either the quantities of IFN made were low or the compounds were too toxic.

A number of double-stranded (ds) RNAs, both natural and synthetic, were reported by Field et al.[4] to be effective IFN inducers in rodents. The most effective was the synthetic ds RNA polyinosinic: polycytidylic acid. It was shown to be a good antiviral agent[5] as well as a reasonably good antitumor agent[6] in rodents, but it proved ineffective in man.[7]

111

MODIFICATION OF POLY I: POLY C

In experiments done in collaboration with several groups, it was shown that primate serum contains relatively high concentrations of enzymes that hydrolyze and inactivate poly I: poly C.[8,9] The poly I: poly C is pyrogenic in rabbits, as shown in Fig. 1. If one incubates poly I: poly C with human serum or with ribonucleases, this pyrogenicity is abolished, as seen in Fig. 2.

Mouse serum contains much less of such hydrolytic activity. A derivative of poly I: poly C that resists such enzymatic hydrolysis was prepared as follows. Solutions (in pyrogen-free 0.85% NaCl) were prepared as indicated: (1) 500 ml

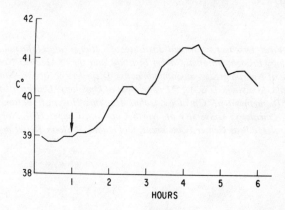

Fig. 1.   Fever response in rabbits (mean of 3) after I. V. injection of 30 μg poly I: poly C in 0.17 ml of 0.15 M pyrogen-free saline.

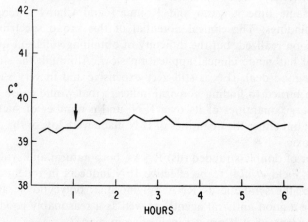

Fig. 2.   Fever response in rabbits (mean of 3) after I. V. injection of 30 μg poly I: poly C in 0.15 ml of 0.15 M pyrogen-free saline that had been treated with 20 μg/ml pancreatic ribonuclease plus 30 units/ml T$_1$ ribonuclease.

of poly I: poly C (4 mg/ml); (2) 250 ml of poly-L-lysine (6 mg/ml); and (3) 250 ml of 2% carboxymethyl cellulose (CMC). The poly-L-lysine was poured slowly, with stirring, into the CMC. A precipitate was formed which redissolved after stirring for 2 additional days. The poly I: poly C was then poured into the poly-L-lysine-CMC complex. Such a preparation contained 2 mg of poly I: poly C/ml and 1.5 mg of poly-L-lysine/ml in 0.5% CMC. This new complex is referred to as poly (ICLC).[9]

A comparison of the hydrolysis by RNase of poly I: poly C with that of poly (ICLC) is shown in Fig. 3, from which it can be concluded that the new complex is 8 to 10 times more resistant than is poly I: poly C.[9] Another piece of evidence showing that poly (ICLC) is more stable thermodynamically than poly I: poly C is the finding that the thermal denaturation temperature, the T_m, of poly (ICLC) is much higher than that of poly I: poly C, as seen in Fig. 4. There is approximately a 38°C difference in T_m's.[9]

Poly (ICLC) retains the ability to induce IFN in mice. Actually, it induces a bit more IFN in mice than does the parent poly I: poly C. The big difference between the two is found in primates. Poly I: poly C, in our hands, did not induce IFN in monkeys or chimpanzees, whereas poly (ICLC) does. Figure 5 shows the kinetics of IFN induction in 2 monkeys receiving a dose of 3 or 5 mg/kg body weight.[9]

There is a great deal of variation seen from monkey to monkey in the amount

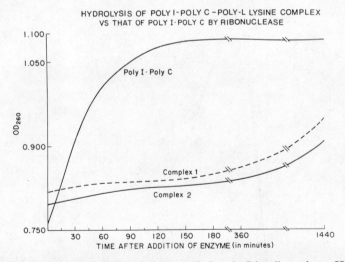

Fig. 3. Hydrolysis of poly (ICLC) complex vs. poly I: poly C by ribonuclease. Hydrolysis of poly I: poly C and two different lots of poly-L-lysine complex by pancreatic RNase. The complexes, at a concentration of 50 μg poly I: poly C/ml in 0.15 M NaCl and 0.01 M phosphate buffer (pH 7.2), were exposed to 5 μg pancreatic RNase/ml at room temperature (about 24°C). A_{260nm} readings were taken at 10 min intervals.

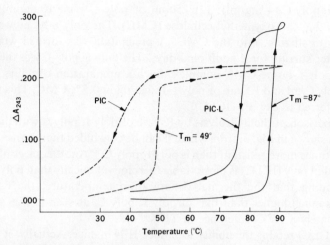

Fig. 4. Thermal denaturation of poly I:poly C and the poly-L-lysine complex of poly I: poly C [poly (ICLC)]. The compounds, at a concentration of 50 μg poly I: poly C/ml in 0.1 $\times$ standard saline-citrate, were heated to the indicated temperatures in a recording spectrophotometer set at 260 nm (melting temperature [T_m]).

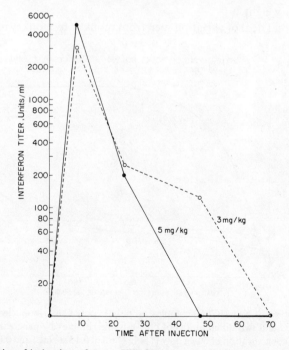

Fig. 5. Kinetics of induction of serum IFN in rhesus monkeys by I. V. administration of 3 or 5 mg/kg poly (ICLC) (one monkey per dose).

of IFN induced by poly (ICLC). At 1–3 mg/kg, peak levels of 500–2,000 units of IFN/ml of serum are induced. At levels of drug of 40 mg/kg, which is lethal to monkeys, we have seen up to 200,000 units of IFN/ml produced before the animal died.

The route of injection affects to some extent the kinetics of IFN production. Figure 6 compares the I.M. and I.V. routes of injection. It will be noted that the peak level induced is somewhat less when the I.M. route is used but that higher levels of IFN persist longer. This has been so in three independent

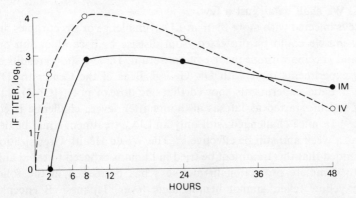

Fig. 6. Effect of route of injection on kinetics of IFN production. Three monkeys were injected with 1 mg/kg body weight by the indicated route. Titers represent mean values of the indicated times.

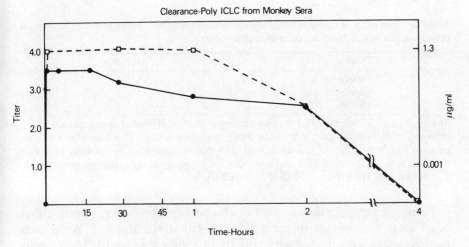

Fig. 7. Clearance of poly (ICLC) from the blood of monkeys injected I. V. Samples were withdrawn at the indicated times and assayed on primary rabbit kidney cells, which are relatively insensitive to monkey IFN.

experiments, with 3 different monkeys for each route, each drug, and each experiment—a total of 9 monkeys for each route.

The drug is cleared fairly rapidly from the blood's circulation. Figure 7 shows that within 2 hours after injection, the drug is decreased to 10% of its initial value and is gone by 4 hours.

ANTIVIRAL STUDIES

Poly (ICLC) is effective in controlling a number of serious viral diseases in primates. We shall detail just a few.

Monkeys injected with more than an LD_{100} challenge of street rabies virus in the neck muscle could be protected from disease by a combination of poly (ICLC) and vaccine without the use of antiserum. Table 1 shows results of one of many experiments done with Dr. George Bear of the Center for Disease Control.[10] Later experiments showed that one dose of poly (ICLC) plus two doses of vaccine started as late as 48 hours after severe challenge is equally effective.[11] In mice challenged with only an LD_{50}, treatment could be delayed as long as a week and still be effective.[12] The World Health Organization has recommended that this treatment be tried in humans exposed to rabid animals. Partial to complete protection in monkeys has been seen in the following diseases: yellow fever, simian hemorrhagic fever, Japanese B encephalitis, vaccinia encephalitis, and Russian spring summer encephalitis. However, the drug was not effective against Machupo virus and perhaps worsened the disease.[13,14]

Table 1. Mortality of rabies-infected rhesus monkeys treated 6 hours after challenge with rabies vaccine plus IFN or rabies vaccine plus inducer.

Treatment	Mortality
Vaccine	7/8
Vaccine + poly (ICLC)	0/8
Vaccine + IFN	1/8

Monkeys were challenged with 1 ml of a predetermined lethal dose of skunk salivary gland rabies virus (0.5 ml into each side of the neck). Beginning 6 hours after injection, monkeys received one dose of 1 ml of human diploid cell strain of vaccine (antigenic value = 5) into the right arm. At the same time and every day for 5 injections, they received either saline, 1×10^6 units of HuIFN-α, or 2 mg of poly (ICLC).

There is a model in chimpanzees of chronic hepatitis B virus infection that bears some resemblance to human disease but is not identical. When such carrier chimps were treated with poly (ICLC), they produced IFN, and tests for the presence of virus were negative. Figure 8 shows the relationship of treatment to IFN production and the presence of the DNA polymerase that is in the virus. During the time when the drug was being given, IFN was produced and evidence of the virus disappeared. However, when treatment was stopped, the virus reappeared.[15] Whether very prolonged treatment would permanently remove the virus has not been determined.

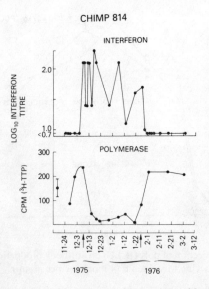

Fig. 8.   Treatment of chronic hepatitis in young chimpanzees with poly I: poly C. The IFN titer is shown above and the virus-associated polymerase activity is shown below. The beginning and end of the treatment period are indicated by arrows on the abscissa. The dot and bar on the graph of DNA polymerase response indicate the mean ($\pm$ 1 SD) of polymerase activity detected in 6 serum samples obtained during the 5 weeks immediately preceding the experiment.

IMMUNE ADJUVANT STUDIES

In addition to being an IFN inducer, poly (ICLC) is an immune adjuvant when used with certain weak antigens. Monovalent influenza virus subunit vaccine designated A/swine X-53, prepared from A/NJ/76 (New Jersey, swine), is only moderate to weakly effective when given as a single dose to young people. When the vaccine was given to monkeys simultaneously with one dose of poly (ICLC), HAI antibody titers in the serum were detectable earlier and rose to higher levels than in monkeys receiving vaccine alone. Four monkeys were used per group, each receiving 200 CCA units. The adjuvant activity of poly (ICLC) was particularly pronounced in young monkeys, in which as little as 10 μg of drug/kg of body weight was effective, as seen in Fig. 9. This level of poly (ICLC) does not induce detectable levels of serum IFN, and no fever was produced.[16]

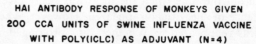

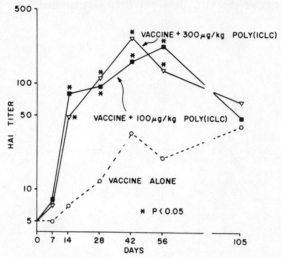

Fig. 9.   Effect of one injection of poly (ICLC) on antibody production by rhesus monkeys in response to a subunit vaccine to swine flu (4 monkeys per group).

Analogous results were obtained in monkeys using inactivated Venezuelan equine encephalomyelitis virus vaccine.[17] Figure 10 shows some of the data. A comparison of the levels attained after administration of vaccine and poly (ICLC) with those attained with vaccine alone indicates that antibody levels in serum were boosted about 40-fold after primary immunization, and perhaps 200-fold after a secondary immunization. There was no alteration in the progression of IgM and IgG development. At the peak of antibody levels, most of the antibody was IgG. Polylysine complexed to carboxymethyl cellulose without poly I: poly C had no adjuvant action.

A polysaccharide vaccine made from *Haemophilus influenzae* is a poor vaccine in very young children in whom the disease threat is maximum. The vaccine is also poor in young monkeys, as shown in Table 2.[18] The data presented are normalized values obtained by radioimmunoassays done by Dr. Porter Anderson. The value of 100 was assigned in each case to the amount of radioactivity found prior to immunization. The vaccine alone caused a minimum boost, but when given with poly (ICLC), there was a more pronounced boost. Polyadenylic:polyuridylic acid complexed to CMC and polylysine was not as effective as poly (ICLC).

It is important to emphasize that the adjuvant effects can be seen at low levels

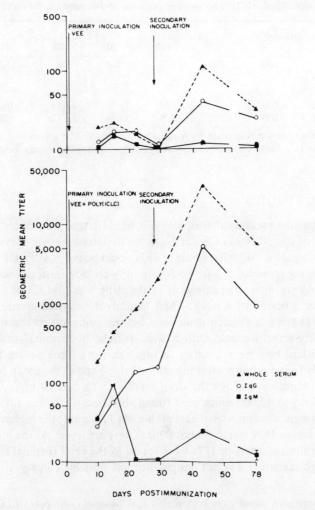

Fig. 10. Serum-neutralizing antibody response by immunoglobulin class of rhesus monkeys inoculated on days 0 and 28 with (A) inactivated VEE virus vaccine (n = 4), or (B) vaccine combined with 200 μg of poly (ICLC)/kg (n = 4). ▲: whole serum antibody titers; ○: antibody from IgG fractions; ■: antibody from IgM fractions.

of drug, below those that induce IFN and below those in which toxicity has been seen.

Comparable effects have been seen from vaccine prepared with Herpes virus envelope antigen[19] and Rift Valley fever virus.[20] However, poly (ICLC) is not a universal adjuvant. Inhibition of antibody production has been seen with albumin and pneumococcal type III polysaccharide.[21]

Table 2.   Effect of poly (ICLC) on monkey response to *Haemophilus* flu vaccine.

Treatment	Pre-injection	Day					
		7	14	20	28	34	42
Vaccine	100	590	348	286	225	187	113
Vaccine + poly (ICLC)							
(0.3 mg/kg)	100	5,643	5,040	3,340	2,063	2,162	780
(0.03 mg/kg)	100	6,589	3,904	1,884	1,132	839	721

Antibody determination was done by a radioimmunoassay. The amount of radioactivity in the pre-injection blood was assigned a value of 100, and the other values were normalized to this level.

CLINICAL STUDIES

After extensive preclinical toxicology, a phase I trial was undertaken with Dr. Levine of the National Cancer Institute to determine what levels of drug would be acceptable and what levels of IFN could be induced.[22] Doses of poly (ICLC) ranging from 0.5 mg/m^2 to 24 mg/m^2 were administered according to the following regimen: one injection of the drug was given, and the patient observed for a period of a week. Then 14 daily doses were given. At least 3 patients were treated at each drug level before going on to the next higher level. Twenty-seven patients with a wide variety of terminal cancers were studied; all had become refractory to other therapy. Peak serum IFN levels were usually found 8 hours after injection. Table 3 shows the mean peak serum IFN level found for each of the drug levels. At 18 and 24 mg/m^2, levels of serum IFN up to 15,000 units were found, but because of the toxicity noted those doses were not considered acceptable. At 12 mg/m^2, the highest tolerated dose, peak serum IFN levels of about 2,000 were achieved. At the higher levels of drug, significant levels of IFN were found in the cerebrospinal fluid (Table 4). Although the study was not designed to test possible efficacy, it was noted

Table 3.   Mean peak serum titers in man after I. V. treatment with poly (ICLC).

Dose level (mg/m^2)	Mean reference units/ml serum[a]
0.5	15 (0–25)[b]
2.5	15 (0–25)
7.5	198 (25–250)
12.0	1,940 (200–5,000)
18.0	4,473 (500–15,000)
27.0	5,820 (2,000–10,000)

a) VSV-CPE assay (international reference units), 8 hours after first dose, greater than or equal to 3 trials at each level.

b) Numbers in parentheses indicate range.

that one case of acute lymphoblastic leukemia did have a complete temporary remission.

Table 4.   Mean peak cerebrospinal fluid (CSF) titers in humans after I. V. treatment with poly (ICLC).

Dose level (mg/m^2)	Mean reference units/ml CSF[a]
0.5	5 (0–10)[b]
12.0	34 (5–63)
18.0	55 (0–115)
27.0	515 (79–1,000)

a) VSV-CPE assay (international reference units), 8 hours after first dose, greater than or equal to 3 trials at each level.
b) Numbers in parentheses indicate range.

There were a number of toxic manifestations associated with administration of the drug in this study. They are summarized in Table 5. Fever was always seen, although the degree tended to decrease with repeated administration. Fever, myalgia, and leukopenia are reminiscent of what is seen with administration of exogenous IFN. Hypotension was sometimes seen and appeared to be dose-related. Variations from this pattern of toxicity have been seen in some of the other clinical studies and will be mentioned later.

Table 5.   Poly (ICLC) toxicity–human.

Manifestation	Number/total (%)
Fever	25/25 (100)[a]
Nausea	11/25 (44)
Thrombocytopenia and leukopenia	17/25 (68)
Hypotension[b]	7/25 (28)
Syndrome of erythema, polyarthralgia, and polymyalgia[b]	4/25 (16)
Renal failure[b]	1/25 (4)
Trial aborted[c]	5/25 (20)

a) Number in parentheses is the percentage of the patients showing the symptoms.
b) Related to dose level and/or magnitude of IFN induction.
c) Three for hypotension; one for renal failure; and one for the syndrome of erythema, polyarthraligia, and polymyalgia: all at higher doses.

There are several ongoing clinical studies with sufficient results to justify a preliminary report. I shall present the more negative studies first. The Children's Hospital Cancer Testing Group has looked at the effect of poly (ICLC) on far advanced cases of the null type of acute lymphoblastic leukemia in children. No remissions have been induced, although antileukemic effects have been observed, as evidenced by a marked decrease in the absolute number of lymphoblasts in the blood of 4 patients and in the bone marrow of at least one. These children were very ill and showed toxicity at lower levels of drug than seen in the study with Dr. Levine.[23]

Similarly, a phase I toxicity study with Drs. Krown and Oetgen at the Sloan-Kettering Institute on patients with a wide variety of malignancies also revealed toxicity at lower levels of drug than reported by Dr. Levine.[24]

In contrast, in studies done with Dr. Leventhal at Johns Hopkins and Dr. Whiznant at the University of North Carolina on healthy children with juvenile laryngopapilloma, toxicities were less than those seen by Dr. Levine. Fever, mild myalgia, and occasional rises in liver enzymes were seen. These patients also were able to tolerate even higher levels of drug than did the patients seen by Dr. Levine. There was also marked improvement in the clinical condition of 7 out of 7 patients. A typical course is seen in Fig. 11.[25] Each dot represents a surgical intervention. It can be seen that surgery was required less and less frequently after treatment with poly (ICLC) began. This patient returned to Peru in September and has required no further surgery. The regimen for these patients consisted of initiation at 4 mg/m², working up to 12 or even 15 mg/m² over several weeks.[25]

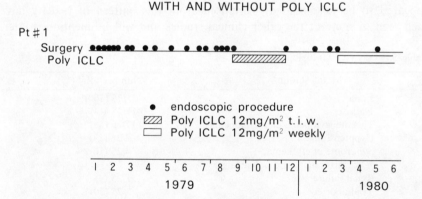

INCIDENCE OF SURGERY
WITH AND WITHOUT POLY ICLC

Fig. 11. Effect of poly (ICLC) on frequency of surgical intervention in juvenile laryngopapilloma in a child. Each dot represent a surgical intervention.[25]

Less dramatic but of some interest are the results being obtained with Drs. Durie and Salmon of the University of Arizona, summarized in Table 6.[26] These are patients who have become refractory to all other therapy. There was subjective and objective improvement in these people but only of a modest degree. (It is planned to study patients with less advanced disease.) They received about 4–6 mg/m² of the drug, once or twice a week, and produced IFN levels ranging from 100 to 2,000 units/ml serum. Their toxic manifestations consisted

Table 6. Poly (ICLC) in patients with multiple myeloma.

M-component type	Comments
Kappa light chains	67% decrease in B-J excretion, plus correction of hypercalcemia and disease stabilization with first period of treatment. 44% decrease in B-J excretion when poly (ICLC) restarted 2 months later. Normocalcemic for 5 months.
IgG kappa	M-component decrease from 5.2–3.9 gm. Improved bone pain and performance status (became ambulatory) for 2–3 months.
IgG lambda	Trial stopped because of toxicity (malignant hypertension).
IgM kappa	Plasmaphoresis requirement decreased from every 14 days to every 28 days.
IgG kappa	Stable disease parameters for 2 months.
Lambda light chains	Died 1 week after initiation of poly (ICLC).
IgG	50% Decrease in serum IgG M-component, plus symptomatic benefit.

of fever, some transient leukopenia, no hypotension, but one incident of hypertension, and transient myalgia.

Possibly the most encouraging results have been in patients with paralytic neurologic diseases. Those studies are ongoing with Drs. Engel and Salazar of the National Institute of Neurological and Communicative Diseases and Stroke. The first patient we studied was a 29-year-old man who had chronic relapsing polyneuropathy since the age of 15.[27] For a while the disease responded somewhat to steroids, but for the 3 years prior to poly (ICLC) therapy, he had been steadily deteriorating until he could not turn over in bed and had to be carried to an electric wheel chair. He received 4 $\mu g/kg$, once or twice weekly. Within 4 weeks he began to show slightly increased muscular strength. It is now over 3 years since treatment started, and he is out of the hospital, has received job training, and is working. He needs to receive poly (ICLC) about every 5 weeks; otherwise, he starts to get weak again. Eight patients with dysimmune neurological diseases refractory to high prolonged doses of prednisone plus azathioprine or cyclophosphamide have been treated so far. Their conditions included chronic dyschwannian neuropathy, chronic dysneuronal neuropathy, chronic myopathy (polymyositis), acute dysneuronal neuropathy, post-infectious demyelinating encephalomyelitis involving cerebellum, cerebrum, and brainstem. These patients were all totally paralyzed. They all benefited by poly (ICLC) treatment to the point where they were able to approximate a normal life.[28] The first 7 cases involved peripheral nerve neuropathies; the last one was a central nervous system neuropathy resembling an acute phase of multiple sclerosis. The patient was completely paralyzed and unresponsive to other therapy. Two days following each weekly treatment with poly (ICLC), there was a definite increase in muscular strength. After 9 months of therapy, he was dismissed and was able to walk with a cane for balance.

In summary, preliminary clinical results with poly (ICLC) suggest that there may be some disease situations hitherto rather poorly accessible to therapy in which the inducer may be useful. More needs to be done to evaluate and control toxic manifestations. Obviously, more extensive, controlled studies are needed before firmer conclusions can be drawn.

REFERENCES

1. Isaacs, A. and Lindemann, J.: Virus interference. I. The interferon. *Proc. R. Soc. Lond.* [*Biol.*], **147**: 258, 1957.
2. Nagano, Y. and Kojima, Y.: Inhibition de l'infection vaccinale par un facteur liquide dans le tissu infecté par le virus homologue. *C. R. Soc. Biol. (Paris)*, **152**: 1627, 1958.
3. Chany, C.: An inhibiting factor of intracellular multiplication of viruses called interferon originating from cancer cells. *C. R. Acad. Sci. [D] (Paris)*, **250**: 3903, 1960.
4. Field, A. K., Tytell, A. A., Lampson, G. P., and Hilleman, M. R.: Inducers of interferon and host resistance. II. Multistranded synthetic polynucleotide complexes. *Proc. Natl. Acad. Sci. USA*, **58**: 1004, 1967.
5. Worthington, M. and Baron, S.: Late therapy with an interferon stimulator in an arbovirus encephalitis in mice. *Proc. Soc. Exp. Biol. Med.*, **136**: 323, 1971.
6. Levy, H. B., Law, L. W., and Rabson, A. S.: Inhibition of tumor growth by polyinosinic-polycytidylic acid. *Proc. Natl. Acad. Sci. USA*, **62**: 357, 1969.
7. Robinson, R. A., Devita, V. T., Levy, H. B., Baron, S., Hubbard, S. P., and Levine, A. S.: A phase I-II trial of multiple-dose polyriboinosinic-polyribocytidylic acid in patients with leukemia or solid tumors. *J. Natl. Cancer Inst.*, **57**: 599, 1976.
8. Nordlund, J. J., Wolff, S. M., and Levy, H. B.: Inhibition of biologic activity of poly I: poly C by human plasma. *Proc. Soc. Exp. Biol. Med.*, **133**: 439, 1970.
9. Levy, H. B., Baer, G., Baron, S., Buckler, C. E., Gibbs, C. J., Iadarola, M. J., London, W. F., and Rice, J.: A modified polyriboinosinic-polycytidylic acid complex that induces interferon in primates. *J. Infect. Dis.*, **132**: 434, 1975.
10. Baer, G. M., Shaddock, J. H., Moore, S. A., Levy, H. B., and Baron, S.: Successful prophylaxis against rabies in mice and rhesus monkeys. The interferon system and vaccine. *J. Infect. Dis.*, **136**: 286, 1977.
11. Baer, G. M., Moore, S. A., Shaddock, J. H., and Levy, H. B.: A single dose of interferon inducer and vaccine: An effective rabies treatment in exposed monkeys. *Bull. WHO* (in press).
12. Moreno, J. A., Bareghcum, S. D., Levy, H. B., and Baer, G. M.: Further studies on rabies postexposure prophylaxis in mice. A comparison of vaccine with interferon and vaccine. *J. Gen. Virol.*, **42**: 219, 1979.
13. Stephen, E. L., Scott, S. K., Eddy, G. A., and Levy, H. B.: Effect of interferon on togavirus and arenavirus infection of animals. *Tex. Rep. Biol. Med.*, **35**: 449, 1977.
14. Levy, H. B.: Induction of interferon *in vivo* by polynucleotides. *Tex. Rep. Biol. Med.*, **35**: 91, 1977.
15. Purcell, R. H., London, W. T., McAuliffe, V. J., Palmer, A. E., Kaplan, P. M., Levy, H. B., Gerin, J. L., Wagner, J., Popper, H., Lvovsky, E., and Wong, D. O.: Modification of chronic hepatitis-B virus infection in chimpanzees by administration of an interferon inducer. *Lancet*, **2**: 757, 1976.

16. Stephen, E. L., Hilmas, D. E., Mangaefico, J. A., and Levy, H. B.: Swine influenza vaccines: Potentiation of antibody responses in rhesus monkeys. *Science*, **197**: 1289, 1977.
17. Harrington, D. G., Crabbs, C. L., Hilmas, D. E., Brown, J. R., Higbef, G., A., Cole, F. B., and Levy, H. B.: Adjuvant effects of low doses of a nuclease resistant derivative of poly I: poly C on antibody responses to inactivated VEE vaccine. *Infect. Immun.*, **24**: 160, 1979.
18. Levy, H. B., Lvovsky, E., Rulez, F., Harrington, D., Anderson, A., Inoe, V., Hilfenhaus, J., and Stephen, E.: Immune modulatory effects of poly ICLC. *Ann. N. Y. Acad. Sci.* (in press).
19. Hilfenhaus, J., Christ, H., Köhler, R., Moser, H., Kirchner, H., and Levy, H. B.: Effect of poly ICLC on the efficacy of herpes simplex virus envelope antigen against herpes simplex infections in mice. *J. Infect. Dis.* (in press).
20. Harrington, D. G., Stephen, E., Peters, J., and Levy, H. B.: Unpublished observations.
21. Levy, H. B., Lvovsky, E., and Baker, P.: Unpublished observations.
22. Levine, A. S., Sivulich, M., Wiernick, P. H., and Levy, H. B.: Initial clinical trials in cancer patients of polyriboinosinic-polyribocytidylic acid stabilized with poly L-lysine in carboxymethyl cellulose (poly ICLC)—a highly effective interferon inducer. *Cancer Res.*, **39**: 1645, 1979.
23. Lamphen, B. and Levy, H. B.: Unpublished observations.
24. Krown, S., Oetgen, H., Stewart, W., and Levy, H. B.: Phase I trial of poly ICLC in cancer patients. In: M. Chirigos (ed.), Proceedings of Symposium on Biological Modifiers in Treatment of Cancer, March 1980.
25. Leventhal, B., Whiznant, J., and Levy, H. B.: Unpublished observations.
26. Durie, B., Salmon, S., and Levy, H. B.: Unpublished observations.
27. Engel, W. K., Cunes, R. A., and Levy, H. B.: Poly ICLC treatment of neuropathy. *Lancet*, **1**: 503, 1978.
28. Engel, W. K., Salazar, A., and Levy, H. B.: Unpublished observations.

Discussion

Dr. NAGANO: I have two questions to Dr. Levy. First, I believe that poly ICLC was repeatedly injected for a number of times. Did you observe the production of interferon in blood at every injection? Is there any concern about the tolerance? Second, concerning the clinical aspect, how serious was the renal damage seen in certain patients? Was it treatable with possible total recovery?

Dr. LEVY: In response to the question about the frequency of injection, there is, with poly ICLC, a hyporesponsive period. That is to say, repeated injections do cause something of a decrease in the amount of interferon that is made. But we have given some of the neurologic disease patients the drug for well over a year, and they still continue to produce interferon. There has been no long-term toxicity that we have seen. The toxicity all disappears when the treatment is stopped. Renal failure was seen only in one patient, and that was at a very high level of drug. So this is not a common feature that we see. I forgot to mention before, and I apologize, that Dr. Machida and Dr. Kuninaka of Yamasa Shoyu Company have prepared poly ICLC here in Japan with their own chemicals and have given it to people, and seem to get about the same levels of interferon that we have seen.

Dr. MACHIDA: I'd like to ask Dr. Levy three questions. First, what do you think is the reason the toxicity of poly ICLC was higher in the patients with acute lymphoblastic leukemia? Second, do you have some evidence or findings that host immune responses such as NK activity or macrophage activity are augmented after the administration of poly ICLC? Third, what is the rationale for using poly ICLC for disimmune neurological disease?

Dr. LEVY: The reason for using poly ICLC in the disimmune neurologic diseases was to see whether or not there would be any modification of the immune system. If indeed these were diseases that were caused by bad immune reactions, by enhancing the immunoreactivity we could modify the disease. Well, we have modified the disease, but we cannot say for certain that this was because of modification of the immune system. That was the hypothesis on which it was tried. The NK cell activity is indeed enhanced by poly ICLC in patients that have received the drug. We have seen this in the study in Arizona and in the study at the National Cancer Institute. To your first question, as to why the children with acute lymphocytic leukemia show more toxicity, I cannot really say. The only thing that I can correlate things with is if the patient is very, very ill to begin with, then we see more toxicity. The patients with the juvenile laryngeal papilloma who really were in good general health showed relatively little toxicity, and the lymphocytic leukemia children were very, very ill. There also is one other item that may be related to this. In studies with Dr. Stringfellow in the U.S., we showed that if you take the serum from the children who are acutely ill with leukemia and put their serum onto human tissue culture cells, and then stimulate those cells to produce interferon, either with poly ICLC or virus, the serum from the leukemic children is able to inhibit fairly strongly the ability of such cells to produce interferon. If, on the other hand, you take serum from some of the other patients who did not have leukemia, their serum did not show this inhibitory action. It may be that there are factors present in the leukemic children which interact badly with the interferon produced or with the drug. Also it could be that their general health was so poor that they could not take any additional stress.

Dr. KOJIMA: I'd like to address two questions to Dr. Levy. I am also engaged in the development of interferon inducer using plant components, and we are currently using rabbits. We have observed seasonal variation in the yield of interferon. Have you seen any seasonal variations in the production of interferon by using poly ICLC? We also found that the seasonal variation decreases when interferon is simultaneously administered. We normally give the inducer orally. If the drug is given in combination with interferon, it works better. Have you looked at the combination with interferon?

Dr. LEVY: We have not done combination therapy of that type. We have been thinking of doing it and I think we will get to do it, but it is more difficult to mount this combination experiment in people than it is in rabbits. We see a great deal of variation from patient to patient, in how much interferon they produce in response to a given level of drug, even in patients who have the same disease; and patients who have different diseases also show big differences. So whether or not we see a seasonal variation, I think it will be very difficult for us to determine, because we don't have enough cases to be able to analyze such matters.

Dr. KOJIMA: Have you conducted any animal study?

Dr. LEVY: Well, we have conducted many animal studies, monkey studies, rabbits, in virus diseases. And the Cancer Institute has looked at the effect of the drug in some of their standard tumor models in mice. In mice, there is very little advantage of poly ICLC over plain poly IC. Poly ICLC produces a little bit more interferon than plain poly IC. The big difference comes in primates—monkeys and people. And we have not looked at any tumor models in monkeys. In various virus diseases that I've mentioned, we have had a moderate amount of success. Much of that material, I think, has been published.

Therapeutic Effect of Human Fibroblast Interferon on Dendritic Keratitis

Yukio UCHIDA,* Michiko KANEKO,* Ritsuko YAMANISHI,* Shusaku KITANO,[2]*
Tatsuko UEDA,[2]* Naohiko TANAKA,[3]* Takatoshi SASAKI,[3]* Koji KAMATA,[3]*
Motokazu ITOI,[4]* Yoshio AKAGI,[4]* Reizo MANABE,[6]* Tsuneji SUDA,[5]*
Shunsaku KOBAYASHI,[6]* Hideto TERANISHI,[6]* Hiroshi SHIOTA,[7]* and Shinta
YAMANE[7]*

*Department of Ophthalmology, Tokyo Women's Medical College, Tokyo, [2]*Department of
Ophthalmology, Nihon University School of Medicine, Tokyo, [3]*Department of Ophthalmology, School of Medicine, Yokohama City University, Yokohama, [4]*Department of Ophthalmology, Kyoto Prefectural University of Medicine, Kyoto, [5]*Department of Ophthalmology,
Osaka University Medical School, Osaka, [6]*Department of Ophthalmology, Yamaguchi University School of Medicine, Ube-city, Yamaguchi-Pref., [7]*Department of Ophthalmology,
School of Medicine, Tokushima University, Tokushima, Japan

SUMMARY

Our study group carried out a randomized, double-blind clinical trial comparing
the effect of 2 concentrations of human fibroblast interferon eye drops in 68 patients
with dendritic keratitis. The therapeutic effect of 10^6 IU/ml appeared to be superior
to that of 10^3 IU/ml, but a statistically significant difference was not noted. It is suggested that interferon eye drops are clinically useful in combination with debridement
of the lesion.

INTRODUCTION

Following the discovery of interferon (IFN), application of the drug to the
medical treatment of viral infections was long awaited. Recently, highly
purified preparations of human IFN have become available for clinical trials
in man. Viral keratoconjunctivitis is a unique disorder for the evaluation of
antiviral agents because it can be treated by topical administration, which

129

requires only a small amount of drug and which induces minimal systemic side-effects. Herpes simplex keratitis is particularly suitable for tests because the dendritic lesion of the cornea indicates the etiology and the morphological changes caused by the drug can be easily observed by a slitlamp microscope.

The effect of topically applied human IFN on dendritic keratitis has been studied by several investigators.[1-8] Most of their results have suggested that IFN works mainly as a prophylactic and has little clinical usefulness in the treatment of established dendritic keratitis, unless other therapeutic measures such as debridement or antiviral drugs are combined. Until recently, it was primarily human leukocyte interferon (HuIFN-α) that was used for studies. It was found to have the ability to suppress lesion formation of herpes simplex keratitis in the rabbit. This result suggested an optimal dose schedule in clinical trials.[5,9]

In contrast, human fibroblast interferon (HuIFN-β), an antigenically different IFN, has appeared in only a few reports.[4,7,10] Previously, we reported that drops of HuIFN-β reduced the severity of herpetic keratitis in rabbits.[11] In a pilot study, we saw the therapeutic effect of HuIFN-β drops on dendritic keratitis in human without additional antiviral measures. A subsequent double-blind study showed a significant difference in the effect between high and low concentrations of HuIFN-β.[10] The number of patients was small, however, and therefore we performed the present study to evaluate the effect of HuIFN-β in a large-scale double-blind test.

SUBJECTS AND METHODS

Seven ophthalmology clinics participated in this study (those with which the authors are affiliated). Patients with dendritic keratitis were admitted to investigation. Diagnosis was made clinically, but the etiological confirmation by immunofluorescence or virus isolation was carried out when laboratory facilities were available. On such occasions, epithelial scraping materials were taken from a small part of the dendritic lesion and were used for virus examination. Unscraped areas of the lesion were subjected to observation.

Preparations of HuIFN-β were provided from Basic Research Laboratories, Toray Industries, Inc. Two concentrations of HuIFN-β, 10^6 IU/ml and 10^3 IU/ml, were compared in this study. Samples to be tested were coded in a randomized manner on the basis of a double-blind test. The code was kept by the National Institute of Health, Tokyo, and broken after the results had been evaluated. One drop (0.04 ml) of a sample was instilled into the conjunctival sac 4 times a day. In every case, gentamicin eye drops were instilled 3 times a day to prevent bacterial infection. Patients were examined daily or every other day under a slitlamp microscope after staining the cornea with fluorescein. The results were documented with photographs and drawings at each visit.

The protocol called for administration of samples to continue for 2 weeks. However, when healing was not apparent after one week of treatment and conditions became worse, the regimen was changed to other methods such as debridement or idoxuridine. Cure was defined as the disappearance of gross staining areas with fluorescein. The results were divided into 5 grades as follows: marked improvement (cured in 4 days), moderate improvement (cured in 7 days), slight improvement (lesion regressed), no change, and aggravation. Before breaking the code, the records of each patient were reviewed by all investigators.

RESULTS

Out of 73 patients, 5 were excluded from the final evaluation; 3 patients did not follow the medication schedule, and 2 were considered to have dendrites with coexisting metaherpetic alteration before treatment. In 44 patients subjected to virus examination, 41 showed positive results for herpes simplex virus by either immunofluorescence or virus isolation. Thirty-six patients were treated with 10^6 IU/ml IFN-β, and 32 were treated with 10^3 IU/ml IFN-β.

The results of treatment are shown in Table 1. The number of patients whose results were judged as marked and moderate improvement was larger in the 10^6 IU/ml group than in the 10^3 IU/ml group. The effect of 10^6 IU/ml HuIFN-β seemed superior to that of 10^3 IU/ml, but when gradings were divided between moderate improvement and slight improvement, the difference was not statistically significant (χ^2 test, $0.2 > p > 0.1$). In most patients admitted to virus examination, scraped areas of the dendritic lesion showed a rapid healing in 2 to 3 days.

Table 1. Results of a double-blind study comparing the effect of two concentrations of HuIFN-β on dendritic keratitis.

	Grade[a]	3+	2+	1+	0	1−	Total
10^6 IU/ml HuIFN-β	No. of patients	7	11	8	6	4	36
	Cumulative percent	19.4	50.0	72.2	88.9	100	
10^3 IU/ml HuIFN-β	No. of patients	3	8	11	1	9	32
	Cumulative percent	9.3	34.3	68.8	71.9	100	

a) 3+: marked improvement; 2+: moderate improvement; 1 +: slight improvement; 0: no change. 1−: aggravation.

DISCUSSION

Our previous placebo-controlled pilot study showed that 5 cases of dendritic keratitis treated with 10^6 IU/ml HuIFN-β 4 times a day showed improvement.

Therefore, this frequency of application was thought to be appropriate. We then used 12 patients as subjects in a double-blind study comparing two concentrations of HuIFN-β, 10^6 IU/ml and 10^3 IU/ml. All 6 patients treated with 10^6 IU/ml showed a favorable response, and the effect of 10^6 IU/ml was significantly superior to that of 10^3 IU/ml. These results demonstrated that HuIFN-β has a therapeutic effect on dendritic keratitis without the additional use of other antiherpetic measures, but, from our experience, its effect appeared to be milder than that of IDU or trifluorothymidine.

The present study conducted on a larger scale also showed that 10^6 IU/ml was more effective than 10^3 IU/ml, but there was no statistical significance. This might be due to a slight therapeutic action by 10^3 IU/ml HuIFN-β.

Jones and coworkers demonstrated a reduction in the recurrence rate of herpetic epithelial lesions when a topical administration of HuIFN-α was combined with minimal wipe debridement.[2,5] Sundmacher and associates reported favorable results by combining HuIFN-α application with thermocautery[1,6,7] and with trifluorothymidine drops.[8] They found no differences in the therapeutic effect on dendritic keratitis between HuIFN-β and HuIFN-α.[7] Our experiment using rabbits showed HuIFN-β to be more effective as a prophylactic agent than as curative one for dendritic keratitis.[10] We have observed that the scraped area of the dendritic lesion healed promptly. Therefore, HuIFN-β would be of practical benefit in the treatment of dendritic keratitis when supported by debridement.

REFERENCES

1. Sundmacher, R., Neumann-Haefelin, D., and Cantell, R.: Successful treatment of dendritic keratitis with human leucocyte interferon. *Albrecht V. Graefes Arch. Klin. Exp. Ophthal.*, **201**: 39–45, 1976.
2. Jones, B. R., Coster, D. J., Falcon, M. G., and Cantell, K.: Topical therapy of ulcerative herpetic keratitis with human interferon. *Lancet*, **2**: 128, 1976.
3. Kaufman, H. E., Meyer, R. F., Laibson, P. R., Waltman, S. R., Nesburn, A. B., and Shuster, J. J.: Human leucocyte interferon for the prevention of recurrences of herpetic Keratitis. *J. Infect. Dis.*, **133** (Suppl.): A165–A168, 1976.
4. McGill, J. I., Cantell, K., Collins, P., Finter, N. B., Laird, R., and Jones, B. R.: Optimal usage of exogenous human interferon for prevention or therapy of herpetic keratitis. *Trans. Opthal. Soc. U. K.*, **97**: 324–326, 1977.
5. Coster, D. J., Falcon, M. G., Cantell, K., and Jones, B. R.: Clinical experience of human leucocyte interferon in the management of herpetic keratitis. *Trans. Ophthal. Soc. U. K.*, **97**: 327–329, 1977.
6. Sundmacher, R., Cantell, K., Haug, P., and Neuman-Haefelin, D.: Role of debridement and interferon in the treatment of dendritic keratitis. *Albrecht V. Graefes Arch. Klin. Exp. Ophthal.*, **207**: 77–82, 1978.
7. Sundmacher, R., Cantell, K., Skoda, R., Hallermann, C., and Heuman-Haefelin, K.: Human leucocyte and fibroblast interferon in a combination therapy of dendritic keratitis. *Albrecht V. Graefes Arch. Klin. Exp. Ophthal.*, **208**: 229–233, 1978.

8. Sundmacher, R., Cantell, K., and Neumann-Haefelin, D.: Combination therapy of dendritic keratitis with trifluorothymidine and interferon. *Lancet*, **2**: 687, 1978.
9. McGill, J. I., Collins, P., Cantell, B. R., and Finter, N. B.: Optimal schedule for use of interferon in the corneas of rabbits with herpes simplex keratitis. *J. Infect Dis.*, **133** (Suppl.): A13–A17, 1976.
10. Uchida, Y., Kaneko, M., Yamanishi, R., and Kobayashi, S.: Effect of human fibroblast interferon on dendritic keratitis. In Herpetic Eye Diseases. pp. 409–413. Editor: R. Sundmacher, Bergman, Munchen, 1981.
11. Kaneko, M., Yamanishi, R., Uchida, Y., and Kobayashi, S.: Topical administration of human fibroblast interferon in herpes simplex keratitis of the rabbit. *Microbiol. Immunol.*, **25**: 85–87, 1981.

Discussion

Dr. REVEL: I have a question to Dr. Uchida. Dr. Romano at the Tel Aviv Hospital, who has been conducting with us studies on the use of the fibroblast interferon for herpes keratitis, has observed that repeated administration of the interferon in cases that are resistant to iodo-dexy-uridine (IDU) can lead to improvement and disappearance of the ulcer. However, one of the problems seems to be inhibition of the re-formation of epithelium. And she has found that if you stop interferon, then the re-epithelization is very fast. I want to ask, Dr. Uchida, if you have similar observations.

Dr. UCHIDA: In the studies that we have carried out, we have not seen any delay in the re-epithelization. But after the ulcer, when there is a trophic ulcer unrelated to virus proliferation, interferon might obstruct re-epithelization. However, in herpetic keratitis we have not observed any delay in the re-epithelization.

Effect of Human Leucocyte or Fibroblast Interferon on Hepatitis B Virus Infection in Patients with Chronic Hepatitis

Toshitsugu ODA and Hiroshi SUZUKI

Department of Medicine, University of Tokyo, Bunkyo-ku, Tokyo 113, Japan

INTRODUCTION

This paper will discuss therapy for chronic hepatitis type B with interferon (IFN) as presently practiced in Japan. The effect of IFN on chronic hepatitis type B is now being investigated in a unified system by the research group of the National Project on Viral Hepatitis subsidezed by a grant-in-aid from the Ministry of Health and Welfare. The members of this Interferon Research Committee, Hepatitis Division, are as follows: T. Oda, University of Tokyo (Chief); R. Kono, NIH, Japan; H. Suzuki, Yamanashi Medical University; F. Ichida, Niigata University; N. Hattori, Kanazawa University; S. Furuta, Shinshu University; T. Takino, Kyoto Prefectural Medical University; Y. Yana, National Nagasaki Hospital; A. Ohbayashi, Metropolitan Komagome Hospital; K. Nishioka, Tokyo Metropolitan Clinical Research Institute; M. Mayumi, Jichi Medical University; and T. Shikata, Nippon University.

MATERIALS

In June 1980 the research group received $1,000 \times 10^6$ IU of IFN-β, which was developed by Toray Co. and authorized by NIH Japan (R. Kono), and 300×10^6 IU of IFN-α, which was produced from human leukocytes and purified by the Japan Red Corss Blood Center. One vial of IFN-β contained 3×10^6 IU, and the specific activity was 10^7 IU/mg protein or more. The contamination with bovine serum albumin (BSA) was 0.5 μg/vial or less. One vial of IFN-α contained 2×10^6 IU, and the specific activity was 1×10^6

135

IU/mg protein. The contamination with egg albumin was 0.2 μg/vial or less.

SUBJECTS, METHODS, AND TEST ITEMS

The subjects were patients who had been diagnosed as having chronic active hepatitis type B in seven facilities (1st Dept. of Medicine, University of Tokyo; 3rd Dept. of Medicine, Niigata University; 2nd Dept. of Medicine, Shinshu University; 1st Dept. of Medicine, Kanazawa University; 3rd Dept. of Medicine, Kyoto Prefectural Medical University; and Metropolitan Komagome Hospital), who were positve in hepatitis virus (HBV)-related DNA polymerase (DNA–P), and who had undergone a liver biopsy within the 3-month period before the initiation of interferon treatment.

A total dose of 36×10^6 IU of IFN-β was administered intramuscularly (I. M.); the daily dose was 3×10^6 IU on the 1st day, 6×10^6 IU on the 2nd day, and 9×10^6 IU from the 3rd to the 5th day. After a 2-day interval, a daily dose of 3×10^6 IU was given intravenously (I. V.) for 2 to 3 weeks. The patients who received treatment with IFN-α were given a dose of 5×10^6 IU I. M. on the 1st day and then a daily dose of 5×10^6 IU I. M. on the following days.

Measurements of serum DNA-P, HBs antigen, and HBe antigen were carried out before administration, on the 1st, 3rd, 5th, and 7th days, and then twice a week during the administration periods, while hematologic examinations and liver functional tests were performed twice a week.

RESULTS AND DISCUSSION

IFN-β

IFN-β was given only to female subjects, as suggested by the report of Merigan *et al.*, and therfore only 3 patients received it. The results of the DNA-P and ALT measurements in these 3 cases are shown in Fig. 1. In all of the patients even I.M. injection of IFN-β caused an obvious reduction of serum DNA-P, which clearly rose again after a 2-day interruption of treatment. This finding indicated that IFN-β inhibited the replication of HBV even though I.M. injection of IFN-β has been said to be virtually ineffective. The effect was recognized rather early in the treatment, and in 2 cases more than a 50% reduction of the activity was observed on the 2nd day.

I.V. injections produced a similar effect on DNA-P, although the effect depended on the dose. However, in 2 of these 3 cases DNA-P never became completely negative even with continuous administration of IFN-β. In the third case DNA-P became completely negative in the 2nd week of I.V. IFN-β injections.

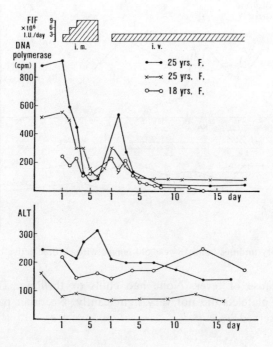

Fig. 1. Effects of IFN-β on chronic hepatits type B.

Serum ALT in the 3 cases varied considerably, elevating in one case, declining in another, and showing little variation in the third.

Figure 2 shows a case in which IFN-β induced a negative DNA-P. The
patient was a 18-year-old female in whom the DNA-P became negative 2 weeks
after the beginning of IFN-β I.V. injections, as described above. IFN-β was
given for 5 days and then discontinued. For about 2 months the DNA-P
remained negative, while HBs antigen declined and HBe antigen turned negative (as determined by the immunodiffusion method). After discontinuing the
IFN-β injections the serum ALT improved, but in the 2nd month after termination of treatment, both the DNA-P and the HBe antigen reverted to positive.

These findings indicate that all 3 cases belonged to type 3 of the classification by Merigan *et al.*, and although HBV replication in the host was inhibited,
IFN-β treatment could not interrupt continuous HBV infection completely.

The patients experienced a temporary rever of 37–39°C after administration that was more sever after I.V. than I.M. injections, but therapy was never

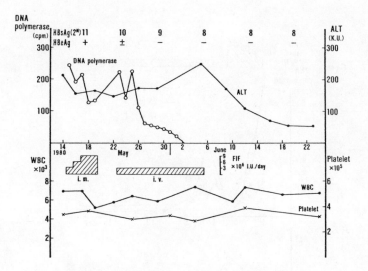

Fig. 2. Laboratory findings in an 18-year-old female with chronic active hepatitis type B.

terminated because of fever. None had chills or thrilling. The counts of leukocytes and platelets did not vary significantly. No other particular side-effects were observed.

IFN-α

IFN-α was given to 2 cases of chronic hepatitis type B. Case 1 was a 30-year-old male whose test results are shown in Fig. 3. DNA-P rapidly fell from 2,047 cpm before administration to 234 cpm 2 days afterward, about 10% of the former value. The level did not decline further despite continuous administration. After the discontinuation of IFN-α DNA-P abruptly increased and after 2 week it had returned almost to the pre-injection level. Serum ALP was about 200 and gradually diminished after IFN-α treatment; this tendency continued after the injections were stopped, and reached an almost normal value. HBs and HBe antigens showed no significant variations. During treatment the counts of leukocytes and platelets markedly declined by rapidly recovered when therapy was terminated. The reduction of leukocytes was mostly due to the reduction of neutrophils.

Figure 4 presents the findings in the other patient who received IFN-α, an 18-year-old male. When he was given 3×10^6 IU of IFN-α, DNA-P tended to elevate, but it rapidly fell when the dose was increased to 10×10^6 IU, although it did not become negative completely. HBs antigen did not vary, but HBe antigen tended to decline. After giving the administration of 10×10^6 IU, leukocyte count was greatly reduced. When the dose was lowered to

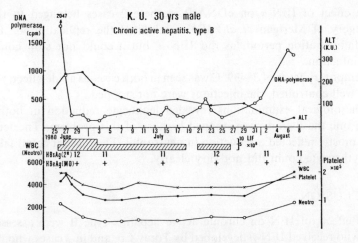

Fig. 3. Laboratory findings in a 30-year-old male with chronic active hepatitis type B.

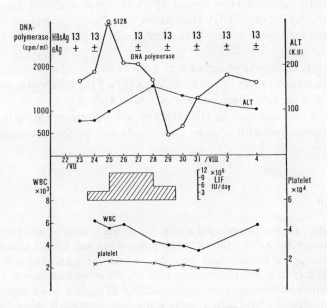

Fig. 4. Laboratory findings in an 18-year-old male with chronic active hepatitis type B.

5×10^6 IU, the drop in leukocytes continued, so the therapy was terminated after a total dose of 42×10^6 IU in 6 days. DNA-P subsequently increased rapidly. The leukocyte count fell for 2 days after the last injection, but after one week it returned to the pretreatment level.

The effect of IFN-α on eDNA-P in these 2 cases belonged to the type 3 category of Merigan *et al.*: IFN-α inhibited the replication of HBV in the administration period, as did IFN-α, but it could not stop continuous HBV infection.

A temporary fever of 38–39° C was seen in both cases as a side-effect, but since it was well controlled, the injections were not stopped.

Hematological examinations revealed leukocyte reduction in both cases, and in one the therapy was stopped because of this problem. The leukocyte count mostly reflected a reduction in neutrophil. The platelet count fell, while the erythrocyte count did not vary clearly.

CONCLUSION

The effects of IFN on chronic active hepatitis type B were assessed in 3 cases who received IFN-β developed by Toray Co. and in 2 cases who received IFN-α prepared by Red Cross Blood Center. The daily dose ranged from 3 $\times$ 10^6 IU to 10 $\times$ 10^6 IU, and the total dose given was 100 $\times$ 10^6 IU.

With both types of IFN, serum DNA-P declined during treatment, indicating the inhibition of NBV replication, but after the therapy was terminated, the level increased; neither IFN could completely control HBV continuous infection.

Temporary fever was observed with both IFNs, but the injections were not stopped because of fever in any case. With IFN-β the leukocytes and platelets declined, but his side-effect was not seen with IFN-β.

The dose and duration of IFN therapy will be researched further, and its use in combination with adenine arabinoside will be also investigated.

Discussion

Dr. GALASSO: I'd like to comment a little bit on the toxicity of adenine arabinoside monophosphate. As was shown in the slides, when you looked at toxicity in the chimpanzees, the dosages used were 25, 50 and 75 mg/kg. And it was dose-dependent: there was less toxicity seen with 25. We agree that there is toxicity seen with adenine arabinoside monophosphate. But 25 mg is a much higher dose than has been used. We have used adenine arabinoside extensively in the United States against herpes infections. It is currently licensed, for instance, against herpes encephalitis, and I expect that it will soon be licensed against neonatal herpes, but at dosages of 10 and 15 mg/kg. We have found very little toxicity unless the patients have a problem with renal function. So you must be careful in use of these drugs and the state of the renal impairment of the patients. Also in the studies it was shown that 5 mg/kg did not have much of an effect in chronic hepatitis patients. Perhaps this is too low a dose, so that if studies are to be done, the dosage should be between 10 and 15 mg/kg of body weight. In addition, studies are currently being conducted to evaluate adenine arabinoside monophosphate in Lyon, France, with Dr. Trepo and in the U.K. with Dr. Thomas and Dr. Sherlock. And They are having very good results using these drugs.

Dr. ODA: Our group is concerned with the dosage of 15 mg/kg being slightly higher than it should be, but we would like to try that dose if possible. 10 mg/kg per day appear to be an appropriate dose in Japan. But it seems desirable to increase the dose.

Dr. SHIOTA: I would like to ask Dr. Oda and probably Dr. Merigan a question concerning the combination therapy of interferon with ara Amp. In my animal experiment, ara Amp showed a very toxic effect. If you apply it in the rabbit cornea, it produces erosion within 4 days. And according to your abstract, Prof. Oda, you mention that ara A and ara Amp are also being studied by this committee. But I do not advise you to use ara Amp, because it is toxic. Now I'd like to ask Dr. Oda why you have picked up ara Amp. Let me explain one more thing. After ara A, it is advisable to use ara Hx. Because ara A is easily deaminized into ara Hx. And the solubility of ara Hx is much greater than that of ara A. Dr. Merigan, I understand that you did not use ara Hx. But have you ever tried the combination therapy of interferon with ara Hx instead of ara Amp?

Dr. MERIGAN: At present, I believe ara Hx is not an investigational drug in the U.S., because in tissue culture, in animal systems against herpes viruses, it has a lower activity by about 30-fold as compared to ara A in virus inhibition. So we do not consider it a desirable choice, because of its lower activity.

Dr. SHIOTA: Yes. Ara Hx has lower activity. But the fact is, ara A is deaminated into ara Hx.

Dr. MERIGAN: But on the other hand, we have a number of clinical experiences which allow us to use ara A without a limiting side effect. So I think our experience in people with ara A has led to its licensing as a drug in the U.S. for both encephalitis and perhaps, as Dr. Galasso mentioned, for neonatal herpes in the near future. We've given about 30 courses of ara Amp, but we had only one patient with toxicity, and this was a patient to whom we gave interferon at the same time and who had some accumulation of the ara Hx. So I personally think that as long as you stay on a low dose with ara Amp, it is a safe drug. This is a clinical experience. Admittedly we did not have your tissue culture experience to prevent us from using it. And there had been a fair amount of experience in herpes simplex and zoster lesions in immuno-suppressed patients that showed good pharmacokinetics and safety of the material in phase I testing before we did the hepatitis patients, it has good activity in the eye, at least in the experimental animal models. Ara Amp is licensed where we had good safety information in other disease settings for man. That's why we went ahead with it in hepatitis.

Dr. GALASSO: There have been extensive studies with ara Amp ointment against herpes keratitis. Its efficacy has been proven; no toxicity has been seen, and it is licensed in the U.S. for clinical treatment of herpes eratitis patients. It is considered to be somewhat better than IDU, but perhaps not as good as trifluoro thymidine.

Dr. MERIGAN: So our clinical experience has been good with ara Amp. But I am sure, on the other hand, there are some systems where a given dose would give toxicity. It sounds like you had a toxic dose for your system.

Dr. Shiota: I would like to ask Dr. Revel about epidemic kerato-conjunctivitis. Based on Prof. Jones and McGill's work on interferon activity against herpetic keratitis, it seems that effective concentration of the interferon lasts for about 24 hours by a drop of interferon. Therefore they say that in order to keep an adequate level of interferon just one drop is enough. But I am not quite sure how often you applied it. If my memory is correct, you applied 6 times a day. Do you have any comments on how often we should apply it on topical application?

Dr. Revel: We have observed the work of Dr. Romano, the ophtalmologist; even in the case of herpetic keratitis, multiple drops give much better results than a single administration per day of a high dose. And this was quite clear in the case of the adenovirus conjunctivitis. The multiple drops—6 times per day—are much better. The reason for that is not very clear. I think we'd have to measure the response of tissue to interferon, and it is very difficult at the present time to say that the antiviral state induced by interferon last for 24 hours, as was claimed by Dr. Jones and Dr. McGill in the beginning.

Dr. Uchida: From the ophthamologist's standpoint, epidemic erato-conjunctivitis is a very troublesome disease for which there is no effective treatment. I am very gratified to hear that Dr. Revel has obtained such good results by using fibroblast interferon for such a troublesome disease. In Japan, Dr. Kishida, Dr. Imanishi, Dr. Negoro and others studied epidemic keratoconjunctivitis using leukocyte interferon. They have seen a prophylactic effect of leukocyte interferon on this disease, and they have also published reports on the therapeutic effect in the Japanese Journal of Ophtalmology. We would like to try to use this fibroblast interferon, but it is difficult for us to collect a sufficient number of control patients. I hope that we will have the opportunity to test the fibroblast interferon.

Some Trials to Treatment of Viral Diseases with Human Leukocyte Interferon

Tsunataro Kishida,[2]* Motoharu Kondo,* Toshikazu Yoshikawa,* Naoyuki Matsumura,* Tadashi Sawada,[2]* Tetsuo Hashida,[2]* Akio Matsuo,* and Hiroshi Nitta[3]*

*Departments of Microbiology, Medicine and Pediatrics, [2]*Kyoto Prefectural University of Medicine, Kamikyo-ku, Kyoto 602, [3]*Kyoto Red Cross Blood Center, Kyoto, Japan

INTRODUCTION

Interferon (IFN) has been reported to have high therapeutic efficiency in hepatitis B virus infection and other viral diseases. However, in addition to the need for a large amount of an IFN preparation for clinical use, neither details of the mode of action nor a therapeutic schedule has been established. In this paper, the effect of human leukocyte interferon (HuIFN-α) on 10 adults and 4 children with hepatitis B virus infection is reported.

PATIENTS AND METHODS

Six adults with liver diseases (3 with liver cirrhosis and one each with chronic active hepatitis, chronic inactive hepatitis, and acute hepatitis) and one healthy adult carrier of HB$_s$Ag for over a year received 4 intramuscular injections every week of HuIFN-α, scheduled as 100×10^4 U, 50×10^4 U, 20×10^4 U, and 10×10^4 U (180×10^4 U total). Four children with HB$_s$Ag-positive chronic active hepatitis were given a large dose of HuIFN-α ($1,780 \times 10^4$ U, $3,200 \times 10^4$ U, $5,000 \times 10^4$ U, and $5,395 \times 10^4$ U in total, respectively) daily or weekly.

HuIFN-α was prepared by the method of Matsuo et al.[1] HB$_s$Ag titer was determined in a reversed passive hemagglutination test and radioimmunoassay (Ausria II, Abbott). Anti-HB$_s$ was assayed with radioimmunoassay (Ausab, Abbott). Anti-HB$_c$ was measured in a immune adherence hemagglutination

143

test. HB$_e$ and anti-HB$_e$ were determined with the micro-Ouchterlony method.

RESULTS

HuIFN-α showed a significant effect in case 1, a patient with HB$_s$Ag-positive liver cirrhosis for over 5 years. After the treatment, HB$_s$Ag declined rapidly, disappeared 2 months later, and never returned to positive during 5 months of observation. At the same time, anti-HB$_s$, which was initially negative, appeared gradually, and the serum transaminase also decreased to a normal level (Fig. 1). Case 2 of chronic active hepatitis showed a marked reduction in HB$_s$Ag titer after 4 injections of HuIFN-α, and there was a decrease of serum transaminase during treatment, although anti-HB$_s$ did not appear (Fig. 2).

Among the 10 adults, a constant or transient depression of HB$_s$Ag was observed in 5 cases, as well as a disappearance of HB$_e$Ag in 2 of 3 cases. In the children, HB$_e$Ag in one of 3 cases disappeared, HB$_s$Ag in one of 4 cases was markedly reduced, and all cases showed significant decrease of serum transaminase after IFN treatment.

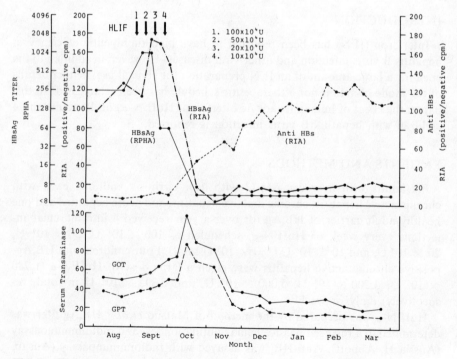

Fig. 1. Clinical course in Case 1.

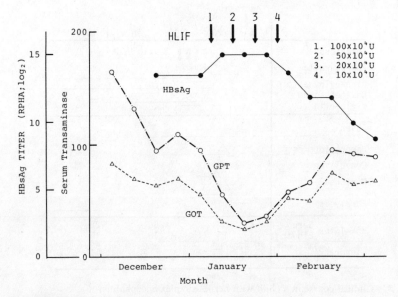

Fig. 2.   Clinical course in Case 2.

In addition to hepatitis, 11-month-old boy with herpes simlex encephalitis was treated by intravenous IFN 229 × 10⁴ U/day for 4 successive days. His clinical diagnosis was made by the rising antibody titer to herpes simplex virus. By the use of IFN, his clinical symptoms showed a rapid improvement as shown in Fig. 3, suggesting that systemic use of IFN may be effective in the treatment of herpes simplex encephalitis.

DISCUSSION

Greenberg et al.[2] administered 0.6 to 17 × 10⁴ U/kg body weight/day of IFN-α intramuscularly to 3 patients with HB$_s$Ag-positive chronic active hepatitis. Desmyter et al.[3] and Kingham et al.[4] gave 10⁷ U and Dolen et al.[5] 10⁶ U per patient per day in similarly documented cases. In all these previous studies, a very large amount of IFN was administered. In our study of children positive in HB$_s$Ag, a marked fall in the titer of HB$_s$Ag and a disappearance of HB$_e$Ag were found in certain cases, also after a large dose of IFN. However, in the study of adults with HB$_s$Ag-positive liver diseases, the effect of a smaller dose of IFN on HB$_s$Ag, HB$_e$Ag, and serum transaminase could be demonstrated. It is concluded that even a smaller doses of IFN can exert an effect on HB$_s$-antigen and HB$_e$-antigen in a short period, and in some cases results in the reduction of HB$_s$-antigen as well as the appearance of HB$_s$-antibody.

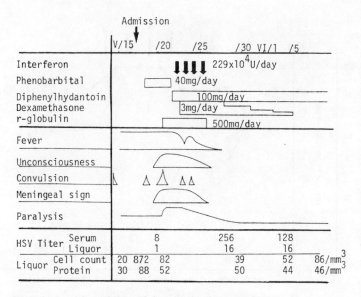

Fig. 3.   Clinical course in a child with herpes simplex encephalitis.

REFERENCES

1. Matsuo, A., Hayashi, S., and Kishida, T.: Production and purification of human leukocyte interferon. *Jap. J. Microbiol.*, **18**: 21–27, 1977.
2. Greenberg, H. B., Pollard, R. B., Lutwick, L. I., Gregory, P. B., Robinson, W. S., and Merigan, T. C.: Effect of human leukocyte interferon on hepatitis B virus infection in patients with chronic active hepatitis. *N. Engl. J. Med.*, **295**: 517–522, 1976.
3. Desmyter, J., Ray, M. B., Degrotte, J., Bradburne, A. F., Desnet, V. J., Edy, V. G., Billiau, A., Desomer, P., and Mortelmans, J.: Administration of human fibroblast interferon in chronic hepatitis-B infection. *Lancet*, **2**: 645–647, 1976.
4. Kingham, J. G. C., Ganguly, N. K., Shaari, Z. D., Mendelson, R., McGuire, M. J., Holgate, S. J., Cartwright, T., Scott, G. M., Richards, B. M., and Wright, R.: Treatment of HBsAg-positive chronic active hepatitis with human fibroblast interferon. *Gut*, **19**: 91–94, 1978.
5. Dolen, J. G., Carter, W. A., Horoszewicz, J. S., Vladutiu, A. O., Leibowitz, A. I., and Nolan, J. P.: Fibroblast interferon treatment of a patient with chronic active hepatitis. *Am. J. Med.*, **67**: 127–131, 1979.

Discussion

Dr. Galasso: I am interested in the encephalitis patients. In the U.S., we have done extensive studies with encephalitis using ara A. And we have come to the conclusion that the only way to properly diagnose herpes encephalitis is by brain biopsy. Was a brain biopsy done? That is the first part of the question. Second part of the question is, even though we have found that ara A to be effective and it is currently licensed against herpes encephalitis, once the patient was unconscious, the prognosis was very bad, and in almost 100% of the cases it was fatal even with ara A. If we are going to discuss herpes encephalitis, we have to be very sure that it is indeed herpes encephalitis, and it is our contention that the only way you can properly diagnose it is by brain biopsy.

Dr. KISHIDA: I agree with your statement, Dr. Galasso, but we feel resistance against conducting a brain biopsy on an 11-month-old baby in Japan. I'd like to know whether there is such resistance in the U.S. The baby was unconscious and we could not do a proper diagnosis. We wanted to save the baby's life at any cost. Because we found that the antibody of herpes virus in the cerebrospinal fluid and the blood circulation has risen and also that CT showed focal symptoms, we concluded that this was herpes encephalitis. But we did not conduct a brain biopsy because the baby was only 11 months old.

Dr. GALASSO: I would agree on the 11 months part. But I do want to clarify one point. When I say brain biopsy, we do not do a brain biopsy and wait until the diagnosis is made. We do a brain biopsy and start treatment immediately. If the brain biopsy is positive we continue. If the brain biopsy is negative, we discontinue.

Dr. BARON: In the treatment of virus diseases with interferon or inducers, I believe we all agree that the interferon administered for therapy must exceed the interferon being produced within the body due to the virus infection. In a case which we studied with Dr. Bellarti at Georgetown University many years ago, a child with herpes encephalitis, we administered poly I: poly C and collected all the specimens to see what the interferon response would be. The child did recover. However, in the spinal fluid, levels of endogenously produced interferon induced by the virus far exceeded any level that we could achieve by the inducer. And so the recovery was probably spontaneous, and the amounts of interferon which we could administer even today would probably not exceed those levels which were induced within the patient. Did you study the level of interferon in the spinal fluid or the blood prior to therapy?

Dr. KISHIDA: No, we did not study it. As you pointed out, many reports say that a considerable amount of interferon is produced in the spinal fluid in case of virus infection of the brain, and I think it is very difficult to administer an amount of interferon which exceeds the endogenously produced amount of interferon. However, some reports say that when interferon is exogenously administered to SSPE patients, their conditions will improve. So I'd like to ask, Dr. Baron, whether you think it is totally meaningless to give interferon exogenously when it cannot exceed the endogenously produced interferon.

Dr. BARON: It is difficult to argue with success. I think, however, that the success must be established in a very well-controlled experiment. Then perhaps the mechanisms of success will be unexpected mechanisms. However, if you achieve true clinical success as demonstrated in the control trial—what do they say, "victory has 1,000 fathers"—then I will join you in applauding.

Dr. KISHIDA: On the other hand, herpes simplex encephalitis is one of viral infections difficult to be treated. At present adenine arabinocide is mainly used under the established diagnosis by brain biopsy, while there is no report treated by HuIFN. In our case presented here, although clinical diagnosis was made by the rising anti-body titer to herpes simplex virus alone, IFN could be given relatively in the early course of disease and resulted in favorable clinical outcome. Thus, systemic administration of IFN might be effective in herpes simplex encephalitis when it is used in the early stage of the disease.

Interferon Treatment of Viral Warts and Some Skin Diseases

Kenichi Uyeno and Akira Ohtsu

Department of Dermatology, Institute of Clinical Medicine, The University of Tsukuba, Sakura-Mura, Ibaraki-Pref., 305, Japan

INTRODUCTION

Several reports of therapeutic attempts to treat viral diseases of the skin such as viral warts and herpes with interferon (IFN) have recently appeared in the literature.[1-18] We have conducted clinical trials of human fibroblast interferon (HuIFN-β) preparations (supplied by Toray Industries, Inc.) for the treatment of patients with viral warts and with malignant or premalignant skin tumors. This report presents the results.

INTERFERON THERAPY FOR VIRAL WARTS

Subjects

Patients with viral diseases of the skin or skin tumors examined at the Outpatient Clinic of the Department of Dermatology, Tsukuba University Hospital, Ibaraki Prefecture, during the period from March 1979 to September 1980 were treated in the study (Table 1).

Drugs

IFN preparations with the following lot numbers and with the potencies indicated in parentheses were used: 78004 (1.0×10^6 U per vial), L002 (0.7×10^6 U), L002 (1.4×10^6 U), L0063 (2.5×10^6 U), L0061 (1×10^6 U), L0083 (3×10^6 U), L0093 (3×10^6 U), and L0103 (3×10^6 U).

These were dissolved in distilled water, physiological saline solution, 0.5% xylocaine solution, or 0.5% procaine solution, as directed for the individual lot number, for local administration. They were used at concentrations of 0.3, 1.0, or 2.5×10^6 U/ml, varying with the patient, but in most cases at 0.3×10^6 U/ml. Finally, 0.5% procaine solution was used as a solvent for all lots throughout the latter portion of the study.

149

Table 1.   Cases of viral warts treated in the study.

Diagnosis	No. of cases studied	No. of lesions treated
Verruca vulgaris (VV)	49	111
Verrucae planae juveniles (VPJ)	8	21
Condyloma acuminatum (CA)	2	2
Molluscum contagiosum (MC)	2	2

Administration

The prepared IFN solutions were stored in a refrigerator at 4° C and used within 3 weeks; hence there was no conspicuous loss in potency during storage.

The solution was injected intratumorally or subtumorally in volumes of 0.05 to 0.1 ml per week. The treatment was generally continued until the wart disappeared.

Therapeutic Results

As can be noted from the data summarized in Table 2, the clinical responses to the IFN therapy were remarkably encouraging. The treatment produced a significant clinical improvement in more than 95 % of the cases of verruca vulgaris (VV) and condyloma acuminatum (CA), and an excellent therapeutic response in the only case of molluscum contagiosum (MC). Patients with verrucae planae juveniles (VPJ) showed a notably lower rate of clinical improvement than those with VV; it may be said that the local IFN therapy is not necessarily apporpriate in cases of VPJ where local injections must be given one after another into a large number of lesions.

Table 2.   Therapeutic results.

	No. of patients	No. of lesions	Clinical response to treatment				Recurrence	Under treatment	Drop-outs
			Excellent	Good	Fair	Poor			
VV	49	111	85	6	2	1	1	13	3
VPJ	8	21	2	1	1		8	6	3
CA	2	2	2						
MC	2	2	1						

Table 3 shows the distribution of frequencies of local IFN injections to the excellent responders. They required an average of 8 injections to achieve a cure.

Patients described a fairly intense pain at the injection site when the drug was administered as a solution in distilled water or physiological saline. With the subsequent use of 0.5 % xylocaine or procaine solution in place of water or saline, the pain at the injection site became substantially reduced to a level nearly comparable to that usually associated with corticosteriod or bleomycin injection, thus posing no particular clinical problem.

Table 3. Distribution of excellent responders (VV) by total number of local IFN doses given per lesion.

No. of injections	1	2	3	4	5	6	7	8	9	10	11	12	13	15	18
No. of lesions		1	7	6	3	4	7	1	13	9	9	6	1	5	3	1

Systemic Effects

Each patient was assessed for routine hematologic and serum biochemical parameters, serum immunoglobulin levels, and so on before and at 2 hours after injection and on the 14th day after initiation of therapy. These examinations did not reveal any significant changes in any of the patients studied (Fig. 1 A-J).

None showed any appreciable rise in plasma IFN titer during this period. We saw no case of systemic clinical manifestations such as fever, arthralgia, or nausea that could be associated with the local IFN injections.

One patient (42 years of age, female, facial VV) developed generalized multiple eruptions, consisting mostly of serous papules and papules and thus resembling lesions of prurigo acuta, after the sixth dose of IFN; these disappeared about 2 weeks afterwards. The eruptions did not recur despite further continuation of the local IFN therapy. It remains unknown whether the episode represented toxic exanthema due to the administration of IFN; further investigation is necessary.

While transient erythematous reactions commonly occur at the site of injection following the local administration of a drug, there were 3 cases in which the skin at the injection site became moderately edematous. Two of these cases had a lesion in the eyebrow region or prepuce, respectively, where a coarse dermis normally lies and is liable to edematization by local injection of a drug. The reactions in these cases, therefore, were considered not to be side-effects of the IFN administration. The third patient had a skin lesion over the malar bone, and was the one who developed the toxic exanthema described above. This episode occurred after one out of 15 local injections; again, significance of the local edematous reaction remains unknown. It may be concluded that no serious adverse reaction which could be associated with the local IFN injection therapy was encountered in the present series.

However, the local injections of IFN were followed in practically all cases by far more pronounced and longer persisting bleeding from the punctured skin than is usual with local injections of other drugs. The reason is under investigation; a possible enhancement of plasmin activity by the introduction of IFN is suspected.

Description of Cases

Figures 2 through 12 provide brief illustrations of representative cases.

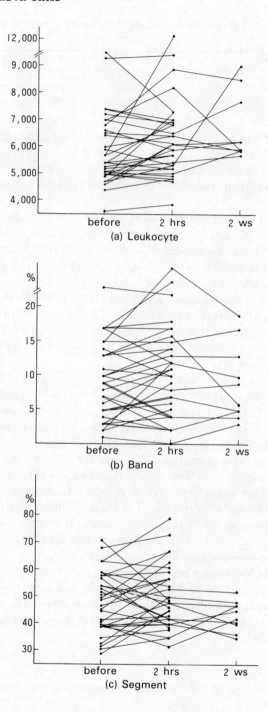

(a) Leukocyte

(b) Band

(c) Segment

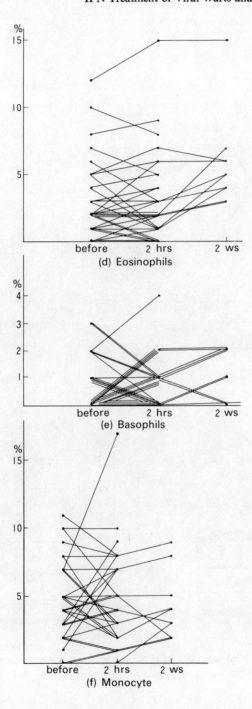

(d) Eosinophils

(e) Basophils

(f) Monocyte

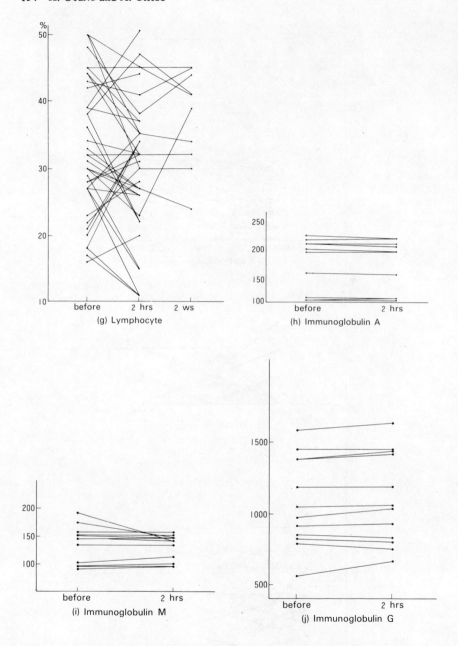

Fig. 1 (a-j).   Effects of local injections of IFN on hemogram and serum immunoglobulin level.

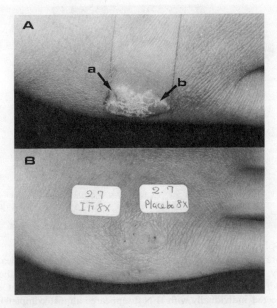

Fig. 2. 19-year-old female with VV.
A: Finding before therapy. Local injections of IFN at *a* and placebo at *b* weekly. B: After the eighth dose. Disappearance of wart is evident at *a* whereas the lesion at *b* remains virtually unchanged.

Comment

The present clinical trial of local IFN injections in patients with viral warts (49 cases of VV, 111 lesions; 8 cases of VPJ, 21 lesions; 2 cases of CA, 2 lesions; and 2 cases of MC, 2 lesions) has demonstrated that the treatment was remarkably effective.

Lesions disappeared after a minimum of one or two local injections or, in a case requiring the longest course of therapy, after as many as 22 doses. Excellent responders required an average of 8 serial weekly injections to achieve a complete cure. This indicates that the local IFN therapy is somewhat inferior to local bleomycin therapy (average number of doses; 3 to 5) or cryosurgery (2 to 4 times) in that it requires a notably greater number of doses.

However, there is no specific treatment for VV and other viral warts at present and effective therapeutic measures vary with the case. The greater the variety of effective therapeutic measures, the more optimistic can we be in treating viral warts under these circumstances. It is of great significance to add to the list local IFN injection therapy, which has proven to be reliably effective, yielding an improvement rate of over 95%, at least for VV.

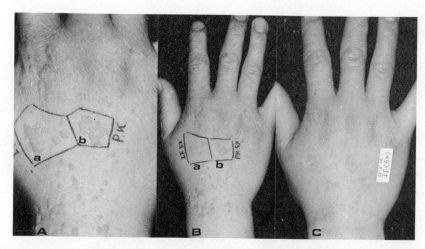

Fig. 3. 30-year-old female with VPJ.
A: Finding before therapy. Local injections of IFN at *a* and physiological saline solution at *b*, respectively, at weekly intervals. B: After the fifth dose. Note the wart at *a* has disappeared, leaving scales, whereas the lesion at *b* remains unchanged. C: Warts over the back of hand injected individually with IFN disappeared almost completely after the fifth dose. The condition recurred subsequently, however, and proved intractable with local IFN injections, IFN ointment, and 5FU ointment.

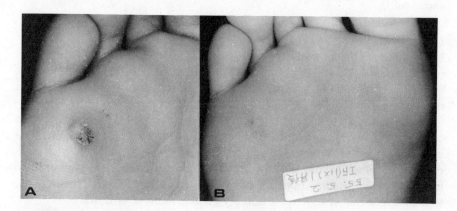

Fig. 4. 19-year-old female with VV.
A: Finding before therapy. Local injection of IFN weekly. B: After the eleventh dose. Completely cured.

The treatment was less efficacious in patients with VJP than in those with VV, as has generally been the rule with other treatments. The local injection therapy for VJP is usually laborious, and the patient himself has to tolerate the

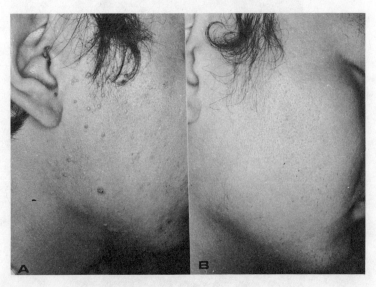

Fig. 5.   20-year-old male with VV.
A: Finding prior to treatment. B: After the fourteenth dose of weekly local IFN injections.
Completely cured.

injection of a dozen to several tens of warts one after another with the drug.
Consequently, dropouts were more frequent in this group and therapeutic
responses slower, as compared to the group of patients with VV. Niimura
et al.[18] reported that treatment with intramuscular IFN injections in doses of
0.3×10^6 U produced a noticeable clinical improvement in occasional cases
of VPJ, and a clinical study to assess the effectiveness of such treatment is
in progress at our clinic.

The local IFN injection therapy was remarkably effective in both cases of CA
in the present series, although the data from such a small number of cases does
not permit any conclusions.

It has been generally agreed that there is no definitive treatment for MC except for removal of lesions by means of trachoma forceps. Cryosurgery with
liquid nitrogen has recently become recognized as an effective measure, but it
does not invariably provide sufficient clinical benefit. One patient with CM
treated with IFN injections into 3 lesions showed a favorable therapeutic response. However, this local injection therapy may not always be advisable for
the treatment of patients with this disease who, in many instances, are infants.

In summary, the results have demonstrated that local IFN injections in
viral warts, especially in VV, are remarkably effective.

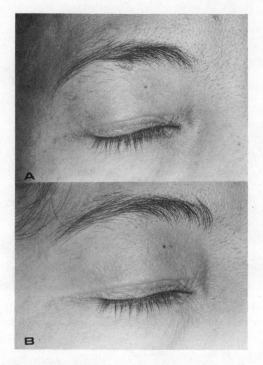

Fig. 6.   49-year-old female with VV.
A: Before treatment. IFN was injected locally at weekly intervals. B: After the ninth dose of IFN.

A complete cure was accomplished after 9 weekly injections of IFN (Lot No. 78004 on one occasion, Lot No. L002 on 4 occasions, and Lot No. L0063 on 4). On a total of 4 occasions with Lot Nos. L002 and L0063, the patient experienced right upper palpebral edematous swelling following injection, the episode occurring singly or consecutively. Skin tests with IFN solutions revealed no significant difference in immediate type reaction from the control, and the patient said a small induration at the injection site persisted for about 3 days.

EFFECTS IN OTHER DISEASES OF THE SKIN

It is natural for the clinician to cherish a desire to apply the antitumor activity of IFN clinically. In the course of treating viral warts by local IFN injections, we decided to try the drug in cases of skin tumors on the assumption that intralesional injection of the substance might be efficacious. As these trials are still at the pilot study stage, cases we have treated will be described only briefly.

Cutaneous Metastases of Malignant Melanoma (acral lentiginous melanoma)

An 80-year-old man had developed patches of skin pigmentation in the area

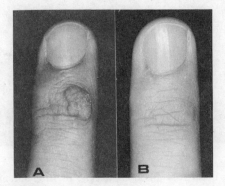

Fig. 7. 20-year-old female with VV.
A: Before treatment. IFN was injected locally at weekly intervals. B: After the eleventh dose.

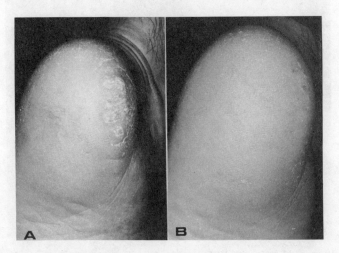

Fig. 8. 36-year-old male with VV.
A: Before treatment. Local IFN injections weekly. Marked cornification occasionally hindered the insertion of an injection needle, requiring application of 50% salicylic acid ointment for softening prior to local injection. B: Finding after the tenth dose.

extending from the instep to the sole of the right foot when he was 31 years of age, and 3 years ago he noticed black-colored masses growing over the right leg and thigh. The tumors recurred after surgical removal. The patient had 8 metastatic skin lesions, which were injected individually with 0.1 to 2.0×10^6 units of IFN 3 times a week. Each lesion received a total of 5 to 13 doses, and all skin tumors were totally resected 10 to 25 days after the final injection and examined

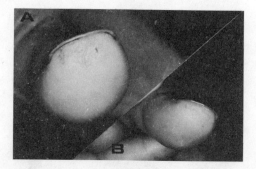

Fig. 9.   36-year-old male with subungual VV.
A: Before treatment. Local IFN injections weekly. B: After the ninth dose. Completely cured.

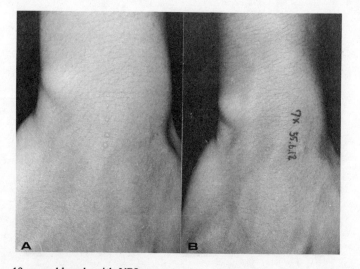

Fig. 10.   19-year-old male with VPJ.
A: Before treatment. IFN was injected locally at weekly intervals. B: After 6 local injections. The lesion has almost completely disappeared.

microscopically. Peritumoral lymphocytic infiltration and degeneration of tumor cells were prominent in 7 of the 8 lesions, whereas in the other lesion which was resected at 9 weeks after therapy, melanophages, alone were sporadically seen with no microscopic evidence of tumor cells.

Skin Metastasis of Gastric Cancer
A 65-year-old woman had a number of hen's egg-sized metastatic skin lesions

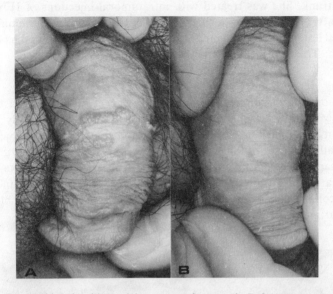

Fig. 11. 40-year-old male with condyloma accuminatum. A: Before treatment. Local IFN injections weekly. B: After 22 local injections. Note that the lesion has disappeared.

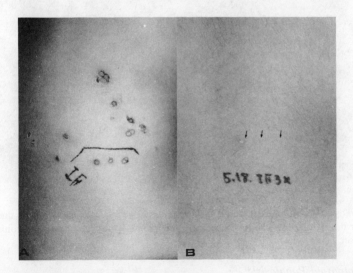

Fig. 12. 6-year-old boy with molluscum contagiosum.
A: Finding before therapy. The lesions had superficial encrustment due to the previous use of a domestic medicament (corrosive?). Three lesions were injected with IFN twice weekly, and the rest of the lesions removed with trachoma forceps.

over the trunk. She was treated with intratumoral injections of IFN weekly but died after having received the third dose. Histopathologic examination of the treated lesions disclosed a modest lymphocytic infiltration in the peritumoral region. The treatment was practically ineffective in this case.

Carcinoma Erysipelatodes (skin metastasis of breast cancer)

Nine months after surgical treatment of a cancer in the left breast of a 43-year-old woman, an erythema the size of a hen's egg with slightly palpable infiltration developed in the left precordial region. IFN was injected intratumorally in doses of 0.4×10^6 units twice a week, and the erythematous lesion disappeared almost completely after 8 doses. Histologic examination revealed a complete disappearance of tumor cells with swollen and homogeneous collagen fibers and lymphohistiocytic infiltrations around blood vessels, sweat glands, and piloerector muscles (Fig. 13).

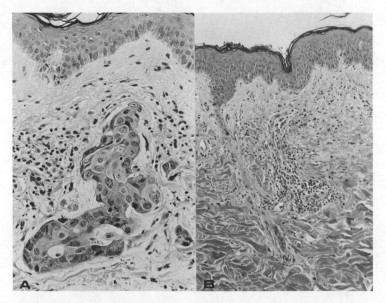

Fig. 13. 43-year-old woman with carcinoma erysipelatodes.
A: Histologic finding before therapy. Nests of metastatic adenocarcinoma cells in the dermis.
B: After the eighth dose. Disappearence of tumor cell nests. Perivascular lymphohistiocytic infiltration.

Lymphomatoid Papulosis[19]

A 28-year-old man had been suffering from episodic development of prurigo-like papules over all areas of his body except the face, palms, and soles during the previous 3 years. He was treated with weekly local injections of 0.1×10^6

units of IFN into the lesions. Each lesion received one to 8 doses in all. Following the treatment, there was microscopic evidence of complete disappearance of atypical lymphoid cells with perivascular lymphohistiocytic infiltration.

Porokeratosis Mibelli

A 76-year-old man with erythrodermia developed approximately 10 lesions of porokeratosis over his trunk and extremities. Injections of 0.1 to 0.3 × 10⁶ units of IFN were administered into each of 6 lesions daily or every other day; each lesion received a total of 8 doses. In four of 5 lesions examined on biopsy, the cornoid lamella and the underlying atypical keratinocytes were found to have disappeared and lymphohistiocytic infiltrations were seen perivascularly (Fig. 14). The cornoid lamella was still present in the other lesion examined. The findings in this case suggested that the administration of IFN

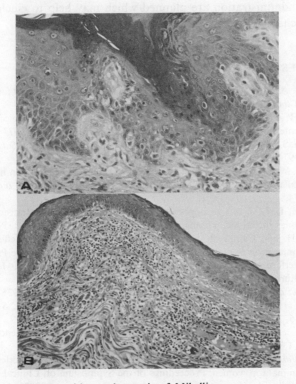

Fig. 14. 76-year-old man with porokeratosis of Mibelli.
A: Histologic finding before therapy. c: cornoid lamella; a: atypical keratinocytes. B: After the eighth dose. Disappearance of cornoid lamella and dyskeratotic cells. Perivascular lymphohistiocytic infiltration.

might prevent the lesions of porokeratosis from progressing into squamous cell carcinoma.

Cutaneous T-cell Lymphoma

About a year ago, eczema-like eruptions appeared on the trunk of a 42-year-old woman and thereafter became gradually enlarged. The lesions were characterized histologically by patchy infiltrations with atypical lymphoid cells. The patient was injected with 0.1 to 0.2×10^6 units intralesionally at weekly intervals. After a total of 8 doses the exanthema exhibited a trend to regressive retraction and, 2 months later, almost completely disappeared. Afterwards, she developed enlarged lymph nodes with a histologic diagnosis of Hodgkin-pattern lymphoma, which prompted treatment with 3×10^6 units of IFN by intravenous drip daily.

Local IFN injection therapy was reasonably effective in these cases of malignant or premalignant skin tumors. Further studies with modifications in dosage and administration are planned which may help to elucidate the underlying mechanisms of antitumor actions.

REFERENCES

1. Stevens, D. A. and Merigan, T. C.: Interferon, antibody and other host factors in herpes zoster. *J. Clin. Invest.*, **51**: 1170–1178, 1967.
2. Strander, H. *et al.*: Clinical and laboratory investigation on man, Systemic administration of potent interferon to man. *J. Natl. Cancer Institute,* **51**: 733–742, 1973
3. Sotomatsu, S. *et al.*: Interferon treatment of viral diseases of the skin. *Saishin-Igaku*, **24**: 726–729, 1974 (in Japanese).
4. Jordan, G. W. *et al.*: Administration of human leukocyte interferon in herpes zoster, I Study, circulating antiviral activity and host responses to infection. *J. Infect. Dis.*, **130**: 56–62, 1974.
5. Rasmussen, L. E. *et al.*: Lymphocyte interferon production and transformation after herpes simplex infections in human. *J. Immun.*, **112**: 728–736, 1974.
6. Strander, H. and Cantell, K.: Studies on antivaral and antitumor effects of human leukocyte interferon *in vitro* and *in vivo*. In: Waymouth, C. (ed); The Production and Use of Interferon for the Treatment and Prevention of Human Virus Infections, The Tissue Culture Assoc., 1974, pp. 49–56.
7. Ueda, K. *et al.*: Anti-viral drugs—Interferon—. *Hifu*, **17**: 310–319, 1975 (in Japanese).
8. Emödi, G. *et al.*: Human interferon therapy for herpes zoster in adullts. *Scand. J. Infect. Dis.*, **7**: 1–5, 1975.
9. Kobza, K. *et al.*: Treatment of herpes infection with human exogenous interferon. *Lancet*, **1**: 1343–1344, 1975.
10. Ikić, D. *et al.*: Preliminary study of the effect of human leukocyte interferon on condyloma accuminata in women. Proceedings of the Symposium on Clinical Uses of Interferon. Yugoslav Academy of Sciences and Arts, Zagreb, pp. 223–227, 1975.
11. Ikić, D. *et al.*: Double-blind clinical study with human leukocyte interferon in therap yof condylomata accuminata. *Ibid.*, pp. 229–233, 1975.

12. Merigan, T. C. *et al.*: Clinical experiences with human interferon application in man. Presented at Fifth Aharon Katzir-Katchalsky Conference, Rehovot, Israel, 1977.
13. Merigan, T. C. *et al.*: Human leukocyte interferon for the treatment of herpes zoster in patients with ceacer. *New Engl. J. Med.*, **298**: 981–987, 1978.
14. Scott, G. M. and Csonka, G. W.: Effect of injection of small doses of human fibroblast interferon into genital warts. A pilot study. *Brit. J. Verer. Dis.*, **55**: 442–445, 1979.
15. Pazin, G. J. *et al.*: Prevention of reactivated herpes simplex infection by human leukocyte interferon after operation on the trigeminal root. *New Engl. J. Med.*, **301**: 225–230, 1979.
16. Uyeno, K.: Clinical use of interferon in dermatological field. *Nihon-Iji-Shimpo*, **2994**: 25–30, 1981 (in Japanese).
17. Uyeno, K. and Ohtsu, A.: Treatment of viral warts with human fibroblast interferon. Presented at the 44th East Japan Dermatological Society, October 1980.
18. Niimura, M. and Uyeno, K.: Clinical application of human β-IFN for viral wart treatment for Cancer, October, 1981.
19. Ohtsu, A. and Uyeno, K.: Treatment of lymphomatoid papulosis with human fibroblast interferon. Presented at the 31st Middle Japan Dermatological Society, August 1980.

Discussion

Dr. ISHIHARA: You have obtained a very good efficacy against warts. I'd like to ask three questions concerning warts. First, have you observed any difference in efficacy of treatment between old and new lesions? Second, the local administration of bleomycin to warts near the finger nail is likely to produce deformation of the nail. Have you observed the same phenomenon with local administration of interferon? Third, for melanoma, we locally administer interferon at a high concentration—that is, 3 million units dissolved with 1ml. Could you kindly tell us what is the optimal concentration of interferon?

Dr. UYENO: For the first question, I do not have specific statistics to answer this question, but as I showed you previously, we observed about 100 lesions, and we did not see much difference between old and new lesions. As for the second question, we have also repeatedly administered bleomycin to warts near the fingernails, but we did not observe deformation of the nail. Deformation was produced by the administration of 5 FU ointment, but not by bleomycin or interferon. As for the third question, we have tried a number of concentrations, although I did not show you the list. Finally we selected the concentration of 300,000 units per ml for common warts.

Results of Clinical Trials with Human Fibroblast Interferon (HuIFN-β)

Dietrich NIETHAMMER, Jörn TREUNER, and Günther DANNECKER

Division of Hematology, Department of Pediatrics, University of Tübingen, Tübingen, Germany

INTRODUCTION

Despite the worldwide publicity interferon has gained recently as an anti-tumor drug, there is very little known as yet of its real value. Strander *et al.* have introduced leukocyte interferon (IFN-α) into clinical use as an adjuvant therapy in osteogenic sarcoma.[1] The same IFN is used in most clinical trials by other groups. Only few reports have been published that describe the use of fibroblast-derived interferon (IFN-β).[2-5] The two types of IFNs differ both in structure and in antigenicity. At present IFN-β is the only IFN available in Germany for clinical use. This report will review the pharmacokinetic studies and clinical results obtained so far with this IFN.

INTERFERON

The IFN-β used in Germany was prepared in Germany from human fibroblast cultures by Rentschler Co., Laupheim (supported by the German Ministry for Research and Technology). The interferon was purified and stored in a lyophilized form at $-4°C$. The specific activity was $1-2 \times 10^6$ IU/mg protein. It was dissolved in physiological saline immediately before injection. Serum collected for the determination of plasma levels was immediately frozen and stored at $-70°C$ until use. IFN concentrations were determined by two different cytopathic effect inhibition assays.[6,7] The IFN-α given to a few patients was a gift from Dr. K. Cantell, Helsinki, and Dr. H. Strander, Stockholm. This IFN was administered intramuscularly.

Supported by the Deutsche Forschungsgemeinschaft (Forschergruppe Leukämieforschung, Projekt C3/4), Federal Ministry of Research and Technology, and Dr. Rentschler Co., Laupheim, Germany.

In general, 1×10^6 IU/10 kg body weight IFN-β were given in children and 6×10^6 IU in adults over 30 min by intravenous infusion. The highest dose used was 10.8×10^6 IU in a boy weighing about 40 kg ($= .27 \times 10^6$ IU/kg body weight).

PHARMACOKINETIC STUDIES

The first problem was to determine the best route of administration of IFN-β. Table 1 summarizes the data obtained in one patient when serum concentrations were measured after different routes of injection. In contrast to IFN-α, detectable serum levels could only be achieved after intravenous (I.V.) injection. These data confirm observations in animals that no serum levels are found when IFN-β is injected intramuscularly (I.M.) and that it can only be traced for a short time in the serum when given I.V.[8] It can be seen that, after I.V. push injections, measurable IFN concentrations were only detectable after 45 min. This time can only be prolonged by I.V. infusions.[9,10] This is in contrast to the results obtained with IFN-α which produces long-lasting serum levels after I.M. injection. An increase in the dose led to higher peaks, and a clear linear relationship could be established between the achieved peak levels and the body weight of the patients.[10]

Table 1.   Serum interferon levels after different routes of administration of 0.1×10^6 IU/kg body weight (IU/ml).

Time (min)	Route of administration		
	Subcutaneous	Intramuscular	Intravenous
5	n.d.	n.d.	128
10	0	0	96
15	n.d.	n.d.	32
30	0	0	24
45	n.d.	n.d.	12
60	0	0	0
120	0	0	n.d.
360	0	0	n.d.

n.d.: not done

It was concluded from these observation that short-term infusions over 30 min seemed to be the best compromise between duration of measurable IFN levels and the peak values achieved in the serum.

Regular controls of the serum levels were performed in most patients. In one boy, serum levels could no longer be detected after 5 months of treatment with IFN-β. Further investigations showed that this patient had developed antibodies (IgG) against IFN-β,[11] 50 μl of his serum neutralized up to 10^4 IU IFN-β, whereas the antiviral activity of IFN-α was not inhibited at all. This was the first observation of homologous antibodies against IFN and of the development of antibodies in a human. It was shown previously by others that human IFN-α and IFN-β have different antigenic properties and that antibodies induced in animals against IFN-β do not react with IFN-α.[12] No such antibodies have been detected by us in other patients.

SIDE-EFFECTS

A test dose of 1×10^5 IU was given subcutaneously on the first day. If no marked skin or general reaction was seen, 5×10^5 or 1×10^6 IU were administered I.V. If this dosage was tolerated, the patient received the full dose. Fever, chills, and, occasionally, shaking chills were common side-effects at the beginning of treatment but they soon lessened and frequently disappeared after the first week. It could be suppressed in most cases by the administration of aspirin or paracetamol 30 min before the start of the infusion.

Only a slight decrease of thrombocyte and/or leukocyte values was seen in a few patients, but no changes of other laboratory parameters were observed. General fatigue was more frequently observed in adult patients than in children. IFN-α seemed to induce longer lasting periods of fatigue than IFN-β. In only one child the use of IFN-β had to be stopped because of severe shaking chills and depression of the blood pressure. In another child, both types of IFN were injected directly into the ventricle system by the means of an Omaja shunt. In this case the fatigue was pronounced but disappeared when the IFN therapy was stopped.

ANTITUMOR STUDIES

Nasopharyngeal Carcinoma

Nasopharyngeal carcinoma (NPC) is a rare tumor in children in all parts of the world. It is a common cause of death in adult males coming from southern China. In Taiwan, it is the leading cancer cause of death.[13] Following the first successful treatment of a patient with this Epstein-Barr virus-related tumor,[9] we have treated 5 other children with NPC. The results have been reported elsewhere.[14]

Table 2 summarizes the data from these 6 children. All patients were between 9 and 14 years of age at the time of initial diagnosis. Involvement of the cervical lymph nodes was observed in 5 of them at that time. Four patients had received extensive radio- and chemotherapy. One child was treated only for a short time before leaving the hospital. When he returned after 3 months, multiple bone lesions were detected. One patient received IFN as an initial treatment, but it was stopped after 9 days because of severe side-effects and because of rapid progression of the tumor. This case is therefore not evaluable. One

Table 2. Summary of 6 children with nasopharyngeal carcinoma treated with IFN-β.

Case	Age (years)	Localiation at onset cervical lymph nodes	Metastases	No. of relapses	Previous therapy	Time of onset to IFN-therapy (years)	Location before IFN treatment	Duration of IFN therapy (days)	Evaluation
1	11	+	–	2	Rad.,[a] chem.[b]	6.0	Local, right sinuses, right orbita, retina, brain	237	Complete remission for 12+ months; 8+ months without IFN therapy
2	12	+	–	1	Rad.; chem.	1.5	Local, right sinuses, right orbita, left humerus	308	Halt of the rapidly growing tumor for months. Rapid progression after end of IFN-therapy
3	14	+	right sphenoid sinus	2	Rad.; some chem.	2.4	Local, pulmonary metastases in both lungs	49	Rapid progression and death
4	11	–	–	1	Some chem.	0.75	Local, multiple bone lesions	46	No therapy over 3 months after some initial chemotherapy; rapid progression; died in spite of chemotherapy after IFN therapy
5	14	+	right hilus	–	–	–	Same	9	Initial treatment stopped after 9 days because of side-effects. Only partial regression after chemotherapy and radiation
6	9	+	–	2	Rad.; chem.	3.0	Local, right sinuses, brain	135	Stop of tumor growth for over 4+ months

a) Rad.: radiation therapy,   b) Chem.: Chemotherapy.

patient had a complete remission of the tumor which had already penetrated all the sinuses and the orbita of the right side as well as the brain during the second relapse.[9] In 2 other patients the rapid growth of their tumors was stopped for 4 and 8 months, respectively. In the latter patient an increase in the dose and treatment with IFN-α did not change the behavior of the tumor. Table 3 summarizes the modes of treatment in this patient. The tumor resumed its initial rapid growth a week after the IFN therapy was stopped. No effect could be observed in the 2 children with extensive metastatic lesions. In summary one can say that therapy with IFN-β was effective in 3 out of 5 evaluable patients. All children had high titers against the Epstein-Barr virus and they had relapsed at least once before. It is impossible to say whether the positive effects were induced by the antiviral activity of IFN or were due to its antiproliferative or immunoregulatory function.

Table 3. IFN doses given to one patient with NPC (weight, 40.0 kg). Tumor growth was stopped throughout the treatment but regression could not be induced. In addition, IFN was injected twice into the right maxillary sinus (6.0×10^6 IU IFN-α, 5.2×10^6 IU IFN-β).

Dose (IU) $\times 10^6$	Type of IFN	Schedule	Duration (days)
2.7	IFN-β	Daily	5
5.4	IFN-β	Daily	34
10.8	IFN-β	Daily	28
10.8	IFN-β	Every 2nd day	31
6.0	IFN-α	Daily	12
3.0	IFN-α	Daily	21
6.0	IFN-β ⎫	Daily	17
+3.0	IFN-α ⎭		
6.0	IFN-β	3x/week	160

Laryngeal Papilloma and Multiple Myeloma

It has been shown that juvenile laryngeal paillomas respond well to IFN-α, but that they come back when IFN therapy is stopped.[15] A positive response in about half of the patients has been observed in multiple myeloma who were also treated with IFN-α.[16] We wanted to see whether IFN-β could induce a similar response. Together with H. Strander and K. Cantell we developed a therapeutic regimen which allowed us to determine whether a failure of treatment with IFN-β was due to the unresponsiveness of this kind of tumor to this type of interferon or due to the special patient (Fig. 1).

Figure 2 summarizes the results obtained in 2 patients with laryngeal papilloma in whom no response could be induced with IFN-β. On the other hand, a clear dose-dependent responsiveness was observed to IFN-α.[17] It seems that IFN-β is of no use in laryngeal papilloma. Nevertheless, it yet remains to be seen whether the dose of IFN-β was too low. It has been reported from Israel

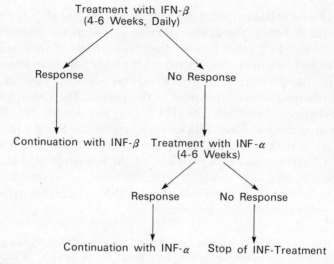

Fig. 1.   Strategy for comparing the clinical effectiveness of the two different IFNs.

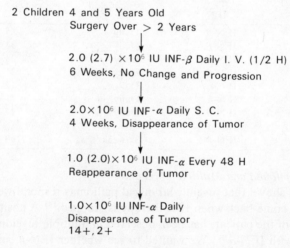

Fig. 2.   Results of treatment of two children with laryngeal papilloma.[17]

that IFN-β can induce a response in this virusrelated tumor when higher doses are used.[18]

Treatment of patients with multiple myeloma led to the following results. The first patient did not respond to either IFN-β to IFN-α. The second patient had a clear-cut positive response to IFN-β, as judged by the disappearance of fever and pain as well as by a decrease of paraproteinemia to far less than 50% of the initial value.

Ongoing Trials in Germany with IFN-β

Several clinical trials have been started in Germany during the last 12 months. They are summarized in Table 4. None of the trials have progressed far enough that clinical results can be evaluated. In stage IV neuroblastoma and osteogenic sarcoma, the patients received chemotherapy and were randomized for additional treatment with IFN. In the trial for gastric cancer, the patients were randomized (IFN treatment alone or no therapy) after the tumor had been resected totally. In low-grade malignant lymphoma, all patients were closely observed for a positive response. The resulting myelomas were described above. A study on nasopharyngeal carcinoma in adults was in the planning phase at the time of this conference.

Table 4. Ongoing trials in Germany using IFN-β as an antineoplastic agent.

Tumor	Randomized	with chemotherapy
Neuroblastoma, Stage IV (children; 1 year)	+	+
Osteogenic sarcoma	+	+
Gastric cancer	+	−
Malignant lymphoma (low grade)	−	−
Myeloma	−	−

Other Tumors Treated with IFN-β

A few patients have been treated with IFN-β in pilot studies (Table 5). They were all patients with end-stage malignant diseases. Most of them had received intensive chemotherapy and/or radiation, and IFN was used as the last possibility. With the exception of one patient with spindle cell sarcoma, who showed a partial response, there was no clear evidence of the effectiveness of IFN-β treatment. This may be related to various causes; (1) end-stage malignomas

Table 5. Other patients with malignant diseases treated with IFN-β.

Tumor	Hospital
Spindle cell sarcoma	Tübingen
CML, blast crisis	Tübingen
Acute lymphatic leukemia child with meningiosis (I. Th. application)	Tübingen
Acute lymphatic leukemia (adult patient)	Dr. Niederle, Essen
Neuroblastoma, Stage IV (relapse)	Tübingen
Colon carcinoma	Dr. Niederle, Essen
Osteogenic sarcoma (2 patients with metastatic lesions)	Dr. Gaedicke, Ulm
Carcinoid (liver involvement)	Dr. Diehl, Hanover
Malignant melanoma	Dr. Riethmüller, Munich
Astrocytoma (intratumerous)	Dr. Mundinger, Freiburg

are certainly a bad choice for a trial of a new therapeutical mode, (2) IFN-β might not be the right IFN in these tumors, or (3) the dosage was too low. In addition, there is more and more evidence that (as in myeloma or nasopharyngeal carcinoma), in a group of patients with the same tumor, not all of them respond to treatment with IFN.

Viral Diseases

Table 6 summarizes the results in viral diseases using IFN-β as an antiviral agent. The results in laryngeal papilloma have already been described. No response was seen in the 2 patients with cytomegalovirus (CMV) infection, which confirms observations by others. The patient with condyloma urethrae had been operated on frequently and the recurrence of condyloma was halted by IFN-β. In one case of a generalized herpes zoster infection after a bone marrow transplant, pneumonia and further spread of the diseases had developed in spite of treatment with adenosine arabinoside (ARA-A). One day after initiation of the IFN treatment, nor more new skin lesions were observed and the pneumonia cleared in a few days.

Table 6. Patients with viral diseases treated with IFN-β.

Disease	No.	Author	Outcome
Laryngeal papilloma	2	Göbel *et al.*[17]	No response to IFN-β; clear response to IFN-α
	1	Tübingen	No response to IFN-β
Condyloma urethrae	1	Dr. Ackermann, Würzburg	response
CMV, chorioretinitis	1	Tübingen	No response
CMV, newborn	1	Tübingen	No response
Generalized herpes zoster with pneumonia	1	Dr. Wilms, Tübingen	Development of pneumonia with Ara-A alone; rapid response in combination with Ara-A
Chronic hepatitis	9	Müller *et al.*[19]	One response

In a controlled multicenter trial, 9 patients with chronic active hepatitis B were treated with IFN-β and the results were compared with the same number of untreated controls. In one patient of the IFN group, HBV-markers (HB$_s$Ag, HB$_e$Ag, DNAP) in the serum and liver were no longer detectable. Disappearance of the markers was followed by a marked clinical, biochemical, and histologic improvement which included normalization of liver enzyme activities and IgG levels. How much of this change was due to a positive effect of IFN-β in this disease cannot be said. No improvement occurred in the other patients.

CONCLUSION

The value of IFN as an antitumor and anti-infectious drug cannot be assessed at the present time. Our results with IFN-β nevertheless suggest that IFN can be of great help in some patients. The future will have to show which role IFN will play in clinical use. Numerous questions will have to be answered before we have a clear idea, such as;

Which tumors or infectious diseases respond to IFN?

Are there differences in the response among patients with the same tumor?

Are there differences in action between the IFNs of various sources?

Which doses do we have to use?

Which time schedule should be used?

How long does it take to see a response to IFN therapy?

What is the value of a combination of chemotherapy and IFN?

What is the action of IFN?

Is there a possibility that IFN has negative side-effects?

Is there the possibility that IFN has a tumor-enhancing effect?

REFERENCES

1. Strander, H., Cantell, K., Carlstrom, G., and Jakobsson, P. A.: Clinical and laboratory investigations on man: Systemic administration of potent interferon to man. *J. Natl. Cancer Inst.*, **51**: 733, 1973.
2. Horoszewicz, J. S., Leong, S. S., Ito, M., Buffet, R., Karakousis, C., Holyoke, E., Job, I., Dolan, J., and Carter, W. A.: Human fibroblast interferon in human neoplasia: Clinical and laboratory study. *Cancer Treat. Rpt.*, **11**: 62, 1899, 1978.
3. Nemoto, T., Carter, W. A., Dolen, J., and Holyoke, D., Horoszewicz, J. S.: Human interferons and interlesional therapy of melanoma and breast carcinoma. *Am. Soc. Cancer Res.*, **20**: 246, 1979.
4. McPherson, T. A. and Tan, Y. H.: Phase-I pharmaraxicology study of human fibroblast interferon in human cancers. *J. Natl. Cancer Inst.*, **65**:75, 1980.
5. Dunnick, J. K. and Galasso, G. J.: Clinical trials with exogenous interferon: Summary of a meeting. *J. Inf. Dis.*, **139**: 109, 1979.
6. Wagner, R. R.: Biological studies of interferon suppression of cellular infection with eastern equine encephalomyelitis virus. *Virology*, **13**: 323–327, 1961.
7. Dake, H. and Degre, M.: A micro assay for mouse and human interferon. *Acta. Path. Mikrobiol. Scand.*, **380**: 863–870, 1972.
8. Hanley, D. F., Wiranowska-Stewart, M., and Stewart, W. E.: II, Pharmacology of interferons. I. Pharmacological distinctions between human leukocyte and fibroblast interferons. *Internat. J. Immunopharmac.*, **1**: 219–226, 1979.
9. Treuner, J., Niethammer, D., Dannecker, G., Hagmann, R., Neef, V., and Hofschneider, P. H.: Successful treatment of nasopharyngeal carcinoma with interferon. *Lancet*, **1**: 817–818, 1980.
10. Treuner, J., Dannecker, G., Joester, K.-E., Hettinger, A., and Niethammer, D.: Pharmacological aspects of clinical stage I/II trials with human beta interferon. *J. Interferon Research*, **1**: 373–380, 1981.

11. Vallbracht, A., Treuner, J., Flehmig, B., Joester, K. E., and Niethammer, D.: Interferon neutralizing antibodies in a patient after treatment with human fibroblast-interferon. *Nature*, **289**: 469–497, 1981.
12. Vilček, J., Havell, E. A., and Yamazaki, S.: Antigenic, physiochemical and biologic characterization of human interferons. *Ann. N. Y. Acad. Sci.*, **284**: 703, 1977.
13. Müller, D., Goldman, J. M., and Gooman, M. L.: Etiologic studies of nasopharyngeal cancer. *Arch. Otolaryngol.*, **94**: 104, 1971.
14. Treuner, J., Niethammer, D., Dannecker, G., Jobke, A., Aldenhoff, P., Kremens, B., Nessler, G., and Börner, H.: Treatment of nasopharyngeal carcinoma in children with fibroblast interferon. In: Nasopharyngeal Carcinoma (Eds.: E. Grundmann, C. R. F. Krueger, D. V. Ablashi). *Cancer Campaign*, **5**: 309–316, Fischer Verlag Stuttgart, New York, 1981.
15. Haglund, S., Lundquist, P. G., Cantell, K., and Strander, H.: Interferon therapy in juvenile laryngeal papillomatosis. *Arch. Otolaryngol.* (in press).
16. Strander, H.: Interferon therapy in myelomatosis. *Lancet*, **2**: 245, 1979.
17. Göbel, U., Arnold, W., Wahn, V., Treuner, J., and Cantell, K.: Comparison of human fibroblast interferon and leukocyte interferon in the treatment of severe laryngeal papillomatosis in children. *Eur. J. Pediatr.*, **137**: 175–176, 1981.
18. Revel, M.: Reported during First Ann. Int. Cong. Interferon Research. Washington, D. C., November 1980.
19. Müller, R., Vido, I., Schmidt, F. W., Deinhardt, F., Fransne, G., Siegert, W., and Hofschneider, H. P.: Long-term treatment with human fibroblast interferon (INF-β) in chronic active hepatitis B: Preliminary data of a controlled trial. (Submitted for publication).

Discussion

Dr. Ogawa: Since we are using the same type of interferon and also since we could not escalate doses enough to make bone marrow suppression, I would like to ask your opinion concerning the optimal dose of fibroblast interferon for clinical phase II trials.

Dr. Niethammer: We don't know yet what will be the optimal dose. I think we have to continue, and as I showed you in one case with nasopharyngeal carcinoma, we increased the dose to 10 million units and we didn't see any regression of tumor. One of our problems in clinical trials is that even if we don't have a response in a trial, it might be necessary to repeat the trial with different doses. It might even be necessary to use fibroblast interferon twice a day.

Dr. Yamazaki: Your report on the possibility of antibody to human interferon being formed is quite shocking. In the interferon study group in Japan, we studied sera from the patients before and during the treatment to see if there is any inhibitor sera from the patients before and during the treatment to see if there is any inhibitor to fibroblast interferon. With the exception of one patient, we did not see any inhibitor formation. In this particular case, the anti-interferon inhibitor activity was already seen in the serum before the interferon administration. As I missed this point, I'd like to ask Dr. Niethammer how many cases were there in which antibody to fibroblast interferon was formed. Also, it is quite difficult to suppose that only intravenous administration produces the antibody. What was the protein content of the interferon that you used when antibody was produced?

Dr. NIETHAMMER: Well, we have treated about 35 patients. We have probably checked about 25 of them for antibody production. And only one patient, whom I have shown, apparently produced antibody. This is very curious: it was exactly the patient with the complete response in nasopharyngeal carcinoma. So he has had clearcut antibody since almost a year ago, and the tumor has not come back. I really do not know why this child produced antibody. There are a lot of possibilities to explain the cause of the antibody production. First of all, this patient had quite extensive injections subcutaneously and intramuscularly to begin with. Some of the studies which I showed had been done with this patient. Then he had 4 weeks of regular daily treatment intravenously. So from that point on, he was not different from the other patients. Of course you can speculate a lot; he might be genetically different. One thing which always comes to my mind is when you look at the history of production of growth hormone, there have been some patients who got very crude human growth hormone and produced antibody against growth hormone. It might be the impurities that helped to induce the antibody; this is supported by Paucker's data and animal data. When you first give crude interferon and then boost with cleaner interferon, you get much higher antibody titer in animals than if you just use pure interferon.

Dr. BARON: Has the child with antibody to fibroblast interferon had any viral infections? How were the viral infections handled by the child and what type of interferon was produced?

Dr. NIETHAMMER: I think that's a very good question. He had two episodes of viral infections; just a common cold. We checked the interferon levels: during one episode he had 80 I.U. of interferon in his plasma, and it was leukocyte interferon. So he was still able to produce leukocyte interferon, and the antibody still did not react with leukocyte interferon.

Dr. BARON: The colds were not unusually prolonged, were they? They were of normal duration?

Dr. NIETHAMMER: Yes, they were of normal duration. There was no evidence of increase of viral infection.

Dr. EZAKI: Did you see any correlation between NK activity and clinical course of the patients after the FIF treatment?

Dr. NIETHAMMER: No. In all patients that we have checked, NK activity goes up very high, to the highest level you can get, so I don't think you can correlate it to the clinical effect.

Dr. EZAKI: So, do you suggest checking any immunological parameter in patients with FIF treatment?

Dr. NIETHAMMER: As far as we know, we don't have any good immunological parameters. Only in myeloma, of course, when, you can see the protein go down. But that's the only thing I know.

Dr. MERIGAN: Weissman has demonstrated and speculated about a single amino acid change in one of his α types of interferon which he has derived from an embryo. He demonstrated a single amino acid producing base change in one of the genes.

And I think it might be interesting to have a skin biopsy of this patient and to stimulate it to make interferon and see if he can block his own interferon, for example.

Dr. NIETHAMMER: That's exactly what we have already done. We have conducted skin biopsy. But we have not stimulated it yet. The other thing we would like to try is to get one of the new fibroblast interferons grown from *E. coli* and to see what is happening there.

Interferon Therapy of Malignant Disease

Hans STRANDER

Radiumhemmet, Karolinska Hospital 104 01 Stockholm, Sweden

INTRODUCTION

Tumor patients have been treated with 3 types of interferon (IFN) preparations in various clinical centers in the world, leukocyte IFN (α), lymphoblast IFN (α), and fibroblast IFN (β). The present status of IFN antitumor therapy is described in a number of reviews.[1-8] At the Karolinska Hospital in Stockholm we have been treating tumor patients for more than 10 years with leukocyte IFN. This communication compiles the results obtained so far and updates the present situation in various clinical trials.

In Vitro Studies

IFNs can exert various effects on an organism. By definition IFNs are able to inhibit the replication of viruses inside the cells. Furthermore, the release of virus particles from cells can be hindered by exposing the cells to IFNs, and IFNs can protect normal cells from undergoing malignant transformation by tumor viruses. Under some circumstances IFNs can also inhibit the growth of tumor cells once the tumor virus has become integrated into the cell. It has also been shown that IFNs can inhibit tumor cells not known to have been transformed by any tumor virus. In general, tumor cells exhibit different sensitivities to IFNs and, within the same tumor type, both extremely sensitive and resistant cells can be found.[9,10]

IFNs display a multitude of effects on various immunologic reactions.[11] This has been shown in both *in vitro* and *in vivo* systems. Whether the effects exerted are beneficial or harmful is unclear because very little is known about the role played by immune reactions under natural conditions in an animal suffering from a tumor disease.

Of the various effects by IFN observed in *in vivo* animal work, we do not know which plays an important role in the antitumor action. Some earlier ex-

179

periments suggest that both direct and indirect effects may have an influence under such circumstances. One could also conclude from the animal work that IFNs can be rather potent antitumor agents, and hence it is fully understandable that clinical work should be now directed toward the evaluation of IFN therapy in tumor disease since more and more IFN has become available for studies.

IFN Preparation

The IFN preparation we have used consists of IFN-α which we obtained from Kari Cantell in Helsinki.[12-14] In 1978, 90,000 buffy coats were employed for IFN production in Helsinki. About 5,000 liters of IFN-α were prepared, and the total production was 2.5×10^{11} international reference units (IU). The 1979 output approached 6,000 liters, with a correspondent rise in IU, and represented a major portion of the global production. The resulting IFN consists of a mixture of several IFN molecules, but recombinant DNA work has not yet revealed how many such molecules are actually present in the preparations.[15]

Purification of the IFN

The IFN-α which we have employed at our clinic has been used at the 0.5% purity level, i.e., the preparations have contained about 99.5% impurities. It is important to emphasize, however, that the same IFN has been purified to homogeneity.[5] Unfortunately, such IFN has not yet been used at the clinical level since the purification loss has been considered too extensive.

Pharmacokinetics

Ten years ago we injected half a million units of human IFN-α intravenously into a patient with melanoma. The patient developed a severe, transient reaction and it was decided not to continue with I.V. injections. Cantell and coworkers were subsequently able to show that intramuscular injections of human IFN-α into rabbits gave rise to good IFN levels in the blood,[16] so we decided to administer IFN by the I.M. route, also. We have continued to do this over the last 10 years. It should be noted, however, that if IFN is more extensively purified than our initial product was, it will become possible to give patients I.V. injections.[17]

Toxicity

The most common side-effects noted after I.M. injection of human IFN-α included fever, fatigue, slight hair loss, transient effects on liver enzyme levels in the blood, and finally granolocyte- and trombocytopenia at higher IFN doses. These side-effects seem to depend at least to some extent on the quantity injected, but it has yet to be decided how much IFN-α actually can be given to a tumor patient.

Clinical Effect on Tumor Diseases

IFNs are able to induce regression of both benign and malignant tumors in man. This has been found for patients with myeloma, Hodgkin's disease, non-Hodgkin's lymphoma, acute leukemia, nasopharyngeal carcinoma, mammary carcinoma, ovarian carcinoma, juvenile laryngeal papilloma, bladder papilloma, and malignant melanoma. The reader is referred to reviews written over the past few years. The following will focus on the studies which have been performed at our hospital.

Osteosarcoma

We have treated 48 patients with nonmetastatic osteosarcoma at the Karolinska Hospital since 1971 in a collaborative study between the Orthopaedic Clinic and Radiumhemmet at the Karolinska Hospital.[18] IFN has been given as adjuvant therapy by the I.M. route, and the dose has been 3×10^6 units a day for one month, then 3 times a week for 17 months. The IFN has been injected immediately after the diagnostic biopsy and hence before surgery. The patients have been operated on for their primary tumors. The present results look encouraging since the 5 year survival rate for the IFN group is 58%, a high rate for a group of classical primary osteosarcoma patients.

Three control groups have been employed in this study. The historical control group collected at the Karolinska Hospital from the preceding 20 years cannot be used at present for evaluation of this study since it consists of patients with tumors that are more malignant than the other groups. All the cases treated in Sweden since 1971 who did not receive IFN therapy have also been collected. This is a contemporary control group, and this group together with the IFN-treated group encompasses all the patients with osteosarcoma in Sweden after 1971, if one subtracts the cases already showing metastatic tumor growth at the time of admission. The contemporary control group has been divided into two. One concurrent group consists of the cases treated between 1971 and 1976, and they have not received any adjuvant therapy. Their 5 year survival is at present 34%. From 1976 all the concurrent cases have been given chemotherapy, and this constitutes another contemporary control group, but too few cases have been followed for 5 years to make meaningful analysis possible. This whole study is still in progress.

It is interesting to note that, in patients who later developed metastases despite undergoing IFN adjuvant therapy, the IFN was unable to prevent subclinical and clinical infections.[19] This is in contrast to the group who never developed any metastases on such therapy and in whom no such infections so far appeared. This finding warrants further study and more data are presently being collected.

Juvenile Laryngeal Papilloma

In 1975 a collaborative study between the Ear, Nose and Throat Department and Radiumhemmet at the Karolinska Hospital was initiated.[20] Ten cases with juvenile laryngeal papillomas have been treated so far. This is a benign tumor probably caused by a papovavirus. IFN-α has been given by I.M. injections, in doses of 3×10^6 units 3 times a week. With these doses regression has been obtained in all 10 patients, but when the total IFN dose per week was reduced and injections were given only once or twice a week, the results were far less convincing. When IFN therapy was completely withdrawn after long-term antitumor therapy in these patients, they have experienced recurrences. On reintroducing the drug, a new response has so far always been observed. We can conclude that, at the higher dose, there is a regular regression of this benign tumor, but we are working rather close to the level where the effects become questionable. The problem of tumor recurrence in this group has to be resolved.

Hodgkin's Lymphoma

A Stage IV lymphocyte-predominant Hodgkin's lymphoma was treated by I.M. injection at a dose of 5×10^6 units daily.[21] A reduction was observed in tumor volume, but later progression took place during ongoing IFN therapy.

Ewing Sarcoma

One patient with Ewing sarcoma has been treated with daily I.M. injections 3×10^6 units of IFN-α. No effect could be demonstrated (unpublished).

Myelomatosis

In 1975 we treated a chemotherapy-resistant patient with myelomatosis and observed a clinical effect. In a collaborative study in Stockholm between Radiumhemmet, Karolinska Hospital, and Seraphimer Hospital in Stockholm, myeloma patients were treated with IFN. A pilot study was undertaken on previously untreated patients. Nine patients were included and IFN was given at a dose of 3×10^6 units daily by I.M. injection. Regression was observed in 5 patients, stabilization in 2 and progression in 2.

In another study in which IFN was given to 6 patients who had previously received chemotherapy, partial regression was observed in 2 patients, stabilization in 2, and progression of the disease in 2.

These studies led to a controlled trial in middle Sweden in which randomized myeloma patients were given IFN-α daily. The dose employed was 3×10^6 units I.M. This was a randomized trial in which conventional Melphalan-Prednisolon therapy was administered to the other arm. In this study the number of responders in the Melphalan-Prednisolon group was 8 out of 33, against 4 out of 31 in the IFN group. Stabilization was recorded in 15 and 19 patients, respectively. It was observed that the results were better for patients receiving nonlyophilized rather than lyophilized IFN-α, perhaps indicating the lower IFN content in the lyophilized preparations. The study is still in progress to investigate possible differences among the various IFN preparations employed.[22,23]

Ovarian Carcinoma

A pilot study was undertaken at Radiumhemmet, Karolinska Hospital, on 5 ovarian carcinoma patients (unpublished). They had all been treated previously with radiation and were all becoming resistant to chemotherapy before IFN therapy was initiated. IFN-α was given by I.M. injection at a dose of 3×10^6 units daily. Two of the patients had extensive ascitic fluid production, and this was arrested in both. Partial regression of solid tumors was observed in only one patient. A randomized study will be started during 1981 in which IFN therapy will be compared to conventional chemotherapy.

Prostate Carcinoma

A randomized study has been initiated at Radiumhemmet in which prostate carcinoma is treated with either IFN or conventional chemotherapy.

Glioblastoma

A pilot study is in progress at the Neurological Department of the Karolinska Hospital and Radiumhemmet with patients who have been operated on for glioblastoma. No results are available as yet from this study.

Mechanism of Antitumor Action

It can be concluded that IFNs under some circumstances display an antitumor effect.[24,25] The reason for this is obscure, and we do not know which of the various effects participate in antitumor action. Much work is needed to clarify whether IFN's main action is direct or indirect.[26] Until we know more about how IFNs act on the patients who do respond to therapy, it will be difficult to construct clinical trials on a theoretical basis. So far, all the clinical trials have had to be formulated on the basis of experience and empirical knowledge.

PROSPECTS FOR THE FUTURE

It is clear that much more basic clinical research has to be undertaken on tumor patients receiving IFN therapy. We have to monitor the patients more in order to identify those who would really benefit from IFN therapy. We need to observe the side-effects, study levels of IFN in the patients' serum, establish different types of tumor cultures and test them for IFN sensitivity, investigate various immunologic variables in IFN-treated patients, do antiviral assays on patients receiving treatment with IFN, and screen for IFN production in patients receiving IFN therapy. Model experiments could be undertaken and enzyme levels determined in the blood of IFN-treated patients.

From the more clinical point of view it would be helpful to be able to vary several factors, e.g., disease, disease stage, dose of IFN, schedule, duration, and the effectiveness of various combination therapies. All this will be possible when more leukocyte IFN becomes available. It is significant that large amounts of IFN-α can now be procued by other means[27] and that in the near future E. coli will also be utilized to provide a large quantity of IFN-α. It will certainly be interesting to study the effects of IFN on tumors when a lack of IFN does not direct the therapeutic routes we have to follow when treating the patients.

Acknowledgments

The research presented in this paper was supported by grants from the Swedish Cancer Society and the Cancer Society of Stockholm.

REFERENCES

1. Cantell, K.: Why is interferon not in clinical use today? *Interferon*, 1: 1–28, 1979.
2. Dunnick, J. K. and Galasso, G. J.: Up-date on clinical trials with exogenous interferon. *J. Infect. Dis.*, 142: 293–299, 1980.
3. Gutterman, J. U., Blumenschein, G. R., Alexanian, A., Yap, H. Y., Buzdar, A. U., Cabanillas, F., Hortobagni, G. N., Hersh, E. M., Rasmussen, S. L., Harmon, M., Kramer, M., and Pestka, S.: Leukocyte interferon-induced tumor regression in human metastatic breast cancer, multiple myeloma and malignant lymphoma. *Ann. Intern. Med.*, 93: 399–406, 1980.
4. Priestman, T. J.: Interferon: An anticancer agent? *Cancer Treat. Rev.*, 9: 223–237, 1979.
5. Rubinstein, M., Rubinstein, S., Familletti, P. C., Gross, M., Miller, R. S., Waldman, A., and Pestka, S.: Human leukocyte interferon purified to homogeneity. *Science*, 202: 1282–1290, 1978.
6. Stewart, W. E., II: The Interferon System. Springer-Verlag, New York, 1979.
7. Strander, H.: Antitumor effects of interferon and its possible use as an antineoplastic agent in man. *Texas Rep. Biol. Med.*, 35: 429–435, 1977.
8. Strander, H.: Interferons: Neoplastic drugs? *Blut*, 35: 277–288, 1977.
9. Adams, A., Strander, H., and Cantell, K.: Sensitivity of the Epstein-Barr virus transformed human lymphoid cell lines to interferon. *J. Gen. Virol.*, 28: 207–217, 1975.
10. Einhorn, S. and Strander, H.: Interferon therapy for neoplastic diseases in man. In: W. R. Strinebring and P. J. Chapple (eds.), Production of Human Interferon and Investigations of Its Clinical Use. Plenum Pub. Corp., 1978, pp. 159–174.
11. Einhorn, S., Blomgren, H., Cantell, K., Strander, H., and Troye, M.: *In vivo* administra-

tion of interferon to man: Studies on the immune system. *Ann. N. Y. Acad. Sci.*, **350**: 580–581, 1980.

12. Cantell, J. and Hirvonen, S.: Preparation of human leukocyte interferon for clinical use. *Texas Rep. Biol. Med.*, **35**: 138–144, 1977.

13. Cantell, K. and Hirvonen, S.: Large scale production of human leukocyte interferon containing 10^8 units per ml. *J. Gen. Virol.*, **49**: 541–543, 1978.

14. Mogensen, K. E. and Cantell, K.: Production and preparation of human leukocyte interferon. *Pharmacol. Ther.* [C], **1**: 369–381, 1977.

15. Nagata, S., Taira, H., Hall, A., Johnsrud, I., Streuli, M., Ecsödi, J., Boll, W., Cantell, K., and Weissman, C.: Synthesis in *E. coli* of a polypeptide with human leukocyte interferon activity. *Nature* (London), **284**: 316–320, 1980.

16. Cantell, K. and Pyhälä, L.: Circulating interferon in rabbits after administration of human interferon by different routes. *J. Gen. Virol.*, **20**: 97–104, 1973.

17. Jordan, G. W., Fried, R. P., and Merigan, T. C.: Administration of human leukocyte interferon in herpes zoster. I. Safety, circulating antiviral activity and host response to infection. *J. Infect. Dis.*, **150**: 56–62, 1974.

18. Strander, H., Aparisi, T., Blomgren, H., Broström, L. A., Cantell, K., Einhorn, S., Ingimarsson, S., Nilsonne, U., and Söderberg, G.: Adjuvant interferon treatment of human osteosarcoma. *Rec. Results Cancer Res.*, **68**: 39–46, 1979.

19. Ingimarsson, S., Cantell, K., Carlström, G., and Strander, H.: Virus infections and recurrence of osteosarcoma in patients receiving human leukocyte interferon. *Intern. J. Cancer*, **26**: 395–399, 1980.

20. Haglund, S., Lundqvist, P.-G., Ingimarsson, S., Cantell, K., and Strander, H.: Interferon therapy in juvenile laryngeal papillomatosis. In: W. Terry (ed.), 2nd Int. Conf. Immunother. Cancer: Present Status of Trials in Man. Nat. Inst. Health, Bethesda, Md. (in press).

21. Blomgren, H., Cantell, K., Johansson, B., Lagergren, C., Ringborg, U., and Strander, H.: Interferon therapy in Hodgkin's disease. *Acta Med. Scand.*, **199**: 527–532, 1976.

22. Mellstedt, H., Aahre, A., Björkholm, M., Cantell, K., Holm, G., Johansson, B., and Strander, H.: Interferon therapy in myelomatosis. *Lancet*, **2**: 245–247, 1979.

23. Mellstedt, H., Aahre, A., Björkholm, M., Strander, H., Brenning, G., Engstedt, L., Gahrton, G., Holm, G., Lerner, R., Lönnqvist, B., Nordenskiöld, B., Killander, A., Stalfeldt, A. M., Simonsson, B., Ternstedt, B., and Wadman, B.: Interferon therapy of patients with myeloma. In: W. Terry (ed.), 2nd Int. Conf. Immunother. Cancer: Present Status of Trials in Man. Nat. Inst. Health, Bethesda, d. (in press).

24. Gresser, I.: Antitumor effects of interferon. In: F. Becker (ed.), Cancer: A Comprehensive Treatise. *Chemotherapy*, **5**: 521–571, 1977.

25. Gresser, I. and Tovey, M. G.: Antitumor effects of interferon. *Bioch. Bioph. Acta*, **516**: 231–247, 1978.

26. Epstein, L. B., Shen, J. T., Abele, J. S., and Reese, C. C.: Sensitivity of human ovarian carcinoma cells to interferon and other antitumor agents as assessed by an *in vitro* semi-solid agar technique. *Ann. N. Y. Acad. Sci.*, **350**: 228–246, 1980.

27. Johnston, M. D., Christofinis, G., Ball, G. D., Fantes, K. H., and Finter, N. B.: A culture system for producing large amounts of human lymphoblastoid interferon. *Develop. Biol. Standard*, **42**: 189–192, 1979.

Pharmacologic and Immunologic Effects of Human Leukocyte Interferon in Patients with Neoplasia: An Interim Report

E.C. Borden, M.J. Hawkins, B.S. Edwards, A.M. Liberati, and K. Cantell

Wisconsin Clinical Cancer Center and VA Hospitals, Madison, Wisconsin, and Central Public Health Laboratory, Helsinki, Finland

SUMMARY

We have been investigating the comparative immunologic and pharmacologic effects of human leukocyte interferon (HuIFN-α) by the intramuscular (I.M.), intravenous (I.V.), and intra-arterial (I.A.) routes in patients with neoplasia. Peak titers are higher after I.V. administration, but titers are more sustained after I.M. administration. Significant hepatic and/or tumor absorption occurred after I.A., intrahepatic administration. Doses to 3×10^6 units I.V. and I.A. and to 9×10^6 units I.M. have been given without problem for durations of 14–21 days. No limiting toxicity by the I.V. or I.A. route has yet been identified. Although serum glutamic oxaloacetic transferase (SGOT) rises in a few patients after I.M. administration, direct intrahepatic infusion by the I.A. route has resulted in no hepatic toxicity.

NK cell activity of normal individuals and individuals with malignancy can be augmented *in vitro* for both fresh leukemia cells and various cell lines (K-562, Chang). Significant augmentation of NK cell activity for allogeneic tumor targets also occurs in patients receiving HuIFN-α.

INTRODUCTION

Interferons are proteins which are defined and assayed biologically by their intracellular inhibition of viral replications. The biologic effects of IFNs include alterations in cell proliferation, immunologic responses, enzymatic activities, and surface characteristics.[1-3] Tumor growth is inhibited and survival prolonged in nonviral-induced, experimental tumor models.[1-3] IFN inducers, such as polyriboinosinic: polyribocytidylic acid (poly I : poly C), produce similar

187

effects. Preliminary results of clinical trials with IFNs as antitumor agents in humans have been encouraging.[4-9] This has resulted in continued commitment of funds to further define the mechanism of antitumor action and optimal conditions for clinical use.

Our clinical studies of IFNs in neoplastic disease have two major objectives. The first is the definition of dose, route, and schedule for optimal serum IFN concentrations, modulation of immunologic responses, and minimal toxicity. The second is the identification of tumor types in which IFNs may have potential therapeutic benefit. We report here the interim results of a continuing investigation of the pharmacokinetics, toxicities, and effects on natural killer (NK) cell activity of IFN-α.

MATERIALS AND METHODS

Interferons

Wet frozen and lyophilized HuIFN-α was obtained from the laboratorie of Kari Cantell and the Finnish National Red Cross, and for the study in Table 1 from the Israel Institute for Biological Research. All were prepared by induction of blood donor buffy coats with Sendai virus and partial purification by potassium thiocyanate precipitation to a specific activity of 10^6 units/mg according to the methods of Cantell.[10] Selected wet frozen and lyophilized vials from each source were checked prior to use and proved to contain the labeled amounts of antiviral activity by comparison to an international standard leukocyte preparation.

IFNs were administered by I.M. injection into the gluteus or biceps. I.V. and I.A. injections were over 10 minutes after dilution into purified human plasma protein fraction (5 % in 0.15 M sodium chloride). I.V. administration was via peripheral vein and I.A. intrahepatic administration in the common hepatic artery. The latter was achieved by a percutaneous catheter in the brachial artery with retrograde placement of the catheter in the common hepatic artery via the celiac axis.[11]

Patients

All patients had recurrent metastatic breast, bronchogenic, or colorectal carcinoma or melanoma. Patients treated by I.A. intrahepatic infusion had tumor metastatic to the liver in addition to other sites. Informed consent was obtained for all investigations.

IFN Assay

IFN was assayed via a quantitative colorimetric assay adapted and refined by our laboratory.[12] Titers were determined on BG9 fibroblasts after challenge with vesicular stomatitis virus. One laboratory unit in this assay is equivalent to 0.46 international leukocyte units and to 0.38 international fibroblast units (results of determinations over 12 months). IFN titers were expressed in international reference fibroblast or leukocyte units by incorporation of an appropriate internal laboratory standard into each assay and repeated comparison of that standard to the reference standard.

NK Cell Cytotoxicity

Human peripheral blood lymphocytes (PBL) were purified by centrifugation (700 g, 30 min, 24°C) through ficoll-hypaque. Mononuclear cells substantially free of contaminating granulocytes and red blood cells were collected at the ficoll-buffer interface, washed 3 times in PBS, and suspended in RPMI 1640 containing 10% fetal bovine serum for subsequent testing. Natural killing (NK) by PBL was measured in a 6-hour chromium release assay in which K-562, a human myeloid leukemia line, and Chang a human liver cell line, were used as targets. K-562 and Chang were labeled by incubating 5×10^6 cells in 1 ml of medium with 100 and 200 $\mu CI/ml$ $Na_2{}^{51}Cr$, respectively, for 40 to 90 minutes. Labeled cells were then resuspended in medium, underlayered with 2 ml fetal bovine serum, and centrifuged at 500 g, 7 min, 24°C, to remove unincorporated isotope. After two such washes, target cells were diluted and added to microtiter wells at 2×10^3 cells per well for the chromium release assay. PBL were then added to the wells at cell concentrations in quadruplicate of 100:1, 50:1, 25:1, and 12.5:1. Spontaneous and maximum chromium release were estimated by incubating targets alone in medium or in a solution of 4% cetrimide, respectively. Percent cytotoxicity due to PBL was calculated according to the following formula:

$$\% \text{ cytotoxicity} = \frac{\text{test well cpm - spontaneous cpm}}{\text{maximum cpm - spontaneous cpm}} \times 100.$$

Spontaneous cpm were usually 10% to 20% of maximum cpm with both targets.

K cell activity (antibody-dependent cell-mediated cytotoxicity) was determined similarly with the use of a 1:10,000 dilution of a rabbit anti-Chang cell serum in the effector cell assay.

RESULTS

Systemic Toxicities

The acute toxicity observed after both I.M. and I.V. administration was mild fever and malaise (Table 1). This usually occurred 3 to 6 hours after administration and persisted for 2 to 4 hours. Malaise was associated with mild myalgia and fatigue. No hypotension was recorded. None of these acute reactions were dose-limiting.

Table 1.   Acute systemic reactions to IFN-α.

Toxicity	3×10^5 units		3×10^6 units	
	I.M.	I.V.	I.M.	I.V.
Fever ($>38°$)	7/11[a]	4/13	11/13	0/2
Malaise ($>$moderate)	3/11	2/13	4/13	0/2
Hypotension ($<90/70$)	0/11	0/13	0/13	0/2

a) Number of patients/number treated.

The major chronic systemic toxicities were anorexia, decline in performance status, and granulocytopenia (Table 2). These were usually associated with moderate weight loss. Inhibition of thyroid-stimulating hormone action *in vitro* by IFN has been reported.[13] Although the free thyroxine index decreased, it remained within the normal range. Thus it probably does not account for the anorexia or weight loss observed. Excess shedding of hair, although not a cosmetic problem, was noted by 14% of the patients. Decreased white count was commonly observed (Table 2). This was predominantly granulocytopenia. In these trials no patient had IFN discontinued. However, the anorexia, fatigue, and decline in performance status were chronic toxicities of sufficient problem that they may prove dose-limiting.

Table 2.   Chronic systemic toxicity of IFN-α.

Toxicity	I.A.	I.M.
Anorexia ($>$ mild)	7/12[a]	3/9
Performance status decrease	9/12	4/9
Hair shedding	0/12	3/9
Mean wt change (kg)	-2.25 (11)[b]	-2.9 (9)
Free thyroxine index (mean nadir decrease)	——	-0.28 (9)
White count decrease (mean nadir $\times 10^3/mm^3$)	-3.36 (11)	-3.22 (9)
Granulocyte decrease (mean nadir $\times 10^3/mm^3$)	-3.18 (9)	-2.15 (8)

a) Number of patients/ number treated.
b) Number of patients.

Similar toxicities were observed after administration of IFN-α by all routes. Although peak serum IFN levels were higher (see below), reactions were no more severe after I.V./I.A. administration when compared to I.M. administration. If anything, systemic reactions were less common with intravascular administration (Tables 1 and 2).

Serum IFN Levels After Various Routes of Administration

Escalation of the I.M. dose from 3 to 9 $\times$ 10^6 units resulted in more persistent and higher peak serum levels (Table 3). Titers were more than 3-fold higher.

Table 3.   Effect of IFN dose on serum titer.

Patient	Serum titer after Given I.M. Dose					
	3 $\times$ 10^6 units			9 $\times$ 10^6 units		
	Hour after dose (day 15)			Hour after dose (day 30–42)		
	0	2	6	0	2	6
PG	0	10	5	30	30	50
GR	10	70	30	50	170	—
FO	1	10	20	20	120	170

Peak I.V. serum titers at 2 dose levels of IFN were approximately 10-fold higher than peak I.M. levels (Table 4). I.M. levels were, however, more sustained, as previously reported by Jordan et al.[14]

Table 4.   Peak IFN serum levels following I.V. and I.M. administration of HuIFN-α.[a]

Dose	Route	Peak level
3 $\times$ 10^5 units	I.V.	30
	I.M.	2
3 $\times$ 10^6 units	I.V.	225
	I.M.	18

a) Data based on 4 patients in each group. Peak titers after I.V. administration within first 5 minutes, after I.M. at 4–6 hours.

Significant hepatic and/or tumor absorption occurred after I.A. intrahepatic administration. Patients received bolus injections over 10 minutes, and blood was collected from a peripheral vein for determination of serum IFN concentration. Serum titers after I.A. administration were significantly lower than after I.V. administration (Fig. 1). These results suggested hepatic and/or tumor extraction of IFN. All patients had metastatic disease in their liver. It is thus impossible to determine from these results whether hepatic or tumor extraction resulted in the first-pass absorption of IFN. Study of other patients with metastatic tumor at nonhepatic sites will allow this distinction to be made in the future.

Despite direct intrahepatic administration at doses of 3 $\times$ 10^5 units daily for 14 or 28 days and 3 $\times$ 10^6 units daily for an additional 14 days, no significant hepatic toxicity was observed. Regular measurement of bilirubin, alkaline pho-

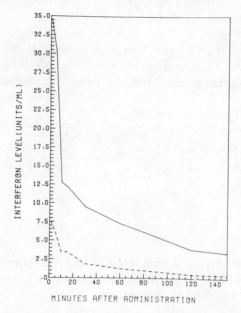

Fig. 1. Comparative IFN serum titers after I.A. intrahepatic (- - -) and I.V. (—) administration of 10^5 units of IFN-α over 10 minutes. Data based on mean titer in 9 patients with hepatic metastases.

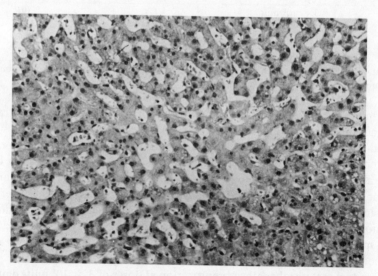

Fig. 2. Histopathology of liver parenchyma in a 34-year-old woman with breast carcinoma after I.A. intrahepatic administration of a cumulative dose of 3×10^7 units of IFN-α over 23 days.

sphatase, and serum glutamic oxaloacetic transferase was performed. No deterioration in liver function, not attributable to progressive hepatic malignancy, was observed. One patient had a liver biopsy performed after 15 days at 3×10^5 units and 8 days at 3×10^6 units. No histologic damage was apparent (Fig. 2).

Natural Killer Cell Activity

NK cell activity is markedly augmented *in vitro* by IFNs and IFN inducers.[15-17] Both NK cell (spontaneous cell-mediated cytotoxicity) and K cell (antibody-dependent cell-mediated cytotoxicity) activities were augmented by treatment of cells from normal donors with the IFN inducer, polyribonosinic: polyribocytidylic acid (Fig. 3). Poly I : poly C resulted in significant enhancement in NK cell activity in 20 of 24 tested individuals. Similarly, both activities were augmented by treatment of effector cells with IFN-α (Fig. 4).

To provide a basis for determination of *in vivo* effects of IFNs on NK cell activity, we have serially measured basal NK cell activity of 11 normal individuals over a period of 18 months. Each subject had a characteristic individual basal level of NK cell activity (Table 5). However, an individual on any single day expressed a variable degree of NK cell and K cell activity (Table 5). To define further the reproducibility of the assay, NK cell activity was measured in a single assay in 10 normal individuals at 4 different times in a 24-hour period (Table 6). Although any single time point could distinctly

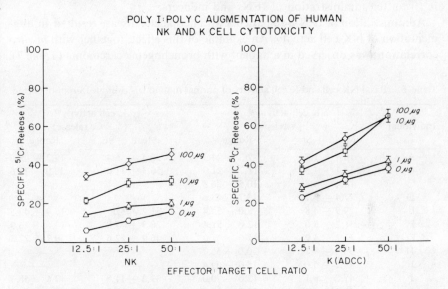

Fig. 3. Stimulation of NK cells and of K cells by poly I : poly C. Effector to target cell ratio = 25:1. Target cells for NK cell assay, K-562; for K cells, Chang with an anti-Chang antibody.

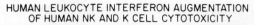

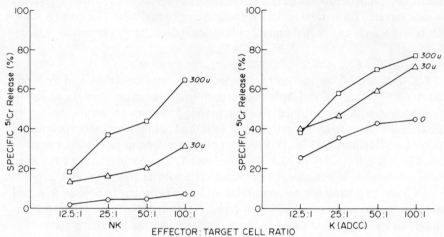

Fig. 4. Stimulation of NK cells and of K cells by IFN-α IFN concentrations: 0 units (○), 30 units (△), and 300 units (□). Target cell line, Chang.

fluctuate, activity at three of four time points was usually relatively constant. These observations provide a basis for defining NK cell and K cell activity *in vivo* after administration of IFNs and inducers.

Administration of IFN-α to patients with neoplastic disease resulted in augmentation of NK cell activity. An example of this effect, together with *in vitro* correlation, was observed in a patient with bronchogenic carcinoma (Table 7).

Table 5.   Basal NK cell and K cell activity of normal individuals over an 18-month period.

Individual	NK cell activity[a] (% ^{51}Cr release) Mean ± SE	Range	K cell activity[b] (% ^{51}Cr release) Mean ± SE	Range
A	16.4 ± 1.8	7.2 − 24.3	35.4 ± 6.4	19.2 − 48.6
B	17.1 ± 1.5	11.7 − 21.0	50.3 ± 11.0	26.0 − 72.6
C	18.4 ± 4.4	10.5 − 26.5	——	——
D	27.4 ± 4.7	13.7 − 43.6	——	——
E	29.9 ± 4.8	8.0 − 55.4	31.2 ± 5.1	15.9 − 42.5
F	31.2 ± 3.6	12.0 − 51.4	28.3 ± 7.0	13.8 − 46.9
G	33.2 ± 4.9	17.6 − 47.0	46.9 ± 12.6	9.7 − 72.5
H	35.8 ± 9.1	20.0 − 55.7	——	——
I	40.2 ± 5.0	15.0 − 69.4	——	——
J	47.8 ± 8.1	12.0 − 70.0	39.2 ± 11.8	17.6 − 58.3
K	50.6 ± 4.6	31.6 − 62.0	35.3 ± 7.7	9.7 − 70.0

a) Target cell K-562. Effector:target ratio = 50:1. Each individual tested 4–12 times.
b) Target cell Chang. Effector: target ratio = 50:1. Each individual tested 4–6 times.

Table 6. Basal NK cell activity of normal individuals over a 24-hour period.

Individual	NK cell activity (% ^{51}Cr release)[a]				
	0 hr	2 hr	4 hr	24 hr	Mean ± SE
A	8.5	8.0	0.0	7.0	5.9 ± 3.8
B	11.7	13.6	12.8	18.1	14.1 ± 1.4
C	25.7	18.4	18.5	11.0	18.4 ± 3.0
H	55.8	50.3	63.8	49.8	54.9 ± 3.3
I	30.7	21.4	25.9	32.0	27.5 ± 2.4
J	51.6	61.1	62.7	53.5	57.2 ± 2.7
L	23.3	43.8	28.7	13.8	27.4 ± 6.3
M	9.4	23.1	22.2	16.8	17.8 ± 3.1
N	32.7	24.8	43.0	23.1	30.9 ± 4.6
O	17.3	21.1	21.6	13.4	18.3 ± 2.0

a) Target cell K-562. Effector: target ratio = 50:1.

Table 7. Effect of IFN-α *in vivo* and *in vitro* on NK cell activity in a patient with bronchogenic carcinoma.

In vitro[a]	Specific release (% ^{51}Cr)
No IFN	3.8 ± 0.7
100 units IFN	11.2 ± 1.1
In vivo[b]	
Day −1	3.2 ± 0.9
Day 0	3.9 ± 0.7
Day +1 (9×10^6 units I.M.)	29.2 ± 2.1
Day +7 (9×10^6 units I.M.)	30.6 ± 1.6

E:T = 50:1 by linear regression for K-562 target cells.
a) For *in vitro* assay, 24 hours of incubation with IFN-α.
b) For *in vivo* determinations, NK cell activity was assessed 6 hours after IFN administration.

DISCUSSION

Further studies will be required to correlate IFN serum levels with observed toxicities and biological response modification. Ultimately, correlations will be made between these parameters and therapeutic effects. Our preliminary findings suggest that some individuals are markedly less sensitive to the biological effects of IFNs *in vivo*. If so, further dose escalation may be required for biological response modification and therapeutic activity.

We have demonstrated that, in addition to established tumor cell lines, fresh allogeneic leukemia cells were lysed more effectively by IFN-boosted NK cells.[17] However, IFNs did not augment NK cell cytotoxicity for autologous tumor cells *in vitro*.[18] Clinical studies will make it possible to determine whether augmentation of T-cell cytotoxicity[19,20] or NK cell cytotoxicity will result in inhibition of tumor growth.

Limited supplies have as yet prevented even a determination of what a maximally tolerated and biologically optimum dose may be. Thus, over the near term, clinical trials with IFNs should remain mostly Phase I-II studies. These should focus on definition of dose, duration, route, and schedule for optimal therapeutic effect, biological response modification, and serum levels. They will also result in increased understanding of the mechanism of antitumor action in man.

Randomized Phase III investigations will be required to define the ultimate role of IFNs in cancer management. IFNs may not be the catholicon of cancer therapy. They are, however, completely different kinds of antitumor compounds from those currently in use. This suggests that IFNs will probably prove of greatest value as significant adjuncts to current systemic therapies for primary and metastatic cancer.

Acknowledgments

The assistance and interest of Karen Sielaff, R.N., in patient care and data analysis, Debbie Groveman and Kathy Zaremba in NK and ADCC assays, and Jack McBain in interferon assays were instrumental in the completion of this project. The editorial assistance of Mary Ann Liposcak enabled the manuscript to be completed on time. Studies were supported by NIH CA20432, the American Cancer Society, and research funds from the Veterans' Administration.

Dr. Hawkins was supported by NIH Cancer Education Grant R25-CH18397 and an American Cancer Society Clinical Fellowship.

Dr. Edwards was supported by NIH Grant 5T32-CA-09075.

Dr. Liberati was supported by Lega Italiana per la lotta coutre i Tumori.

REFERENCES

1. Borden, E. C.: Interferons: Rationale for clinical trials in neoplastic disease. *Ann. Intern. Med.*, **91**: 472–479, 1979.
2. Krim, M.: Review: Towards tumor therapy with interferons. Part I. Interferons: Production and properties. *Blood*, **55**: 711–721, 1980; Part II. Interferons: *In vivo* effects. *Blood*, **55**: 875–884, 1980.
3. Gresser, I.: Antitumor effects of interferons. In: (ed.), F. Becker, *Cancer*: A Comprehensive Treatise, **5**: 521–571, 1977.
4. Gutterman, J. U., Blumenschein, G. R., Alexanian, R., Yap, H. Y., Buzdar, A. U., Cabanillas, F., Hortobagyi, G. N., Hersh, E. M., Rasmussen, S. L., Harmon, M., Kramer, M., and Pestka, S.: Leukocyte interferon-induced tumor regression in human metastatic breask cancer, multiple myeloma, and malignant lymphoma. *Ann. Intern. Med.*, **93**: 399–406, 1980.
5. Horoszewicz, J. S., Leong, S. S., Ito, M., Karakousis, C., Holyoke, E., Job, L., Doken, J. G., and Carter, W. A.: Human fibroblast interferon in human neoplasia: Clinical and laboratory study. *Cancer Canver Treat. Rep.*, **62**: 1899–1906, 1978.

6. Merigan, T. C., Sikora, K., Breeden, J. H., Levy, R., and Rosenberg, S. A.: Preliminary observations on the effect of human leukocyte interferon in non-Hodgkin's lymphoma. *New Engl. J. Med.*, **299**: 1449–1453, 1978.
7. Hill, N. O., Loeb, E., Pardue, A. S., Dorn, G. L., Khan, A., and Hill, J. M.: Response of acute leukemia to leukocyte interferon. *J. Clin. Hematol. Oncol.*, **9**: 137–149, 1979.
8. Mellstedt, H., Ahre, A., Bjorkholm, M., Holm, G., Johnansson, B., and Strander, H.: Interferon therapy in myelomatosis. *Lancet*, **1**: 245–247, 1979.
9. Borden, E. C. and Hawkins, M. J.: Interferons for human neoplastic and viral diseases. *Comp. Ther.*, **6**: 6–15, 1980.
10. Cantell, K., Hirvonen, S., Morensen, K. E., and Phyala, L.: Human leukocyte interferon: Production, purification, stability and animal experiments in the production and use of interferon for the treatment and prevention of human virus infections. In: C. Waymouth (ed.), *Proceedings of a Tissue Culture Association Workshop*, **3**: 35–38, 1973.
11. Wirtanen, G. W.: Percutaneous transbrachial artery infusion catheter techniques. *Am. J. Roent.*, **68**: 696–700, 1973.
12. Borden, E. C. and Leonhardt, P. H.: A quantitative semimicro, semiautomated colorimetric assay for interferon. *J. Lab. Clin. Med.*, **89**: 1036–1042, 1977.
13. Grollman, E. F., Lee, G., Ramos, S., Lazo, P. S., Kaback, H. R., Friedman, R. M., and Kohn, L. D.: Relationships of the structure and function of the interferon receptor to hormone receptors and establishment of the antiviral state. *Cancer Res.*, **38**: 4172–4185, 1978.
14. Jordan, G. W., Fried, R. P., and Merigan, T. C.: Administration of human leukocyte interferon in herpes zoster. I. Safety, circulating antiviral activity, and host responses to interferon. *J. Infect. Dis.*, **130**: 56–62, 1974.
15. Herberman, R. B., Ortaldo, J. R., and Bonnard, G. D.: Augmentation by interferon of humam natural and antibody-dependent cell-mediated cytotoxicity. *Nature*, **277**: 221–223, 1979.
16. Einhorn, S., Blomgren, H., and Strander, H.: Interferon and spontaneous cytotoxocity in man. I. Enhancement of the spontaneous cytotoxicity of peripheral lymphocytes by human leukocyte interferon. *Int. J. Cancer*, **22**: 405–412, 1978.
17. Zarling, J. M., Eskra, L., Borden, E. C., Horoszewicz, J., and Carter, W. A.: Activation of human natural killer cells cytotoxic for human leukemia cells by purified interferon. *J. Immunol.*, **123**: 63–70, 1979.
18. Vanky, F. T., Argove, S. A., Einhorn, S. A., and Klein, E.: Role of alloantigens in natural killing. Allogeneic but not autologous tumor biopsy cells are sensitive for interferon-induced cytotoxicity of human blood lymphocytes. *J. Exp. Med.*, **151**: 1151–1165, 1980.
19. Zarling, J. M., Sosman, J., Eskra, L., Borden, E. C., Horoszewicz, J. S., and Carter, W.A.: Enhancement of T cell cytotoxic responses by purified human fibroblast interferon. *J. Immunol.*, **121**: 2002–2004, 1978.
20. Heron, I., Berg, K., and Cantell, K.: Regulatory effect of interferon on T cells *in vitro*. *J. Immunol.*, **117**: 1370–1373, 1976.

Discussion

Dr. OGAWA: When you escalated doses to 9 million, did you find any increase in hematologic toxicity? This is my first question. My second question is that recently we have been thinking that response rate may depend on the tumor volume of the patient. In your breast cancer patient, did you observe such a correlation?

Dr. BORDEN: The first question, in terms of increased toxicity to the escalated dose: this is very difficult to sort out with the duration, and the fact is that the patients were already receiving 3 million units. My impression is that there was no increase in toxicity with the escalation of dose. And I can back that with the finding, for example, that the granulocyte counts did not further decrease with further dose escalation. Further, there did not appear to be any major increase in anorexia or decrease in performance status in the patients. In response to the second question, on the relationship to tumor burden or tumor mass, as to whether that correlates with response, I tried to look at that in terms of the trials and I ended up frustrated because I know of no real way to quantitate that. If you can give me a good way to quantitate that, I would be glad to look at it.

Dr. OGAWA: In the future, if I can, I will do so. Thank you.

Dr. NIETHAMMER: I may have missed the point in your presentation. Dr. Strander has shown in his previous talk that when you give leukocyte interferon intravenously, you get a higher peak, but the duration is much shorter. And we think that one of the disadvantages of fibroblast interferon might be that we have only very short blood levels. Why do you intend now to shift from intramuscular injection to intravenous injection?

Dr. BORDEN: I am not sure I follow the point.

Dr. NIETHAMMER: You said that in the future you will probably change over from intramuscular to intravenous injection, which would means that you will get higher peak levels but with shorter duration. What is the objective of this change?

Dr. BORDEN: I think to try and get an answer to the question that you raised: is the higher peak level more important, or are the more sustained intramuscular levels more important in terms of achieving tumor response as previously shown by Dr. Strander's, Dr. Merigan's and, more recently, our own studies? I don't know if the higher peak is better or the longer duration is more optimum.

Dr. EZAKI: In the proceedings, you showed that increased cytotoxic activity of NK cells against allorgeneic tumor cells are observed. Have you ever conducted any study in which the cytotoxic activity of NK cells was also observed against autologous tumor cells?

Dr. BORDEN: That's obviously a very important and critical question. We are currently just beginning studies along those lines.

Clinical and Immunologic Studies of Human Fibroblast Interferon

Makoto OGAWA, Kohji EZAKI, and Kenichi OKABE

Cancer Chemotherapy Center, Japanese Foundation for Cancer Research, Toshima-ku, Tokyo, 170, Japan

SUMMARY

Human fibroblast interferon (HuIFN-β) was used in 19 patients with various types of malignant disease, most of whom had had previous chemotherapy. They received 3×10^6 IU or 6×10^6 IU of HuIFN-β I.V. daily. Out of 17 evaluable patients, one patient with chronic lymphocytic leukemia showed partial remission and 3 patients with multiple myeloma, stomach cancer, and malignant melanoma indicated stable disease (SD). The majority of patients experienced fever over 38°C and chills, but these side-effects generally disappeared in several days. Other side-effects included general malaise, anorexia, hepatic dysfunction, and renal dysfunction were mild and tolerable.

Lymphocyte natural killer(NK) activity against a culture cell line was measured before and at various times after IFN-β treatment in 8 patients. The majority of patients reached the highest NK activity at 18–24 hours, most at 24 hours, after treatment was initiated; the level declined with daily infusions of IFN-β, but usually remained above the pretreatment level. In contrast, an increase in cytotoxic activity against autologous tumor cells was not observed following IFN-β treatment in all 4 patients whose tumor cells were available. Mixed lymphocyte tumor cell reaction (MLTR) was performed in 4 patients. One of them showed a slight increase after treatment but the rest had no change. In vitro sensitization tests to assess the in vitro generation of cytotoxic cells were negative in all 4 patients, and lymphocyte blastogenic responses to nonspecific mitogens showed no significant change. An increase in the delayed-type hypersensitivity reaction to recall antigens was observed in most of the patients after HuIFN-β treatment.

INTRODUCTION

The antitumor effects of IFN have been established in spontaneous and transplantable animal tumor systems of both viral and nonviral origin. Since the report of activity against osteogenic sarcoma by Strander,[1] there has been much interest in the use of IFN for the treatment of human malignant diseases. Subsequent reports have indicated significant antitumor effects against malignant lymphoma,[2,3] multiple myeloma,[4] acute leukemia,[5] and breast cancer.[6]

The mechanism of antitumor activity by IFN has been interpreted both as a direct cytotoxic effect on tumor cells and as an effect mediated through the immune system. In the present paper, we describe our clinical experience using human fibroblast interferon (HuIFN-β), as well as the immunologic studies done on patients under treatment with the drug.

MATERIALS AND METHODS

IFN was produced from a human fibroblast cell line at Toray Co., Japan, and offered to use for clinical study. Since the supply of HuIFN-β was limited, it was decided that the target tumors to take first priority would be malignant lymphoma and myeloma for systemic administration and maligant melanoma for local injection. As the supply increased thereafter, acute leukemia, osteogenic sarcoma, stomach cancer, breast cancer, and others were included in the study.

The criteria for patient selection were as follows: (1) patients with histologic or cytologic proof of the presence of one of the target tumors and (2) measurable lesions; (3) patients who became refractory to standard treatments, with a minimum 4 weeks from cessation of prior treatment and with life expectancy of more than 2 months; (4) patients who indicated a Karnofsky performance status greater than 50%, (5) adequate physiological functions, (6) age less than 75 years old, and (7) no active double cancers. All patients were treated with HuIFN-β alone. Most of the patients received 3×10^6 IU of IFN daily and in some patients the dose was escalated to 6×10^6 IU. IFN-β was dissolved in 250 ml of 5% glucose and infused intravenously (I.V.) over a period of one hour. This was repeated every day until the tumor progression become obvious.

Immunologic studies included: (1) natural killer (NK) activity of lymphocytes, (2) lymphocyte blastogenic response to nonspecific mitogens: phytohemagglutinin (PHA), Concanavalin A (Con A), and pokeweed mitogen (PWM), (3) skin tests for delayed type hypersensitivity to nonspecific antigens: Varidase, Candida, and PPD. Further studies were also performed in the cases in which autologous tumor cells were available. Tumor cells were collected either from bone marrow or pleural effusion or ascites before starting treatment. Controlled freezing was carried out in a Cryo-Med programmable freezing system, and cells were stored at $-180°C$ in liquid nitrogen. Additional immunologic tests examined lymphocyte cytotoxicity to autologous tumor cells, lymphocyte blastogenic responses to mitomycin C (MMC)-treated autologous tumor cells, and *in vitro* sensitization to assess the generation of cytotoxic lymphocytes induced by autologous tumor cells.

In vitro lymphocyte studies were performed before starting IFN-β treatment and every 6 hours until 24 hours after treatment, and then repeated every 3–5 days. Skin tests were done before treatment and then every 1–2 weeks.

NK Activity and Lymphocyte Cytotoxicity

Peripheral blood lymphocytes from patients were purified from heparinized venous blood by Ficoll-Conrey gradient. After 2 washes with PBS supplemented with 2.5% AB (+) male serum, the lymphocytes were resuspended in RPMI 1640 medium supplemented with 10% AB (+) male serum. The lymphocyte concentrations were adjusted to 5×10^5/ml, 1×10^6/ml, and 2×10^6/ml, and 0.2 ml were added to triplicate wells of Nunc-U-bottomed plate. A ^{51}Cr release assay was applied to detect lymphocyte NK activity and cytotoxicity.

K-562, derived from chronic myeloid leukemia in blast crisis, and Daudi, derived from Burkitt's lymphoma, were used as target cells for NK activity. Frozen tumor cells were thawed rapidly at 37°C, washed 3 times, and counted in a hemocytometer. For target cell preparation, K-562, Daudi, and autologous tumor cells were adjusted to 2×10^6 in 0.2 ml of medium and 50–100 μCi in 0.1 ml of $Na_2\ ^{51}CrO_4$ (New England Nuclear, 200–300 mCi/mg) was added to each cell suspension and incubated at 37°C for 1.5 hours. After the incubation, the cells were washed 3 times, resuspended in medium, and adjusted to 5×10^5/ml. Next, 0.02 ml of ^{51}Cr-labeled target cells (1×10^4) were added to different concentrations of lymphocytes in triplicate wells, giving 10:1, 20:1, and 40:1 effector to target cell ratios. After 6 hours of incubation at 37°C in a 5% CO_2 atmosphere, the supernatant in the wells was harvested with a Titertec supernatant collection system and cpm of ^{51}Cr released into supernatant were measured in a well-type gamma counter. Spontaneous and maximal release were determined by the incubation of target cells with medium alone or 0.5% NP-40, respectively. Percent cytotoxicity was calculated as:

$$\frac{\text{cpm experimental release - cpm spontaneous release}}{\text{cpm maximal release - cpm spontaneous release}} \times 100.$$

Lymphocyte Blastogenic Response

Microculture lymphocyte stimulation assay was employed to monitor lymphocyte blastogenic responses. The lymphocyte concentration was adjusted to 5×10^5/ml for mitogen-treated cultures and 0.2 ml were added to triplicate wells of Nunc-flat bottomed plate. For MLTR cultures, the cell concentration was adjusted to 1×10^6/ml and 0.1 ml was added to triplicate wells.

Nonspecific mitogens were added in 0.02 ml with the following concentrations: PHA 1:100, PWM 1:30, Con A 1:200 of the stock solutions. For MLTR cultures, autologous tumor cells were thawed, washed, and treated with 100 μg/ml of MMC for 1 hour. After 3 washes, the cells were adjusted to 1×10^6/ml and 0.1 ml was added in culture plates to an equivalent number of autologous lymphocytes. Cultures were incubated at 37°C in a 5% CO_2 atmosphere. Mitogen-treated cultures were terminated after 5 days and MLTR cultures were terminated after 7 days of incubation. During the final 7 hours of incubation, 1 μCi/well of ^{3}H-thymidine (New England Nuclear, 11.5 Ci/mM) was added to the cultures. Labeled cells were harvested onto glass fiber filters by a MASH (multiple automated sample harvester) and processed for liquid scintillation counting. Lymphocyte blastogenic responses were taken as cpm per 1×10^5 lymphocytes. The stimulation index (SI) was taken as the cpm in the stimulated culture derived by the cpm in the appropriate unstimulated control.

In Vitro Sensitization

For *in vitro* sensitization, MLTR cultures were performed with minor modifications in the lymphocyte-to-tumor cell ratio. MMC-treated tumor cells were adjusted to 1×10^6/ml, 1×10^5/ml, and 1×10^4/ml, and 0.1 ml was added to Nunc-U-bottomed plates, giving 1:1, 10:1, and 100:1 lymphocyte-to-tumor cell ratios. After 7 days of incubation, well contents were gently pipetted to disperse cell clumps and 1×10^4 ^{51}Cr-labeled tumor cells were added to the wells and assayed for ^{51}Cr release.

Delayed Hypersensitivity Skin Test Reactions

Delayed hypersensitivity was evaluated by a battery of skin test antigens, including Varidase, Candida, and PPD. The induration response was recorded at 24 and 48 hours, and mean diameter was recorded in millimeters.

RESULTS

Nineteen patients with various malignant diseases were subjects of the study: 4 with non-Hodgkin's lymphoma (NHL); 3 with multiple myeloma; 2 each with acute myelocytic leukemia (AML), breast cancer, stomach cancer, and hepatoma; one each with chronic lymphocytic leukemia (CLL), ovarian cancer, malignant melanoma, and common duct cancer. Table 1 summarizes the clinical responses of all the patients under the treatment with HuIFN-β.

One of the multiple myeloma patients and one of the hepatoma patients died within 7 days of treatment, and both were considered as early deaths. One out of 17 evaluable patients achieved partial remission (PR), and 3 out of 17 were considered to demonstrate stable disease (SD). Among 4 previously un-

Table 1.   Evaluation of HuIFN-β in cancer patients.

Case	Age	Sex	Diagnosis	Previous chemotherapy	Dose		Response
					IU	Days	
Y. M.	52	M	NHL[a]	+	3×10^6	$\times 30$	PD[b]
					6×10^6	$\times 12$	
H. Y.	67	F	NHL	+	3×10^6	$\times 23$	PD
N. Y.	34	F	NHL	+	3×10^6	$\times 14$	PD
					6×10^6	$\times 14$	
F. A.	71	F	NHL	+	3×10^6	$\times 15$	PD
S. N.	56	F	Multiple myeloma	−	3×10^6	$\times 38$	PD
S. T.	57	M	Multiple myeloma	+	3×10^6	$\times 80$	SD[c]
I. T.	54	F	Multiple myeloma	+	3×10^6	$\times 7$	NE[d]
Y. Y.	71	F	AML[e]	−	3×10^6	$\times 10$	PD
S. H.	16	M	AML	+	6×10^6	$\times 10$	PD
K. S.	52	F	Breast ca.	+	3×10^6	$\times 21$	PD
					6×10^6	$\times 12$	
K. R.	43	F	Breast ca.	+	3×10^6	$\times 10$	PD
A. K.	59	F	Stomach ca.	+	3×10^6	$\times 55$	SD
S. U.	44	F	Stomach ca.	−	3×10^6	$\times 37$	PD
L. K.	32	M	Hepatoma	+	6×10^6	$\times 16$	PD
I. T.	48	M	Hepatoma	+	3×10^6	$\times 5$	NE
N. T.	73	F	CLL[f]	−	3×10^6	$\times 40$	PR[g]
Y. K.	37	F	Ovarian ca.	+	6×10^6	$\times 30$	PD
O. N.	51	M	Malignant melanoma	+	6×10^6	$\times 102$	SD
K. F.	62	F	Common duct ca.	+	3×10^6	$\times 14$	PD

a) NHL: non-Hodgkin's lymphoma.
b) PD: progressive disease.
c) SD: stable disease.
d) NE: not evaluable.
e) AML: acute myelocytic leukemia.
f) CLL: chronic lymphocytic leukemia.
g) PR: partial remission.

treated patients, 1 achieved PR, but the rest indicated progressive disease (PD). Out of 6 patients who received 6×10^6 IU of IFN-β either from the initial treatment or in the middle of the course of treatment, only one reached SD and the others had PD. One patient who entered into PR had previously untreated CLL. The 3 patients with SD had diagnoses of multiple myeloma, stomach cancer, and malignant melanoma, and all had been previously treated. Among them, 2 patients, one with stomach cancer and the other with malignant melanoma, had a relatively short duration of SD. Their diseases became progressive even while receiving IFN, in about 20 days and 40 days, respectively. A brief description is presented below of the 2 patients who demonstrated PR and SD.

Case 1 (Fig. 1): A 73-year-old female was admitted to the hospital because of the generalized lymphadenopathy. Her initial WBC count was 100,300/cmm, most of which were matured lymphocytes with a B-cell markers. Hepatomegaly was also observed. The diagnosis of CLL was made, and she was placed on a daily I.V. infusion of 3×10^6 IU HuIFN-β. Her WBC count dropped dramatically after starting the IFN; the count fell to 25,600/cmm on the 7th day and to less than 10,000/cmm on the 20th day, with more than 30% neutrophils. During the treatment, no significant change was observed in the levels of hemoglobin and platelet counts, while the proportion of erythroid and myeloid series in the bone marrow increased. Hepatomegaly and lymphadenopathy were still present, although they showed mild decreases in size.

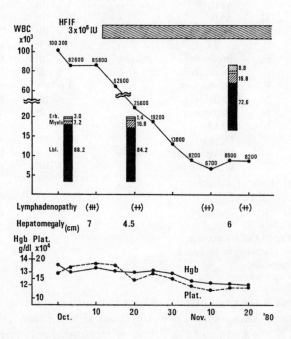

Fig. 1. N.T. 73 y.o. female CLL.

Case 2 (Fig. 2): Hyperproteinemia was found during a regular check-up in a 57-year-old male, and the diagnosis of IgA myeloma was made in March 1980. Serum IgA was 1,980 mg/dl. Bence-Jones protein in the urine was negative and a bone survey was normal. Plasma cell level in the bone marrow was 17.4%. Initially he was placed on melphalan treatment, which was continued until the end of May. Serum IgA was down to 1,250 mg/dl, but about one month later, IgA went up to 1,500 mg/dl and 3×10^6 IU of HuIFN-β was started I.V. daily.

IgA went down to 1,000 mg/dl in 30 days and remained at this level during IFN treatment. Plasma cells in the bone marrow declined to 12–14%. After 43 days of IFN treatment, he was discharged and continued on IFN 3 times a week in the outpatient clinic.

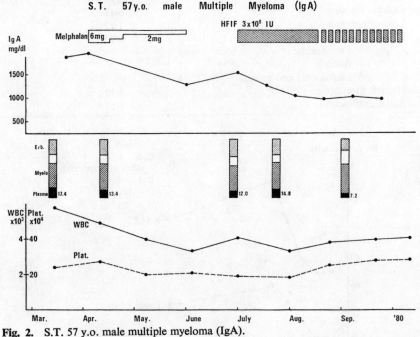

Fig. 2.   S.T. 57 y.o. male multiple myeloma (IgA).

At the beginning of the HuIFN-β therapy, the majority of the patients experienced fever over 38° C and chills. These side-effects usually disappeared after several days' treatment. Out of 17 evaluable patients, 6 complained of general malaise and one had anorexia. Myelosuppression, mainly leukopenia and anemia, was observed in 5 patients, although the degree was mild. Mild and reversible hepatic and renal dysfunction were observed in 3 patients and one patient, respectively. These side-effects were all tolerable and did not require the cessation of IFN treatment. (Table 2).

Lymphocyte NK activity and cytotoxicity in one patient with multiple myeloma are shown in Fig. 3. Among the 3 levels of target to effector ratio used, 1:40 always elicited the highest response, so the data are presented with this ratio. Twelve hours following IFN treatment, NK activity against K-562 and Daudi were slightly higher than the pretreatment level; the level rose much higher thereafter and the highest activity was observed at 24 hours. In contrast, cytotoxicity to autologous tumor cells remained unchanged during IFN treatment.

Table 2. Toxicity.

Symptom	Number affected/number evaluated
Fever (>38°C)	17/19
Chills	15/19
General malaise	6/17
Loss of appetite	1/17
Myelosuppression	5/17
Leukopenia 3	
Anemia 1	
Leukopenia and anemia 1	
Hepatic dysfunction	3/17
Renal dysfunction	1/17

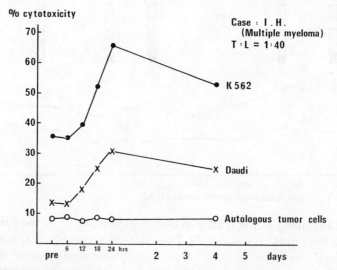

Fig. 3.   Natural killer activity.

NK activity against K-562 in all 8 patients following IFN-β treatment is shown in Fig. 4. After an injection, there was an initial decrease at 6 hours in some patients, followed by an increase above the pretreatment level, and the majority of the patients reached the highest NK activity at 18–24 hours, mainly at 24 hours. Thereafter, NK activity decreased even with daily I.V. infusions of IFN, but usually remained above pretreatment levels.

Autologous tumor cells were stored in 4 patients and lymphocyte cytotoxicity was done in these patients (Fig. 5). Two of them had 5–10% cytotoxicity before IFN treatment, but the other 2 showed almost no cytotoxicity. Following treatment, none of the patients demonstrated an increase of cytotoxicity, although NK activity was enhanced.

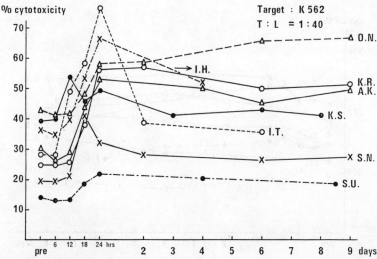

Fig. 4. Natural killer activity.

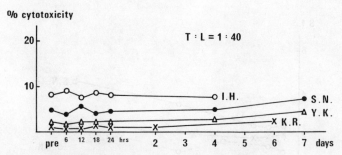

Fig. 5. Autologous tumor cell kill activity.

Tests of lymphocyte blastogenic responses to nonspecific mitogens were done in 8 patients. Because the responses to PWM and Con A were similar, only the results using PHA are shown in Fig. 6. There were slight decreases in some patients at 6 hours following IFN injection, but in general, blastogenic responses remained unchanged before and after treatment.

Figure 7 shows the results of MLTR which were done in 4 patients. One patient indicated a slight increase in SI at 7 and 14 days after IFN treatment, but no change was seen in the others. *In vivo* sensitization was performed in these 4 patients, but *in vitro* generation of cytotoxic cells induced by autologous tumor cells was not observed before or after IFN therapy. Even the patient who showed a slight increase of MLTR after treatment had no change in *in vitro* sensitization.

The changes in skin test reactivity to recall antigens are shown in Table 3.

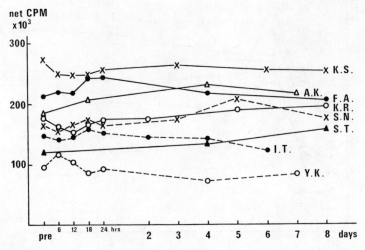

Fig. 6.   Lymphocyte blastogenic response to PHA.

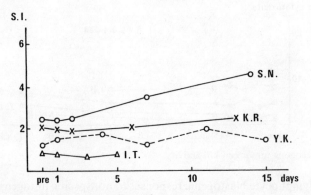

Fig. 7.   Mixed lymphocyte tumor cellr eaction.

Most patients had 100% or more increase in skin test reactivity to all the recall antigens after IFN injections.

DISCUSSION

There have been several reports that leukocyte interferon (HuIFN-α) was useful for various types of malignant diseases, such as Hodgkin's disease, non-Hodgkin's lymphoma, multiple myeloma, acute leukemia, breast cancer, and so on. HuIFN-α is expensive and relatively difficult to obtain in large quantities. HuIFN-β is produced from a human fibroblast cell line and can be relatively

Table 3. Delayed-type hypersensitivity reaction (induration mm).

		Before	1 wk	2 wks	3 wks	4 wks	5 wks
S.N.	PPD	7 × 5	4 × 5	8 × 7	15 × 13	7 × 8	8 × 7
	Candida	14 × 13	10 × 7	13 × 10	12 × 12	15 × 15	10 × 8
	Varidase	8 × 8	15 × 15	35 × 33	33 × 25	23 × 25	25 × 23
A.K.	PPD	0 × 0	3 × 3	2 × 2		4 × 4	
	Candida	0 × 0	3 × 3	0 × 0		4 × 4	
	Varidase	0 × 0	10 × 10	10 × 10		18 × 14	
O.N.	PPD	34 × 42		52 × 57		48 × 38	
	Candida	30 × 22		52 × 40		64 × 50	
	Varidase	23 × 25		80 × 50		100 × 60	
K.S.	PPD	0 × 0				7 × 7	
	Candida	0 × 0				6 × 6	
	Varidase	19 × 18				40 × 32	
S.T.	PPD	10 × 10			20 × 20		
	Candida	11 × 11			20 × 20		
	Varidase	23 × 20			43 × 34		
Y.K.	PPD	5 × 5		0 × 0		0 × 0	
	Candida	9 × 8		0 × 0		0 × 0	
	Varidase	13 × 12		30 × 18		10 × 10	
L.K.	PPD	8 × 8			10 × 10		
	Candida	10 × 11			10 × 10		
	Varidase	20 × 20			40 × 30		

easily obtained in large quantities. If the efficacy of IFN-β in the treatment of malignant diseases is proven, it may become more widely used.

In Canada, in a phase I study of IFN-β, 4 patients with colon cancer and one patient with renal cell carcinoma showed no progression of the disease with this drug.[7] The clinical effect of HuIFN-β in our present study was less impressive. This result may be due to the patients' status, as the majority of the patients had advanced disease when IFN therapy was started. We still do not know the optimal dose and schedule for IFN-β administration, and these factors may also have contributed to our poor response. However, it is interesting that one patient with B-CLL achieved a partial remission with HuIFN-β. The WBC count dropped rapidly after starting IFN, which suggested that there was a direct cytotoxic activity against CLL cells. We must accumulate more cases to confirm the antitumor activity of IFN-β and to evaluate its mechanism of action. We also need to determine the optimal dose and schedule for the best clinical results.

The side-effects were all tolerable and did not require the cessation of IFN treatment.

IFN has been shown to have an antitumor effect mediated by the immune system, in addition to its direct cytocidal effect. From experimental animal studies it has been concluded that the immune mediated antitumor effects of

IFN are due to the enhancement of three factors: NK activity, phagocytosis, and the cytotoxicity of sensitized lymphocytes. Our present study clearly demonstrated the enhancement of NK activity as we observed an increase shortly after IFN administration and the highest activity 24 hours later. Einhorn *et al.*[8] and Huddlestone *et al.*[9] reported a peak NK activity at 12 hours and at 18 hours after HuIFN-α treatment, respectively. Our data using HuIFN-β is similar, although the point of highest activity is a little later.

In contrast to NK activity, lymphocyte cytotoxicity to autologous tumor cells was not enhanced by IFN-β treatment. The reason for this phenomenon is unknown, but there are several possible explanations. First, frozen-stored tumor cells may have a lower NK sensitivity than culture lines do. Vánky *et al.*[10] reported that an enhancement of NK activity against established cell lines was induced after the incubation of lymphocytes with IFN-α *in vitro*, but that auttologous lymphocyte-mediated cytotoxicity using fresh tumor cells or frozen tumor cells was not enhanced. They observed, however, that after 5–6 days of cultivation of the tumor cells, the cytotoxic sensitivity increased. Second, there may be only small number of cytotoxic cells that can recognize tumor-specific antigens. Third, IFN-β may enhance only NK activity without increasing cytotoxic T-cell activity, which means that the IFN will affect only nonspecific tumor cell toxicity.

A mild increase of MLTR was observed in only one patient after IFN treatment but *in vitro* sensitization to study the generation of cytotoxic cells was negative in all patients. These data suggest that IFN-β has limited activity in the stimulation of tumor specific immune reactions. However, the number of patients was small, and we will need more opportunities to investigate the activation of tumor-specific immunity. It is especially important to determine whether generation and/or activation of cytotoxic T-cells are actually induced by IFN-β.

The present study has shown that all the patients had enhanced NK activity after IFN treatment, although most of them experienced a clinical progression of disease. This may suggest that there is no correlation between NK activity and clinical course. However, the majority of the patients had advanced tumors and carried bulky tumor masses, so it is possible that greater NK activity might not induce clinical improvement in the patients with a large tumor burden. Therefore, it is essential to assess the correlation between IFN-β-induced enhancement of NK activity and the clinical course in patients with a small tumor burden, that is, in the early stages of a malignant disease.

Acknowledgment

The authors are grateful to Ms. K. Abe for her excellent technical assistance.

REFERENCES

1. Strander, H.: Interferons: Anti-neoplastic drugs? *Blut*, **35**: 277–288, 1977.
2. Blomgren, H., Cantell, K., Johansson, B., Lagergren, C., Ringborg, U., and Strander, H.: Interferon therapy in Hodgkin's disease. *Acta Med. Scand.*, **199**: 527–532, 1976.
3. Merigan, T., Sikora, K., Breeden, J. H., Levy, R., and Rosenberg, S. A.: Preliminary observation on the effect of human leukocyte interferon in non-Hodgkin's lymphoma. *N. Engl. J. Med.*, **299**: 1449–1453, 1978.
4. Mellstedt, H., Ahre, A., Bjorkholm, M., Holm, G., Johansson, B., and Strander, H.: Interferon therapy in myelomatosis. *Lancet*, **1**: 245–247, 1979.
5. Hill, N. O., Loeb, E., Pardue, A. S., Dorn, G. L., Khan, A., and Hill, J. M.: Response of acute leukemia to leukocyte interferon. *J. Clin. Hematol. Oncol.*, **9**: 137–149, 1979.
6. Gutterman, J. U., Yap, Y., Buzdar, A., Alexanian, R., Hersh, E. M., Cabanillas, F., and Greenberg, S.: Leukocyte interferon induced tumor regression in patients with breast cancer and B-cell neoplasms. *Proc. Am. Assoc. Cancer Res.*, **20**: 167, 1979.
7. MacPherson, T. A. and Tan, Y. H.: Phase I study of human fibroblast interferon in human malignancy. *Proc. Amer. Soc. Clin. Oncol.*, **20**: 378, 1979.
8. Einhorn, S., Blomgren, H., and Strander, H.: Interferon and spontaneous cytotoxicity in man. *Acta Med. Scand.*, **204**: 477–483, 1978.
9. Huddlestone, J., Merigan, T. C., and Oldstone, M. B. A.: Induction and kinetics of natural killer cells in human following interferon therapy. *Nature*, **282**: 417–419, 1979.
10. Vánky, F. T., Argos, S. A., Einhorn, S. A., and Klein, E.: Role of alloantigens in natural killing. Allogeneic but not autologous tumor biopsy cells are sensitive for interferon-induced cytotoxicity of human blood lymphocytes. *J. Exp. Med.*, **151**: 1151–1165, 1980.

Discussion

Dr. LEVY: Dr. Ogawa, I wonder if you could tell me what the source of your interferon was.

Dr. OGAWA: It was fibroblast interferon.

Dr. LEVY: Made here in Japan?

Dr. OGAWA: Yes. By Toray Company.

Dr. KOBAYASHI: In the side effects, you had 3 cases of hepatotoxicity. They were not hepatoma patients, were they?

Dr. OGAWA: Yes, they were. A transient reversible change in SGOT or SGPT was observed, but it did not become any obstacle to the treatment.

Dr. KOBAYASHI: So there was no effect on hepatoma?

Dr. OGAWA: No, no effect at all.

Dr. KOBAYASHI: Now I would like to ask you or Dr. Shimoyama, the next speaker, to comment on the following point. We observed one case of a 50-year old man who had hepatoma with liver cirrhosis. E antigen was positive by the RIA method. We administered 3 million units of fibroblast interferon dissolved in 4 ml per day by continuous arterial infusion using chronofuser for about 30 days. The total amount given was 100 million units. After 40 days, neither angiogram nor CT revealed any change in the size of the major tumor in the liver. The level of AFP decreased from

1700 ng/ml to 900 ng/ml after 2 weeks, and then increased to 1600 ng/ml after 40 days. During that time, neither fever nor pain was observed. I would like to have your or Dr. Shimoyama's comment on this continuous arterial infusion method.

Dr. OGAWA: We have chosen hepatoma patients because we supposed the virus had something to do with the disease. Unfortunately, the treatment was not effective for the 2 cases, maybe because the systemic condition of the patients was not so good. As for your continuous arterial infusion method, I believe it is very attractive. If we compare this arterial infusion method with conventional systemic chemotherapy, the former appears to be more effective. If we can get the direct cytocidal effect of fibroblast interferon, this infusion method will be very attractive.

Dr. SHIMOYAMA: I would like to make a comment on this point. Interferon has cytocidal activity to a certain type of cancer cell. In this case, the higher the concentration of interferon, the more the effect is potentiated. I think the key is how we can sustain the concentration.

Dr. BEKTIMIROV: In your clinical trial, why has the age of patients been limited to under 75? Are there any data concerning a correlation between the age of patients and their response to interferon? And also could you comment, if possible, on the relationship between age and natural killer activity of lymphocytes?

Dr. OGAWA: We thought that older patients might not be able to tolerate the interferon therapy because of its side effects. Therefore we limited the age to 75. Concerning the relation between age and natural killer activity, I do not have the exact answer.

Clinical and Experimental Studies of Antitumor Activ man Fibroblast Interferon

Masanori SHIMOYAMA, Takeshi KITAHARA, Masanori NAKAZAWA, Tohru ISE, Isamu ADACHI, Shigeaki YOSHIDA, and Heizaburo ICHIKAWA

Department of Internal Medicine and Pediatrics, Natinoal Cancer Center Hospital, Tokyo

SUMMARY

Preliminary phase I and II studies of human fibroblast interferon were conducted in 12 patients with malignant disease. In addition, the antitumor activity of HuIFN-β against various tissue culture cell lines and transplantable ascitic tumors derived from malignant human tumors in athymic nude mice was investigated.

HuIFN-β was given daily I.V. in doses of 1.5 to 6.0 $\times$ 10^6 IU for about 6 to 30 days, or by I.T. injections once every 2 to 3 days in doses of 0.6 to 9.0 $\times$ 10^6 IU. The side-effects of IFN included low- to high-grade fever after both I.V. and I.T. injections, fatigue, and slight anorexia. Myelosuppression was minimal. When IFN was given by I.T. injection, tumor regression was observed only at the injection sites in 2 patients, one with cutaneous T-cell lymphoma and another with rhabdomyosarcoma, but regression was not seen in tumors without the injections. Other patients who received I.T. injection of IFN (2 with breast cancer, one each with gastric cancer and lymphoma) had no tumor regression. Four patients with lymphoma, one with brain tumor, and one with rhabdomyosarcoma were treated with I.V. injections of IFN without tumor regression.

The blood levels of HuIFN-β were measured in 3 patients who were given 3 or 6 $\times$ 10^6 IU I.V. The level peaked (at about 200 IU/ml) just after the injection, followed by a rapid decrease for the next few hours. No trace of IFN was detected in the blood of one patient with lymphoma who was given 6 $\times$ 10^6 IU without any side-effects.

The growth activity of most of the 11 tissue culture cell lines derived from hematologic malignancies was inhibited by HuIFN-β at a concentration of more than 1 $\times$ 10^4 IU/ml. However, the concentration required for *in vitro* growth inhibition of cultured leukemia and lymphoma cells were much higher than the blood levels obtained after the I.V. injection of 3 to 6 $\times$ 10^6 IU of IFN. Athymic nude mice bearing transplantable ascitic human breast cancer cells (Hattori) survived for a long time

213

only when they were treated with daily I. P. injections of 1×10^7 IU/kg of IFN for 10 days; both daily injections of 1×10^6 IU/kg and single injections of 1×10^8 IU/kg of IFN were not effective. Similarly, athymic nude mice bearing transplantable ascitic human T-acute lymphocytic leukemia (Ichikawa) survived for a long time only when they were treated with daily I.P. injections of 1×10^8 IU/kg of IFN for 10 days, while both daily injections of less than 1×10^7 IU/kg and single injections of 1×10^8 IU/kg were not effective. These findings indicate that one of the reasons why the I.V. injection of HuIFN-β was not effective at all, while the I.T. injection was effective only at the injection sites in the same patients, may be that tumor cells have a low sensitivity to HuIFN-β and the blood level obtained after I.V. injection is insufficient.

INTRODUCTION

The mechanism of antitumor activity by interferon (IFN) has not yet been fully elucidated. It has been reported that IFN can inhibit cell growth of *in vitro* cultured cells at reasonably low concentrations[1-5] and can cause bone marrow suppression as well as hair loss when given systemically to the patient.[6] These results suggest that the main mechanism of antitumor activity is the direct cytocidal action of IFN rather than its indirect antitumor action through immunologic potentiation.

We conducted experiments to measure the *in vitro* sensitivity of cultured cell lines to human fibroblast interferon (HuIFN-β; Toray Industries, Inc.) and to test *in vivo* the chemotherapeutic effects of HuIFN-β on transplantable ascitic tumors derived from cultured human cancer cell lines in athymic nude mice. We also undertook, preliminary phase I and phase II studies of HuIFN-β in patients with malignant diseases.

MATERIALS AND METHODS

The cultured cell lines used in this experiment were as follows: SEKI/Melanoma[7] derived from melanoma; Okajima/stomach ca.[8] derived from stomach cancer; OAT[9] derived from oat cell caricinoma of the lung; MOLT3,[10] P12/Ichikawa,[11] and RPMI-8402/Sommer[12] derived from T-cell type acute lymphocytic leukemia (ALL); Daudi[13] and P3HRI[14] derived from Burkitt's lymphoma; NALL-1[15] derived from nonTnonB ALL; HL-60[16] derived from acúte promyelocytic leukemia; and K-562[17] derived from chronic myelogenous leukemia in blastic crisis. These were cultured in RPMI 1640 medium supplemented with 10% fetal calf serum (FCS; GIVCO) at 37°C in a CO_2 incubator (Forma Scientific Co.).

Growth inhibition of cultured cells by HuIFN-β was measured quantitatively by the modified extrapolation method of Alexander *et al.*[18] HuIFN-β was dissolved in RPMI 1640 medium supplemented with 10% FCS immediately before use and each cultured cell suspension at a concentration of 10^5/ml was incubated with an appropriate concentration of the IFN at 37°C for 3 days in the CO_2 incubator. After a cell count was made with each culture tube, the cells were washed and resuspended, or diluted if necessary, in IFN-free culture medium for further growth. The culture medium was changed every 3 days, and the cell count was made at least once every 2 to 3 days until a constant exponential cell growth was obtained. The surviving fraction of cells exposed to IFN was calculated from each growth curve by the extrapolation method of Alexander et al.[18]

Animal experiments were performed with two strains: the Ichikawa strain,[19] which is an ascitic T-cell leukemia cell line in athymic nude mice established from an early culture of P12/Ichikawa,[11] and the Hattori strain,[20] an ascitic breast cancer cell line in athymic nude mice which was established from a cultured Hattori/breast cancer[21] cell line. As reported previously,[22] all athymic nude mice inoculated with over 10^6 Ichikawa cells developed ascites and pleural effusion and died of the disease. A distinct correlation between the survival time and the number of tumor cells inoculated was observed.[22] In this experiment, 10^8 cells were inoculated intraperitoneally (I.P.) into athymic nude mice. The treatment was started 48 hours after the inoculation. All the mice inoculated with over 5×10^6 Hattori cells developed ascites and died of the disease.[20] In the present experiment 5×10^7 cells were inoculated I.P. into athymic nude mice and the treatment was started 48 hours after the inoculation. HuIFN-β was given I.P. as single-dose therapy or as daily-dose therapy for 10 days. Athymic nude mice, 6 to 10 weeks old with a BALB/c genetic background, were supplied by the Central Institute for Experimental Animals, Kawasaki, Japan. They were kept in a vinyl isolator under specific-pathogen-free conditions with sterile food and water.

Preliminary clinical phase I and II studies were conducted in patients with malignant lymphomas or solid cancers, who had become refractory to conventional chemotherapy. HuIFN-β was given intravenously (I.V.) daily at a dose of 1.5 to 6×10^6 international units (IU) or intratumorally (I.T.) at a dose of 0.3 to 1.0×10^6 IU in a single site once every 2 to 3 days. The antitumor effect was assesed by regression in tumor size.

Blood concentrations of IFN were measured by Shudo Yamazaki, M.D., at the National Institute of Health. Details of the method are described elsewhere in this book.[23]

RESULTS

Sensitivity of Various Cultured Cell Lines to HuIFN-β

The concentrations of HuIFN-β required for 90% growth inhibition (IC_{90}) are listed in Table 1. Daudi is the most sensitive cell line, with IC_{90} of 1×10^3 IU/ml. P3HRI, RPMI-8402/Sommer, P12/Ichikawa, NALL-1, and SEKI/Melanoma are low-sensitive, with IC_{90} of about 1 to 2×10^4 IU/ml, while the other 5 cell lines, Okajima/Stomach ca., MOLT3, OAT, HL-60, and K-562, are quite resistant, with IC_{90} more than 1×10^5 IU/ml.

Table 1. Concentrations of HuIFN-β required for 90% inhibition of growth in various cultured cell lines.

Cell lines	IC_{90} (IU/ml)
SEKI/Melanoma	2×10^4
OKAJIMA/Stomach ca.	1×10^5
MOLT3	$> 10^5$
P12/Ichikawa	2×10^4
RPMI–8402/Sommer	8×10^3
Daudi	1×10^3
P3HR1	8×10^3
OAT	$> 10^5$
NALL-1	2×10^4
HL-60	$> 10^5$
K562	$> 10^5$

Effect of HuIFN-β on Transplantable Ascitic Human T-cell Type of Acute Lymphocytic Leukemia Cell Line: (Ichikawa) and breast cancer cell line (Hattori) in athymic nude mice

As shown in Table 2, the survival time of athymic nude mice transplanted I.P. with 1×10^8 cells of the Ichikawa cell line was not affected by I.P. single dose therapy of up to 1×10^8 IU/kg of HuIFN-β nor was it influenced I.P. daily injections of 1×10^7 IU/kg or less of IFN administered for 10 days starting 48 hours after the inoculation with cancer cells. But the survival time increased significantly when the mice were treated with daily injections of 1×10^8 IU of IFN for 10 days.

Table 2. Chemotherapeutic effect of HuIFN-β on athymic nude mice bearing ascitic Ichikawa cells.

Treatment schedule	Dose (IU/kg/day)	Total dose (IU/kg)	ILS (%)	100–day survivors
Day 2	1×10^7	1×10^7	4	0/3
(single)	1×10^8	1×10^8	9	0/3
Day 2–11	1×10^6	1×10^7	4	0/3
(daily, 10 days)	1×10^7	1×10^8	30	0/7
	1×10^8	1×10^9	96	0/3

The survival time of athymic nude mice transplanted I.P. with 5×10^7 cells of the Hattori cell line was markedly increased by I.P. daily injections of 1×10^7 IU/kg of IFN for 10 days starting 48 hours after the inoculation, 7 of 8 mice were 100-days survivors, while all of the control mice and mice treated with a daily dose of 1×10^6 IU/kg or less for 10 days were dead within 25 days after the inoculation (Table 3). A single injection of up to 1×10^8 IU/kg of IFN given 48 hours after the inoculation was not effective at all, as shown in Table 3.

Table 3. Chemotherapeutic effect of HuIFN-β on athymic nude mice bearing ascitic Hattori cells.

Treatment schedule	Dose (IU/kg/day)	Total dose (IU/kg)	ILS (%)	100–day survivors
Day 2	1×10^7	1×10^7	16	0/3
(single)	1×10^8	1×10^8	−11	0/3
Day 2–11	1×10^6	1×10^7	−26	0/6
(daily, 10 days)	1×10^7	1×10^8	>526	7/8

Preliminary Phase I and Phase II Studies of HuIFN-β

Two patients with B-cell lymphoma and one each with nonTnonB lymphoblastic lymphoma, Hodgkin's disease, rhabdomyosarcoma, and medulloblastoma were treated daily I.V. with 1 to 6×10^6 IU of HuIFN-β for 6 to 30 days. No antitumor effect was observed in these patients at all. Three patients had a transient fever after the injection. Two patients had leukocytopenia and thrombocytopenia. Slight anorexia and fatigability was observed in 3 patients. (Table 4).

The effect of I.T. injections of IFN was tested in 6 patients with various kinds of malignancies. In 2 of the 6 patients, tumor regression was observed only at the injection sites. In one patient with rhabdomyosarcoma, I.T. injection of IFN was effective, while I.V. injection was not.

Fever was observed in 2 of 3 patients who were given more than 3×10^6 IU of IFN I.T. No other side-effects were observed.

Blood levels of HuIFN-β were measured in a few patients to whom IFN was given I.V. as shown in Fig. 1. The serum concentration of IFN reached a peak, about 200 IU/ml, immediately after the I.V. injection of 3×10^6 IU of IFN. The level decreased rapidly within the first 60 min, then fell off gradually, and was not detected at 6 hours after the injection. Curiously enough, IFN was not detected at all in the serum of one patient with B-cell lymphoma, even though 6×10^6 IU of HuIFN-β was injected I.V.

DISCUSSION

HuIFN-β can inhibit *in vitro* growth of various cultured cells derived from human malignant diseases. However, the concentration required to inhibit cell

Table 4.   Clinical trial of HuIFN-β.

Case	Diagnosis	Dose ×10⁶ IU	Total dose ×10⁶ IU	Anti-tumor effect	Side-effect			Others
					Fever	Before/nadir WBC ×10³/µl	Platelets ×10⁴/µl	
I) S I) Systemic injection (I.V.)								
1. TM:	B-lymphoma	3–6	126	—	—	2.4 → 1.9	10.2 → 5.9	Anorexia, fatigue
2. SS:	B-lymphoma	3	84	—	—	—	—	Anorexia, fatigue
3. FT:	Lymphoblastic-lymphoma	3	24	—	37–38°C	—	—	
4. HH:	Hodgkin's disease	3	75	—	37–38°C	—	—	Anorexia, fatigue
5. UM:	Rhabdomyosar-coma	1.5–3	12	—	38°C	—	—	
6. AM:	Medulloblastoma	1–3	44	—	—	5.3 → 2.1	15.4 → 5.9	—
II) Intratumoral injection								
7. SS:	B-lymphoma	3–6	18	—	38–39°C	—	—	—
8. UA:	Cutaneous T-cell lymphoma	3–6	24	+	38–39°C	—	—	—
9. UM:	Rhabdomyosarcoma	0.6–3	68	+, −	38–39°C	—	—	—
10. HM:	Stomach ca	0.6–1	10	—	—	—	—	—
11. MT:	Breast ca	0.3–1	<10	—	—	—	—	—
12. MY:	Breast ca	0.3–1	<10	—	—	—	—	—

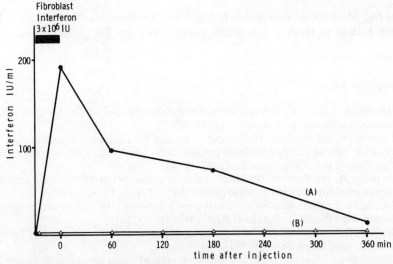

Fig. 1.   Blood level of HuIFN-β after I.V. drip infusion of 3 × 10⁶ IU.

growth by 90 % was much higher than the maximum serum concentration obtained after I.V. injection of 3 × 10⁶ IU of IFN into the patients. Thus, HuIFN-β may be ineffective when it is given intravenously, but effective when it is given intratumorally, because it is thought that the effective concentration is obtained only when HuIFN-β is given intratumorally. This hypothesis was confirmed in one patient with rhabdomyosarcoma who was treated with I.V. and I.T. infections of IFN sequentially; I.T. injection was effective while I.V. injection was not. This finding indicates that one mode of antitumor activity by HuIFN-β is its direct growth-inhibiting action. In animal experiments using athymic nude mice inoculated with a transplantable human cancer cell line, only a massive daily dose therapy of HuIFN-β was effective. Based on this animal experiment, the effective dose of HuIFN-β to adult patients with 50 kg body weight would be 500 × 10⁶ IU or more. This dose is at least 170 times greater than the regular dose used in clinical trials, at the present time, suggesting that systemic administration of IFN would not be effective until massive dose therapy can be given safely to cancer patients. The purity of the IFN is not adequate and is said to be less than 1 %, so that further purification is necessary.

The side-effects we noted were almost the same as those already reported.[6] However, bone marrow suppression was rather mild compared with that observed in leukocyte IFN therapy.

Acknowledgment

This work was supported in part by a Grant-in-Aid for Cancer Research from the Ministry of Health and Welfare, a Grant-in-Aid for Cancer Research from the Ministry of Education, Science and Culture, and the entrusted Research Fund for Human Fibroblast Interferon from Toray Industries, Inc.

REFERENCES

1. Hilfenhaus, J. et al.: Growth inhibition of human lymphoblastoid Daudi cells in vitro by interferon preparation. Arch. Virol., 51: 87, 1976.
2. Einhorn, S. and Strander, H.: Interferon therapy for neoplastic disease in man. In: W. R. Stinebring and P. J. Chapple (eds.), Human Interferon Production and Clinical Use. Plenum Pub. Corp., New York, 1977, p. 159.
3. Strander, H. and Einhorn, S.: Effect of human leucocyte interferon on the growth of human osteosarcoma cells in tissue culture. Int. J. Cancer, 19: 468, 1977.
4. Lee, S. H. S. et al.: Interferon induced growth depression in diploid and heteroploid human cells. Proc. Soc. Exp. Biol. Med., 139: 1438, 1972.
5. Gaffney, E. V. et al.: Inhibition of growth and transformation of human cells by interferon. J. Natl. Cancer Inst., 50: 871, 1973.
6. Gutterman, J. U. et al.: Leucocyte interferon-induced tumor regression in human metastatic breast cancer, multiple myeloma, and malignant lymphoma. Ann. Int. Med., 93: 399, 1980.
7. Shimoyama, M. et al.: Establishment of cultured melanoma cell line (SEKI). Proc. Japan Assoc. Cancer Res., 30: 219, 1971.
8. Minato, K. et al.: Unpublished data.
9. Ohboshi, T. et al.: A new floating cell line derived from human pulmonary carcinoma of oat cell type. GANN, 62: 505, 1971.
10. Minowada, J. et al.: Rosette-forming human lymphoid cell line. I. Establishment and evidence for origin of thymusderived lymphocytes. J. Natl. Cancer Inst., 49: 891, 1972.
11. Shimoyama, M. et al.: Cultured lymphoblastic cell line of T-cell type derived from T-acute lymphocytic leukemia. Acta Haematol. Jpn., 40: 734, 1977. (in Japanese).
12. Sahai Srirastera, B. I. et al.: J. Natl. Cancer Inst., 55: 11, 1975.
13. Klein, E. et al.: Surface IgM-kappa specificity on a Burkitt lymphoma cell in vivo and in vitro derived culture lines. Cancer Res., 28: 1300, 1968.
14. Hinuma, Y. et al.: Cloning of immunoglobulin-producing human leukemic and lymphoma cells in long-term cultures. Proc. Soc. Exp. Biol. Med., 24: 107, 1967.
15. Miyoshi, I. et al.: Human B-cells, T-cells and null cell leukemic cell lines derived from acute lymphoblastic leukemias. Nature, 267: 843, 1977.
16. Collins, S. et al.: Continuous growth and differentiation of human myeloid leukemic cells in suspension culture. Nature, 270: 347, 1977.
17. Lozzio, C. B. et al.: Human chronic myelogenous leukemia cell line with positive Philadelphia chromosome. Blood, 45: 321, 1975.
18. Alexander, P.: Mouse lymphoma cells with different radiosensitivities. Nature, 192: 572, 1961.
19. Kitahara, T. et al.: Establishment of a serially transplantable human acute leukemia cell line in nude mice in ascites form. Acta Haematol. Jpn., 4: 140, 1978.
20. Kitahara, T. et al.: Chemotherapeutic effects of various anticancer agents against nude mice bearing ascitic Hattori cells. Proc. Japan Assoc. Cancer Res., 36: 147, 1977.
21. Minato, K. et al.: Establishment of two cultured human cancer cell lines: Hattori/breast ca. derived from pleural effusion of breast cancer patient and Saito cell line derived from cancer patients of unknown origin. Proc. Japan Assoc. Cancer Res., 33: 5, 1974.

22. Kitahara, T.: Establishment of a human leukemia cell line in nude mice and its application to the screening system of antileukemic agents. *Acta Haematol. Jpn.*, **43**: 1034, 1980.
23. Yamazaki, S. *et al.*: in press.

Discussion

Dr. YAMAMOTO: In my experiments using poly IC, the longer administration was effective but the short administration was not. Could you explain the reason for this?

Dr. SHIMOYAMA: In *in vitro* growth inhibition experiments with fibroblast interferon, longer exposure to the interferon usually results in a stronger growth inhibition of cultured tumor cells than shorter exposure. Therefore, I think that longer exposure to the interferon is essential for better effect.

Dr. VILČEK: I have a question and a comment concerning your experiments in nude mice. My question is how did you administer the fibroblast interferon, and did you check how much of this is demonstrable in the circulation of the nude mice?

Dr. SHIMOYAMA: It was an intraperitoneal injection. We did not measure the concentration in blood nor in the ascites.

Dr. VILČEK: And the tumor also grew intraperitoneally, so that there was certainly direct contact?

Dr. SHIMOYAMA: That's right.

Dr. VILČEK: In that case, my comment is probably not quite appropriate, but I will make it anyway. There is a certain amount of cross-reaction of human interferon into mouse cells. So you at least run the theoretical risk of activating NK cells or perhaps some other defense mechanisms in the mouse if you really inject huge doses of human interferon.

Dr. SHIMOYAMA: Because of lack of data, I cannot comment on this point.

Dr. MACHIDA: In relation to Dr. Vilček's comment, I believe that you used human interferon in the nude mouse because you wanted to see the direct action.

Dr. SHIMOYAMA: Yes.

Dr. MACHIDA: In clinical applications, it appears to me that it is almost impossible to sustain such a high concentration level.

Dr. SHIMOYAMA: Yes, with current products it is quite impossible.

Dr. MACHIDA: However, as was reported this morning, some cases of topical administration showed a good response. In many cases lymphocyte infiltration was also observed. So it might be better if you use mice interferon as well as human interferon to compare them in nude mice.

Dr. SHIMOYAMA: If we can get mouse interferon, I want to do such an experiment.

Effect of Human Leukocyte Interferon on Metastatic Lung Tumor of Osteosarcoma and Primary Lung Cancer

Shinjiro Ban,* Tetsuo Yamagiwa,* Tetsuji Yanagawa,⁴* Kisaburo Sakakida,* Hidemoto Ito,²* Koichi Murakami,²* Akio Matsuo,³* Jiro Imanishi,³* and Tsunataro Kishida³*

*Departments of Orthopaedic Surgery, ²*Radiology, and ³*Microbiology, Kyoto Prefectural University of Medicine, Kyoto, ⁴*Clinic of Orthopaedic Surgery, National Maizuru Hospital, Kyoto, Japan

INTRODUCTION

Human interferon (IFN) was first used clinically as an antitumor agent against osteosarcoma by Strander,[1] who demonstrated that human leukocyte interferon (HuIFN-α) could prevent pulmonary metastasis in cases of osteosarcoma. However there have been no reports dealing with the antitumor effect of human IFN on established pulmonary metastases in such cases. In the present study, IFN was used for the osteosarcoma patients after pulmonary metastases were detected. Four patients were treated with intravenous (I.V.) or intramuscular (I.M.) administration of HuIFN-α. A transient effect from the IFN treatment was apparent in 2 cases, but not in the other 2.

We also injected IFN into 5 patients with primary lung cancer, but there was no apparent inhibition of tumor growth.

MATERIALS AND METHODS

HuIFN-α was induced by Sendai virus (hemagglutinating virus of Japan (HVJ)) in human peripheral leukocytes which had been primed with 100 IU/ml of HuIFN-α for 2 hours at 37°C. Twenty hours later, this preparation was harvested and acidified to pH 2 with HCl in order to inactivate the residual inducing virus.

Two days later, the pH level was adjusted to 3.0 with 1 N NaOH. It was concentrated and purified by means of SP-Sephadex C-25 chromatography, and

223

further purified by means of gel filtration through a Sephadex G-100 column. This preparation was further concentrated by means of SP-Sephadex C-25 chromatography, filtrated with a millipore filter for sterilization, lyophilized, and stored at 4°C. Immediately before administration, it was dissolved in a physiological saline solution. Its specific activity was 3×10^5 IU/mg protein.

Interferon Assay

Interferon activity was assayed by means of microtiter and plaque reduction methods which have been described elsewhere in detail.[2]

Cell Growth Inhibition

The tumor cells from the pleural exudate of the first case were cultivated and examined for the sensitivity of the tumor cells to HuIFN-α. We cultivated together 1.5×10^4 tumor cells/ml and 2,000 IU/ml of HuIFN-α in Eagle's MEM supplemented with 10% fetal bovine serum. The viable cells were counted by means of trypan blue dye exclusion testing at 3, 7, 11, 16, and 23 days after incubation in a 5% CO_2 humidified atmosphere at 37°C.

CLINICAL USE OF HuIFN-α FOR OSTEOSARCOMA: FOUR CASE REPORTS

Case 1

A 29-year old woman suffered from osteosarcoma of the distal femur. Nine months after the transfemoral amputation pulmonary metastases were detected and 8 months later she was admitted to our hospital for interferon treatment. Two or 3 times a week, 3×10^6 IU of HuIFN-α were administered, mainly I.V.

Three months after the interferon treatment, the growth rate of one metastasized tumor mass had declined. About months later, the metastatic lesions were irradiated with a small dose of ^{60}Co which may have had no effect on the tumor mass.

The size of one tumor was reduced by treatment with a total dosage of 58 $\times 10^6$ IU of IFN (Fig. 1). Some of the other tumors were diminished in varying degrees during the IFN treatment and no change was noted in others. The patient finally died of dyspnea by increased pleural effusion.

Elevated serum alkaline phosphatase levels rapidly returned to normal with IFN treatment, but increased again one month before death. The tuberculin skin reaction, which had been negative before treatment, became positive 3 months afterward. Subjective symptoms such as night sweats and anorexia were improved during therapy with 50×10^6 IU of IFN. No side-effects were observed except transient leukopenia.

Tumor cells from the pleural exudate of this patient were isolated and

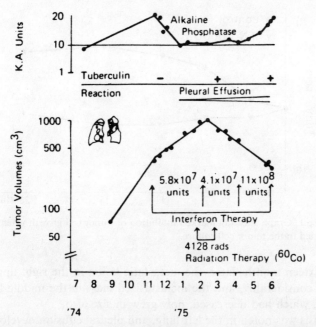

Fig. 1. Case 1. Diagram showing effect of HuIFN-α on pulmonary metastasis from osteosarcoma. Three months after IFN treatment, the growth rate of a metastasized tumor mass lessened, and 3 months later, the size of tumor was diminished. Elevated serum alkaline phosphatase returned to a normal range with IFN therapy, but increased again one month before death.

cultivated. The sensitivity of these tumor cells to HuIFN-α was determined *in vitro*. When 2,000 IU of IFN was added to the tumor cell culture, there was marked inhibition of tumor cell growth. (Fig. 2).

Case 2

An 18-year-old male with osteosarcoma of the right distal femur was transfemorally amputated. Three months later, a metastatic lesion was found in the lower lobe of the left lung. Thirty days later, he underwent treatment with I.M. injections of HuIFN-α, 250,000 IU twice a week; after 170 days the dose was gradually increased to 3×10^6 IU twice a week.

Eight months after the IFN treatment, the growth rate of the metastatic tumor mass in the right pulmonary lobe decreased, but the pleural exudate increased markedly. Two weeks later, the pleural exudate suddenly declined. The size of the metastatic lesion also shrank rapidly. Twenty days later, the volume of metastatic tumor in the right lung had decreased by a third.

One year after the IFN treatment, one particular metastatic tumor was contracting, while other tumors were growing. The pleural effusion gradually im-

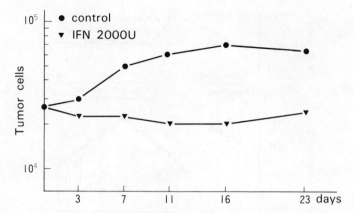

Fig. 2. Case 1. Graph showing marked inhibition of tumor cell growth when 2,000 IU of IFN was added to the tumor cell culture.

proved. Sixteen months later, the metastatic lesion in the right upper lobe a-gain grew considerably, and the metastasized mass in the middle lobe of the right lung, which had decreased, now grew in size also.

Atelectasis was noted in the left lung, and pleural effusion developed again, although the dose of IFN was increased to 5×10^6 IU 6. The left lung did not function at all, and all the metastatic areas grew rapidly. The highly positive tuberculin skin reaction became pseudopositive, suggesting a depression of the host immunity. The patient died about 19 months after the discovery of the pulmonary metastases.

The change of volume in the tumor mass during treatment with IFN is shown in Fig. 3. The size of the metastatic lesion in the lower lobe of the right lung declined 8.5 months after IFN treatment, and by 15 months after the treatment, the volume of the tumor mass had diminished to about one-tenth of the maximum volume. After this, the metastatic lesion grew again, even though the dose of IFN was increased to 5×10^6 IU. The serum alkaline phosphatase level was reduced to a normal level by the IFN therapy. No side-effects were seen except for transient fever.

Case 3

The patient, a 17-year-old boy, was found to have osteosarcoma in the right distal femur, and about a month later, his right femur was amputated. Nine months after the amputation, a metastatic lesion in the left lung as large as 1.5 cm in diameter was detected. The serum alkaline phosphatase level was gradually increasing. Two months after the detection of pulmonary metastases, 3×10^6 IU of HuIFN-α was administered I.M. twice a week.

X-ray examination showed no suppressive effect by the IFN on metastatic

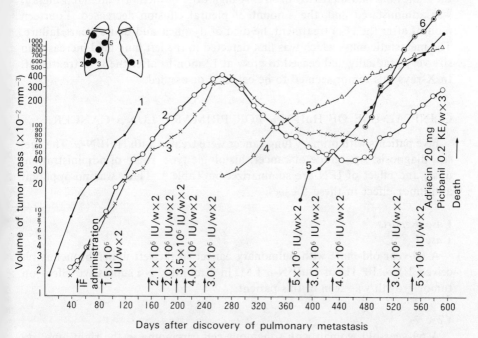

Fig. 3. Case 2. Time course of Changes in the volume of the tumor mass during IFN treatment. Eight and one-half months after treatment, the volume of one tumor mass (No. 2) was reduced and 7 months later, it had diminished to about one-tenth of the maximum volume. Other tumors (Nos. 4 and 5), however, were growing.

tumor growth during treatment until death. Three months after the IFN injections, the number and the size of pulmonary metastase continued to increase. Pleural effusion was also noted. Six months later, this patient died. During the IFN therapy, a negative PPD skin reaction changed to positive, and there was transient leukopenia and fever.

Case 4

A 23-year-old male had osteosarcoma in the right proximal tibia. An amputation above the knee was carried out after the intra-arterial administration of adriamycin. Histologic examination revealed the osteoblastic type of osteosarcoma. Pulmonary metastases were found 8 months after the amputation, and HuIFN-α was administered I.M. At first, the dose of IFN was 5×10^5 IU twice a week, but it was increased to 1×10^6 IU twice a week one month later because of an increase in the number and size of the metastatic masses.

Six months after the IFN treatment, the metastatic mass of the middle lobe of the right lung had increased in size. A high dose of methotrexate (100 mg/kg) was administered and, the amount of pleural effusion decreased. Fourteen months after the IFN treatment, he died of dyspnea and acute heart failure. The metastatic mass which was first detected in the left lung field increased in size very gradually and ceased to grow at 12 months after the IFN treatment. In X-rays this tumor seemed to be calcified or ossified.

CLINICAL USE OF HuIFN-α FOR PRIMARY LUNG CANCER

Five patients with primary lung cancer were treated with HuIFN-α. The age, sex, diagnosis, site, grade of cancer, histologic type, route of administration, dose, and effect of IFN are summarized in Table 1. There was no apparent antitumor effect in these 5 cases.

Case Reports
Case 1
A 69-year-old-male with pulmonary cancer in the left upper bronchus received 1.5 × 10⁸ IU of HuIFN-α I.M. in 3 months. No supressive effect on tumor growth was seen in this patient.

Case 2
A 69-year-old woman with squamous cell carcinoma in the right lung, received a total of 1.11 × 10⁸ IU of HuIFN-α over a 3 month period.

Although a decrease in the growth rate of the tumor mass was observed after the IFN administration, there was no apparent suppressive effect on the tumor growth in this case.

DISCUSSION

The antitumor effect of HuIFN-α on patients with malignancies was first reported by Falcoff *et al.*[3] Since 1972, Strander[1] and his coworkers have treated osteosarcoma patients with HuIFN-α. Their recent work has demonstrated that HuIFN-α was able to prevent the metastasizing of osteosarcoma to the lung and to prolong the survival rate of patients compared with a control group.[4]

In the present study, HuIFN-α was given to 4 patients who alreay had pulmonary metastases. In 2 of the 4 cases, IFN was able to reduce the tumor mass, although the effect was transient. It was observed that there was some reduction of the tumor mass during the treatment.

During the period of reduction, host immunity may also have been at a normal level, as the PPD skin reaction become positive. This may suggest an in-

Table 1. Summary of 5 patients with primary lung cancer treated with HuIFN-α.

Case No.	1	2	3	4	5
Age (Years)/Sex	76/ M	66/ M	69/ M	69/M	70/ M
Site of tumor	Rt. upper bronc.	Rt. B$_3$	Upper bronchus	Rt. B$_6$	Rt. B$_6$
T.N.M.	T$_3$N$_0$M$_0$	T$_3$N$_0$M$_0$	T$_3$N$_0$M$_0$	T$_3$N$_0$M$_0$	
Stage	III	III	III	III	
Pathology	Squamous cell carcinoma	Squamous cell carcinoma	Squamous cell carcinoma	Squamous cell carcinoma	Squamous cell carcinoma
Dose of IFN (IU)	3 × 10^6, 3/Week	3 × 10^6, 3/Week	3 × 10^6, 3/Week	3 × 10^6, 3/Week	3 × 10^5, 3/Week 3 × 10^6,
Route of IFN	I.M.	I.M.	I.M.	I.M.	I.M.
Total dose	5.4 × 10^7 IU	1.98 × 10^8 IU	1.05 × 10^8 IU	1.11 × 10^8 IU	6.12 × 10^7 IU
Effect	(−)	(−)	(−)	(−)	(−)
Skin reaction					
PHA	(±) → (−)	(+) → (−)	(+) → (+)	(±) → (±)	(+) → (+)
PPD	(−) → (−)	(±) → (−)	(+) → (+)	(+) → (+)	(−) → (−)

direct antitumor effect by IFN by the medium from lymphocytes and/or macrophages, but the exact mechanism is still unknown.

We also treated cases of primary lung cancer with HuIFN-α, but there was no apparent evidence of an antitumor effect. Blomgren *et al.*[5] and Strander[1] reported that IFN has a transient effect in Hodgkin's disease and multiple myeloma. It is clear that IFN exerts varying effects on different types of malignancies.

The present study suggests that IFN appliable for the adjuvant treatment of osteosarcoma. Before a complete cure of the cancer can be achieved, a better method of IFN administration will have to be developed. Further studies that examine the mechanism of tumor growth inhibition, side-effects, purification of IFN, and so on will also be necessary for the clinical use of this drug on a large scale.

CONCLUSION

Four patients with osteosarcoma who had pulmonary metastases after the amputation of the affected limb were given HuIFN-α. In 2 cases, the size of the metastasized tumor mass diminished temporarily 6 or 8 months after IFN treatment, and serum alkaline phosphatase levels declined to a normal range. Five other patients with primary lung cancer underwent treatment with HuIFN-α, but there was no apparent evidence of a suppression of tumor growth.

REFERENCES

1. Strander, H., Cantell, K., Jacobsson, P. A., Nilsonne, U., and Söderberg, G.: Exogeneous interferon therapy of osteogenic sarcoma. *Acta Orthop. Scand.*, **45**: 958, 1974.
2. Matsuo, A., Hayashi, S., and Kishida, T.: Production and purification of human leukocyte interferon. *Jap. J. Microbiol.*, **18**: 21–27, 1974.
3. Falcoff, E., Falcoff, R., Fournier, F., and Chany, C.: Production en masse, purification partielle et caractérisation d'un interféron destiné à des essais thérapeutiques humains. *Ann. Inst. Pasteur*, **111**: 562–584, 1966.
4. Adamson, U., Aparisi, T., Bromström, L. A., Cantell, K., Einhorn, S., Hall, K., Ingimarsson, S., Nilsonne, U., Strander, H., and Sönderberg, H.: Interferon treatment of human osteosarcoma. Study week of the Pontifical Academy of Sciences, Vatican City, Oct. 17–21, 1977. "The Role of Non-Specific Immunity in the Prevention and Treatment of Cancer." *Pontificiae Acad. Scient. Scripta Varia*, **43**: 383–406, 1979.
5. Blomgren, H., Cantell, K., Johansson, B., Lagergren, C., Ringborg, U., and Strander, H.: Interferon therapy in Hodgkin's disease. *Acta Med. Scand.*, **199**: 527–532, 1976.

Clinical Use of Human Leukocyte Interferon in Neurogenic Tumors and Other Childhood Tumors

Tadashi SAWADA,* Mutsuhiko TOZAWA,* Takuro KIDOWAKI,* Terufusa TANAKA,* Tomoichi KUSUNOKI,* Yoshio NAKAGAWA,[2]* Kenzo SUZUKI,[2]* Satoshi UEDA,[2]* Kimiyoshi HIRAKAWA,[2]* Tohru OKU,[3]* Masakazu KITA,[3]* and Tsunataro KISHIDA[3]*

Departments of Pediatrics,* Neurosurgery,[2]* and Microbiology,[3]* Kyoto Prefectural University of Medicine, Kawaramachi, Kamikyo-ku, Kyoto, Japan

SUMMARY

Investigations have been undertaken to determine whether human leukocyte interferon (HuIFN-α) exerts therapeutic effects on malignant tumors.[1-3] In this study, we present clinical observations on the results of HuIFN-α administration in human neurogenic tumors, other malignant diseases in childhood, and C1300 A/J mouse neuroblastoma.

HUMAN STUDY

There were 12 patients: 7 children and 5 adults; 5 were males and 7 were females. Their ages ranged from 2 to 55 years. Six cases were brain tumors: 3 glioblastomas, 2 medulloblastomas, and one astrocytoma. Five were abdominal tumors: 2 neuroblastomas, 2 Wilms' tumors, and one malignant teratoma. One was a thoracic rhabdomyosarcoma.

The HuIFN-α used in this study was prepared at the Green Cross Company and Kyoto Red Cross Blood Center in Japan. Its specific activity was 0.5–5.5 × 10^6 IU/mg protein.

The clinical findings in these 12 cases and the effects of IFN administration are shown in Table 1.

231

Table 1.   Clinical findings and effects of IFN-α in 12 cases.

Case	Age	Sex	Tumor	Stage	Dose regime		Total dose	Effect
1. M.T.	42	F	Glioblastoma	Recurrent	5×10^4 IU once/wk I.M.	10 months	200×10^4 IU	+
2. N.T.	10	F	Medulloblastoma	Recurrent		9 months	180×10^4 IU	+
3. U.I.	55	F	Glioblastoma	Recurrent		9 months	180×10^4 IU	−
4. M.I.	51	M	Glioblastoma	Recurrent	300×10^4 IU every 2days I.M.	4 months	$12,900 \times 10^4$ IU	−
5. I.Q.	16	F	Astrocytoma	Recurrent		9 months	$17,850 \times 10^4$ IU	−
6. K.K.	9	M	Medulloblastoma	Recurrent		5 months	$11,370 \times 10^4$ IU	−
7. T.H.	3	F	Malignant teratoma	Terminal	$50-60 \times 10^4$ IU/day I.M.	4 months	$5,000 \times 10^4$ IU	±
8. D.K.	9	M	Rhabdomyosarcoma	Terminal	$10-30 \times 10^4$ IU/day I.T.	1 week	130×10^4 IU	?
9. R.N.	2	F	Wilms' tumor	Pulmonary metastasis	$50-100 \times 10^4$ IU, 3 times/wk I.M.	1 month	$1,310 \times 10^4$ IU	−
10. T.M.	7	M	Wilms' tumor	Terminal	$50-60 \times 10^4$ IU, 3 times/wk I.M.; 50×10^4 IU/day I. T.	2 months	$1,700 \times 10^4$ IU	−
11. M.N.	5	M	Neuroblastoma	Terminal	$10-50 \times 10^4$ IU/day I.T.	15 days	750×10^4 IU	−
12. R.T.	21	F	Neuroblastoma	Terminal	30×10^4 IU every 2 days to 2 tumors I.T.	1 week	200×10^4 IU	?
						20 days	600×10^4 IU	+
					300×10^4 IU every 2 days I.M.	11 days	$1,800 \times 10^4$ IU	?

Study on Brain Tumors

The 6 patients with brain tumors (cases 1–6) had undergone operations and subsequently received adjuvant radiotherapy to the tumor area. More than 6 months after the termination of radiation, the patients experienced the same clinical symptoms as those found at the time of the initial diagnosis, and recurrent masses were detected by brain CT scanning. Thereafter, HuIFN-α was injected intramuscularly (I.M.) into the these patients. The effects of IFN administration on tumor growth were evaluated by the change of tumor volume as detected by a CT scan of the recurrent tumor mass.

Case 1–3 received a single I.M. injection of 5×10^4 IU of IFN weekly for 9–10 months. Their total dosages were 180–200×10^4 IU, a low dose group. Cases 4–6 received an I.M. injection of 300×10^4 IU of IFN every other day for 4–9 months. Their total dosages were $11,370$–$17,850 \times 10^4$ IU, a high dose group. Volumes of the tumor masses in these patients before and during IFN administration are shown on Fig. 1.

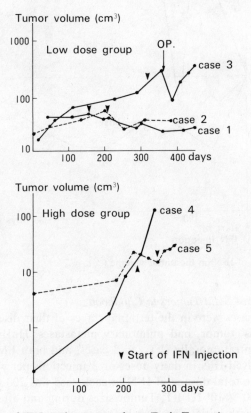

Fig. 1.   The effects of IFN on the tumor volume (Brain Tumors).

Arrest of tumor growth and reduction of tumor size were observed in case 1 with glioblastoma and case 2 with medulloblastoma, in the low dose group. In the remaining patient with glioblastoma from the low dose group, case 3, the volume of the tumor mass increased during the IFN injections. The tumor masses of cases 4 and 5 in the high dose group were not reduced in size. In case 6, with medulloblastoma, the antitumor effect of IFN could not be evaluated because the patient had multiple meningeal dissemination of the disease. The effects of IFN on the tumor volumes are shown in Fig. 2 by the increase or decrease of the initial volumes.

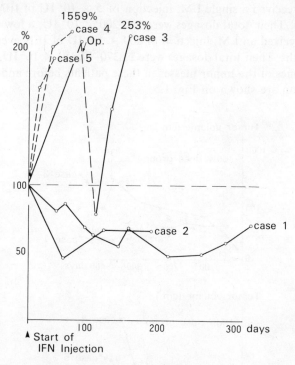

Fig. 2.   The effects of IFN on the tumor volume (%).

Study on Malignant Solid Tumors in Childhood

Five of the 6 cases were in the terminal stages of their diseases. The other case, with Wilms' tumor, had pulmonary metastases. HuIFN-α was given I.M. to 5 cases, intratumorally (I.T.) to 3 cases, and both I.M. and I.T. in 2 cases. They received IFN in daily doses or 3 injections per week for 1 week to 4 months. The total dosage of IFN in each case was 200–5,000 $\times$ 10^4 IU I.M. and 130–750 $\times$ 10^4 IU I.T. Tumor sizes during and after the injections were compared with initial sizes just before treatment.

1. Case 7: T.H., Malignant Teratoma (Fig. 3)

At 10 months of age, the patiant was observed to have a diffuse swelling of the 1-sacrococcygeal region, and her tumor mass was removed subtotally by the second surgery. Her initial serum AFP was extremely high. Six months later, the appearance of 1-hilar masses and elevated serum AFP levels were noted, although she was being treated with radiation therapy and VAC (vincristine, actinomycin D, and cyclophosphamide) chemotherapy.

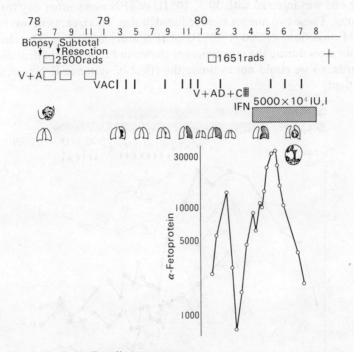

Fig. 3.   Case 7: T. H. 3y. F malignant teratoma.

The hilar masses increased in size, and her serum AFP also rose despite intensive chemotherapy with VAC and/or V-AD-C (vincristine, adriamycin, and cyclophosphamide). At 3 years of age, she received daily I.M. injections of $50–60 \times 10^4$ IU of HuIFN-α, a total $5,000 \times 10^4$ IU, for 4 months. At 1.5 months after beginning the IFN therapy, her AFP levels had decreased and the 1-hilar masses had been transiently reduced in size. Two months later, the masses increased in size and new metastatic masses were seen in the parietal and occipital regions by a brain CT scan. Her disease steadily progressed and she died with massive metastases 4 months after IFN administration.

It is difficult to determine whether the changes in serum AFP levels and in the size of the masses were caused by IFN therapy, VAC, or both.

2. *Case 12*: *R.T., Neuroblastoma (Fig. 4)*

At 16 years of age, an abdominal mass on the right flank of this patient was diagnosed as neuroblastoma. The extent of her disease was stage III. She had 3 operations to remove the primary tumor which originated from the r-adrenal gland. At 21 years of age, multiple metastases to the bone, bone marrow, liver, and cervical, mediastinal, and abdominal lymph nodes were present. One of these cervical masses was injected I.T. and the area surrounding another one was injected with 30×10^4 IU of IFN every other day for a total of 10 times. These two masses were reduced in size. This treatment was followed by 6 I.M. injections of 300×10^4 IU of IFN every other day. The changes in the tumor sizes during the injections are shown in Fig. 4. The patient died soon afterwards, so we could not evaluate the effect of systemic IFN injections on this patient.

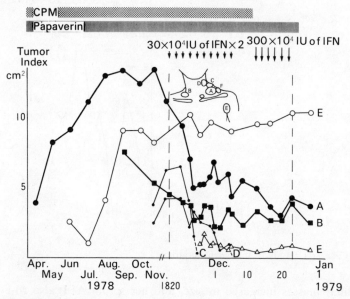

Fig. 4. Neuroblastoma

In this case of neuroblastoma, the two masses were significantly reduced in size by lesional injections of IFN. The details of this case were reported previously.[4] In case 7, the malignant teratoma, the serum AFP level declined and a transient reduction of metastatic pulmonary masses was observed after the IFN injections were begun. The effects of IFN on case 8, with rhabdomyosarcoma, and on case 11, with neuroblastoma, were not evaluated because of short observation periods. In two cases with Wilms' tumor, IFN provided no therapeutic benefits.

Side-Effects of HuIFN-α Administration

A transient high fever was noticed in 5 children and 2 adults after IFN injections, both I.M. and I.T. but it was not necessary to discontinue the therapy. A generalized toxic eruption appeared in case 9 eighteen hours after an I.M. injection. There were no significant changes in the laboratory data of these patients during the periods before and after the IFN injections.

MOUSE STUDY

Inbred A/J mice, 8–12 weeks old, were used for this study. Syngeneic C1300 neuroblastoma tumor was kindly supplied by Dr. Arima (Department of Pediatric Surgery, Kagoshima University School of Medicine) and was maintained by serial transfers *in vivo*.

Mouse interferons (IFNs), B-IFN and L-IFN, were prepared for this study at our laboratory. B-IFN was prepared from the brains of ICR mice inoculated with Japanese encephalitis virus (JaG Ar01). The specific activity of the B-IFN used was 6×10^4 units/mg protein. L-IFN was prepared from L929 cells infected with Newcastle disease virus (NDV, Miyadera strain). Its specific activity was 1.4×10^6 units/mg protein.

IFN and CPM (cyclophosphamide) was administered to A/J mice inoculated with Cl300 neuroblastoma. All mice were inoculated subcutaneously in the interscapular area with 1×10^6 tumor cells. On the 8th day after inoculation, implantation of the tumor was confirmed and tumor-bearing mice were treated with B-IFN, L-IFN, CPM, or a combination of IFN and CPM. The animals received 25,000 IU of IFN given in 3 injections per week and 40 mg/kg of CPM was given by one I.P. injection.

The mean survival time of control mice inoculated with tumor cells was 28 days, and all mice died within 34 days after inoculation. However, each group of mice which received B-IFN, L-IFN, or CPM demonstrated a prolonged survival. Furthermore, a combination of B-IFN or L-IFN and CPM led to a significant prolongation of survival compared to IFN or CPM alone. The surviving mice (3/8 = 37.5%) demonstrated a regression in their tumor masses.

COMMENTS AND SUMMARY

We investigated the effects of HuIFN-α on human malignant tumors such as brain tumors and various tumors in childhood. One glioblastoma and one medulloblastoma out of the 6 recurrent brain tumors were reduced in size by low dose I.M. injections of IFN, and the remaining 4 tumors, one in the low dose group and 3 in the high dose group, were not affected. One weekly I.M. injection with a low dose of IFN produced a greater antitumor effect than 3

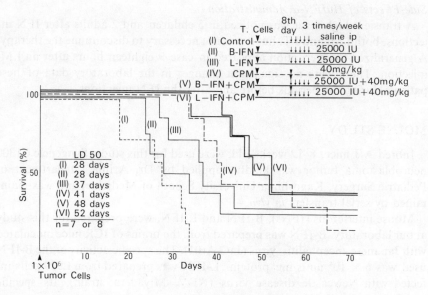

Fig. 5. The effect of IFN on the percent survival of C1300 tumor bearing mice.

weekly I.M. injections with a high dose of IFN. However, one neuroblastoma of the 6 representative malignant tumors in childhood was reduced in tumor size by lesional injections of moderate amounts of IFN, suggesting that a higher IFN level in the tumor mass is required for the reduction of this tumor.

The discrepancy in the response of brain tumors and neuroblastoma to IFN, is not clear. Apparently, the effective dose of IFN differs according to the type of tumor. The IFN did not accelerate tumor growth.

There were no serious side-effects except high fever and skin eruptions.

The study of mouse neuroblastoma demonstrated a favorable response to I.P. IFN administration. The combination of IFN and CPM administration, in particular, affected tumor growth more markedly than IFN or CPM administration alone. The reports of Gresser et al. described the same results in a series of experiments with several transplantable tumors in mice of different strains.[5-7] They concluded that daily I.P. injection of IFN led to a significant prolongation of survival compared to CPM or IFN alone in mice with established spontaneous AKR leukemia.

In conclusion, our study shows a reasonable possibility that IFN is effective in reducing the tumor mass of some human malignant tumors and mouse neuroblastoma.

REFERENCES

1. Strander, H., Cantell, K., Jakobsson, P. A. *et al.*: Exogenous interferon therapy of osteogenic sarcoma. *Acta Orthop. Scand.*, **45**: 958, 1974.
2. Blomgren, H., Cantell, K., Johansson, B. *et al.*: Interferon therapy in Hodgkin's disease. A case report. *Acta Med. Scand.*, **199**: 527, 1976.
3. Merigan, T. C., Sikora, K., Breeden, J. H. *et al.*: Preliminary observations on the effect of human leukocyte interferon in non-Hodgkin's lymphoma. *New Engl. J. Med.*, **299**: 1449, 1978.
4. Sawada, T., Fujita, T., Kusunoki, T. *et al.*: Preliminary report on the clinical use of clinical use of human leukocyte interferon in neuroblastoma. *Cancer Treat. Rep.*, **63**: 2111, 1979.
5. Gresser, I., Maury, G., and Tovey, M.: *Europ. J. Cancer*, **14**: 97, 1978.
6. Gresser, I. and Tovey, M.: Antitumor effects of interferon. *B B A*, **516**: 231, 1978.
7. Priestman, T. J.: Interferon: An anti-cancer agent? *Cancer Treat Rev.*, **6**: 223, 1979.

Clinical Experiences with Human Fibroblast Interferon

Hisashi FURUE

Department of Internal Medicine, Teikyo University School of Medicine, Tokyo, Japan

In patients with malignant tumors, serum interferon levels were measured after administration of 3×10^6 IU of human fibroblast interferon (HuIFN-β) by a single intravenous (I.V.) injection, I.V. drip infusion, or intramuscular (I.M.) injection. Results were as follows:

(1) Single I.V. administration. The serum HuIFN-β level rose to 320 U/ml immediately after the injection then fell rapidly to half the concentration in about 20 minutes. The IFN could no longer be detected in the blood at 6 hours after the injection. Higher doses raised the level and prolonged the persistence of circulating IFN.

(2) I.V. drip infusion. Following start of drip infusion, the IFN concentration gradually increased and reached a level of 120 IU/ml immediately after completion of the infusion. Subsequently, the IFN rapidly cleared from the circulation. The early half-time was 60 minutes. No IFN was detected beyond 6 hours after completion of the infusion.

(3) I.M. injection. IFN could never be demonstrated throughout a period of 24-hour observation following the injection.

It has been deduced from these findings that HuIFN-β will produce therapeutic effects only by I.V. administration.

In our studies, serum IFN assays were performed by measuring the cytopathic effect (CPE) of vesicular stomatitis virus (VSV) in monolayer cultures of human embryonic lung (HEL) cells.

Seventeen patients were treated with HuIFN-β: 4 cases with acute myelogenous leukemia (AML), 4 with malignant lymphomas, 2 with stomach cancer, and one case each of monocytic leukemia (MoL), multiple myeloma, small cell carcinoma of the lung, esophageal cancer, colon cancer, liver cancer, and hepatitis B. Of the 16 patients with malignant tumors, 9 received only IFN, 4 were given IFN subsequent to cancer chemotherapy, and the remaining 3 cases were treated with IFN in combination with chemotherapy.

IFN was administered in doses of 3×10^6 IU daily or 2 to 3 times a week, usually by I.V. drip infusion. The treatment was continued for as long a period as possible. The total doses ranged between 3×10^6 IU and 2.2×10^8 IU.

The HuIFN-β therapy failed to produce any appreciable clinical improvement in the 9 cases treated with a single injection. In contrast, a complete remission (CR) occurred in 3 of 7 cases in which the IFN was administered subsequent to or in combination with cancer chemotherapy, 2 cases of AML and one case of MoL. Therefore, CR was achieved in 3 out of 5 cases of leukemia treated.

In one case of AML, a 5-year-old girl weighing 10 kg, the clinical findings suggested that the I.V. administration of IFN was potentially of value. The girl had become refractory to a variety of anticancer agents, including vincristine (VCR), and was moribund. IFN was initiated at a daily dose of 1.1×10^6 IU following VCR treatment (3 doses of 0.5 mg). Thereafter, the patient responded promptly and attained a complete remission. Her weight increased to 15 kg in 2 months of IFN therapy (total dose, 3.2×10^7 U) and she has returned to a normal daily life.

Various immunologic parameters which included peripheral lymphocyte count, T- and B-cell counts and percentages, lymphocyte blastogenesis stimulated with PHA, and IAP (immunosuppressive acid protein) were assessed during the treatment with IFN. In all 6 cases treated with a single injection of IFN, these parameters did not show any significant improvement and the clinical condition continued to deteriorate as with those undergoing conservative treatment. In contrast, immunologic improvement was observed in the cases that achieved CR following combined treatment with IFN and cancer chemotherapy.

Of the 17 patients treated, including a case of hepatitis B, 10 cases developed fever, with chills in 5 of the patients. In 5 cases, further administration of IFN was discontinued because of fever. None of the patients with the fever reaction became adjusted to the IFN during the full course of medication. However, the degree of fever apparently varied with the lot, which was evident even in the same individual. The fever reaction was controllable by premedication with a nonsteroid anti-inflammatory agent. One patient developed a slight transient neuralgic pain of the extremities in association with fever. Whether all the side-effects will disappear on purification of the IFN remains to be seen. But 7 patients remained completely free of side reactions throughout the treatment. Two patients receiving IFN over extended periods were tested for antibodies to calf serum as well as to IFN, and both proved to be negative.

These preliminary results obtained with HuIFN-β treatment of cancer patients argue for an increase in therapeutic trials. An increased cure rate may be achieved in the treatment of malignant tumors by appropriate combinations of IFN with conventional cancer treatment. More laboratory studies as well as carefully controlled clinical observations in humans are warranted. Steps are being taken towards the purification of IFN and the determination of its chemical structure.

Discussion

Dr. STRANDER: Concerning the side effects, do you find that they subside with time as some other people have found? Also, I am wondering about steroid application to patients on interferon. I think that if the patients are going to be treated for a long time with steroids, it might have some effects on the effects of interferon. Do you have any comments on this?

Dr. FURUE: I have many cases of leukemia in which we use steroids in combination with interferon. Yesterday it was pointed out that use of steroids in combination with interferon is not advisable. But in my case, especially for AML cases, we use steroids with interferon.

Dr. STRANDER: I see. I think there are some studies in mice which could indicate that some of the effects of interferon can be reduced if you give steroids to animals. So one has to keep this in mind. What about the side effects? Do they weaken in time if you repeat the injection?

Dr. FURUE: No, we didn't observe any tolerance. We administered steroid to a patient with a fever for a long period. This is the case of a 32-year-old man with AML in CR. The 38.5°C fever continued almost daily for 2 months, and no tolerance was observed.

Treatment of Malignant Melanoma by Intratumoral A[...]tion of Human Fibroblast Interferon

Kazuyuki Ishihara, Kenichi Hayasaka, and Fumio Hasegawa

Department of Dermatology and Laboratory of Clinical Electron Microscopy, National Cancer Center Hospital, Tokyo, Japan

INTRODUCTION

It is generally known that malignant melanomas are not radiosensitive and are unresponsive to chemotherapy. This type of tumor is prone to metastasize to the skin or subcutaneous tissues before visceral involvement occurs. Effective local treatment is necessary in such circumstances, but since radiotherapy and anticancer chemotherapeutic agents are of little benefit, other treatment modalities have been investigated. Intratumoral administration of viable BCG vaccine and Picibanil have been used for this purpose, but various adverse reactions are usually associated with these preparations, e.g., fever, anorexia, lassitude, and local reactions at the injection site such as reddening and ulceration, which impose a considerable burden on the patient. In view of this, we decided to explore the clinical applicability of interferon and observed its antitumor effects and influence on the patient's condition.

MATERIALS AND METHODS

We used human fibroblast interferon (HuIFN-β) supplied from Toray Industries, Inc., in vials containing 3×10^6 units (U). The content in each vial was dissolved in 1 ml of physiological saline for intratumoral (I.T.) injection. The initial dose was 3–6×10^5 U, depending upon the size of the tumor, and the dosage was increased thereafter up to a maximum level of 6×10^6 U according to the size of the tumor and the number of metastatic lesions. I.T. injections were given every other day as a rule.

Cutaneous and subcutaneous metastatic lesions of malignant melanoma

245

were the main subjects of treatment, although primary lesions were also treated in some of the cases. A large proportion of the patients had multiple lesions; the lesions were excised sequentially at the end of the treatment period and examined histopathologically.

The following criteria were employed for assessment of the clinical response to I.T. IFN therapy: excellent, a complete disappearance of tumor; good, a contraction of tumor by more than 90%; fair, a reduction in tumor size by 50 to 90%; and poor, no or less than a 50% reduction in tumor size.

Light and electron microscopic examinations of lesions were made on specimens obtained before and at various periods during the treatment. The laboratory examinations performed included the PPD skin test, lymphocyte blastogenesis test with PHA, peripheral blood lymphocyte and leukocyte counts, plasma immunoglobulin and complement levels, and hepatic and renal function tests. No other treatment was performed during the I.T. IFN therapy.

CLINICAL RESULTS

Eight patients with malignant melanoma were treated in this study, and the results are summarized in Table 1. The therapeutic response was excellent in 4 cases, good in 2, fair in 1, and unknown in 1. The total number of I.T. injections given ranged from 3 to 67, with the total dose ranging from 9×10^5 to 180×10^6 U. Of the 8 patients, 5 are still receiving the medication, treatment has been discontinued in 1 case in whom a complete disappearance of the tumor was achieved, and the remaining 2 cases have developed a marked metastatic involvement of the viscera despite some antitumor benefit with the cutaneous or subcutaneous metastatic lesions.

In Case No. 1, a male aged 51 years, the patient first noted a black speckle on the bulb of the left second toe 12 months before he was first seen at this hospital, but it was left untreated. The skin lesion began rapidly enlarging with central ulceration about 5 months after the first examination, at which no regional lymph nodes were palpable. The region was amputated at 5 cm distant from the tumor margin, with regional lymphadenectomy. There was microscopic evidence of metastasis in one of 8 excised lymph nodes. The primary lesion was nodular melanoma at level I.V. of the Clark's staging scheme. The patient received 50 mg of pepleomycin prior to the operation, and combination chemotherapy with DTIC, ACNU, and vincristine postoperatively. The combination chemotherapy was repeated one month after the operation. Metastatic lesions developed in the skin and subcutis of the left leg about one year later and grew rapidly in number in 5–6 weeks. These lesions measured 2–10 mm in diameter, and there were approximately 50 lesions in all at the start of I.T. IFN therapy. The treatment was instituted with an initial dose of 6×10^5 U

Table 1. Therapeutic results in individual cases.

Case No.	Name	Sex, age	Primary lesion	Stage	Locations	Metastatic lesions Sites of injection	Number	Size (mm)	No. of doses	Total dose × 10⁴ IU	Response[a]	Remarks
1	Y.A.	M, 51	Toes	IV	Lymph, skin, subcutaneous tissue	Lower extremities, skin, subcutaneous tissue	Innumerable	2–10	67	18,000	Excellent	HuIFN-β regimen being continued
2	S.O.	F, 65	Finger nails	IV	Lymph, skin	Forearm, skin	4	4–10	8	720	Excellent	Metastatic lesions disappeared
3	M.N.	M, 74	Sole	IV	Lymph, lung, pleural effusion, skin	Lower extremities, skin	Innumerable	8–12	4	360	Excellent	Discontinued despite partial regression
4	F.T.	M, 79	Sole	IV	Lymph, lung, skin, subcutaneous cutaneous tissue	Lower leg, skin	12	30–60	3	180	Fair	Discontinued
5	H.K.	M, 37	Sole	II	Lymph	Toes	3	10	3	180	Uncertain	Being continued
6	T.T.	F, 72	Finger-nails	IV	Lymph, skin	Arms, skin	4	10	4	90	Good	Being continued
7	S.I.	M, 56	Back	IV	Lymph, skin	Lower extremities, skin	7	10–15	5	1,500	Excellent	Being continued
8	Y.F.	M, 38	Face	IV	Lymph, skin	Breast	1	8	4	600	Good	Being continued

a) Excellent: complete disappearance of tumor.
   Good: more than 90% reduction.
   Fair: 50–90% reduction.

and the dosage was increased to a maximum level of 6×10^6 U per injection on alternate days.

Figure 1 shows a metastatic lesion seen as a black hemispherical elevation, measuring 9×9 mm, before the start of IFN therapy. A marked reddening was noted around the tumor at 48 hours after the initial I.T. injection of 6×10^5 U (Fig. 2). The tumor disappeared almost completely after the seventh I.T. injection (Fig. 3), at which time a biopsy was carried out. No tumor cells

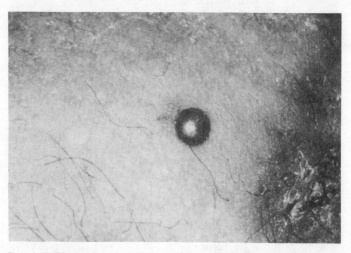

Fig. 1. Case 1 (Table 1, No. 1), malignant melanoma. Metastasis to the skin of lower extremity before therapy.

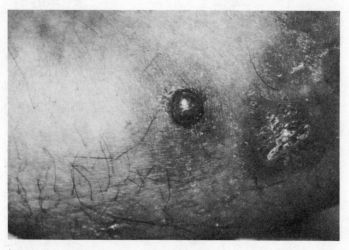

Fig. 2. Case 1. Forty-eight hours after I.T. injection of 60×10^4 IU of HuIFN-β. Note redness surrounding the tumor.

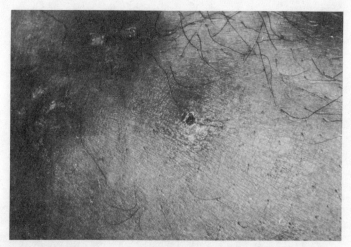

Fig. 3. Case 1. After 7 I.T. injections of IFN the tumor is no longer noticeable.

were found in the biopsy specimen. All other metastatic lesions on the skin of this patient were similarly treated by I.T. injections of IFN, and practically all of the lesions disappeared by the 67th dose, with no development of new lesions. He has been progressing favorably in the 6 months following the conclusion of the IFN therapy. No adverse reactions were observed besides pain and reddening at the sites of injection.

Figure 4 illustrates changes in various immunologic parameters observed in this case following the treatment. As can be seen, there was little or no change in the peripheral blood lymphocyte (Ly) count, whereas the leukocyte count was depressed slightly after initiation of the IFN therapy. The test for blastoid

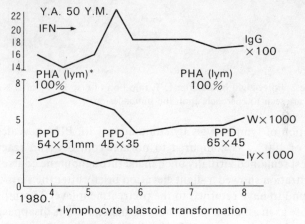

Fig. 4. Lymphocyte blastoid transformation.

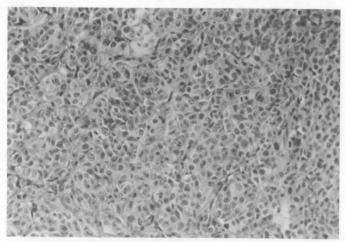

Fig. 5. Case 2 (Table 1, No. 2), before therapy. The affected tissue is replaced almost entirely by tumor cells. Few lymphocytes are seen. H. E. staining.

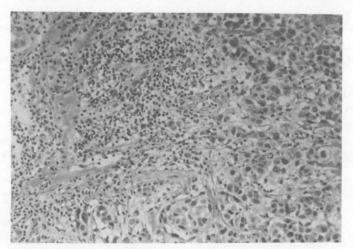

Fig. 6. Case 2. Forty-eight hours after I. T. injection of 6×10^5 IU of IFN, multitudes of lymphocytes are seen to encroach upon the tumor lesion.

transformation of lymphocytes by stimulation with PHA revealed a stimulation index of 100%, as compared to normal controls, and reactivity to the PPD skin test remained virtually unchanged throughout the course. The plasma IgG concentration showed a slight elevation briefly after the start of treatment, but was found to have returned to the pretreatment level 2 months later.

In this case as in all other excellent responders, tumors disappeared after 3–4 injections at the earliest or after 7–10 injections at the latest.

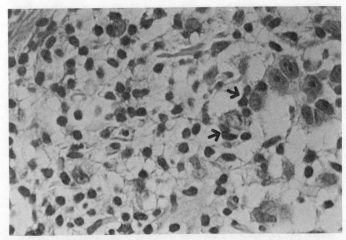

Fig. 7. Case 2. After 2 injections of IFN. Lymphocytes are seen coming into contact with tumor cells (arrow).

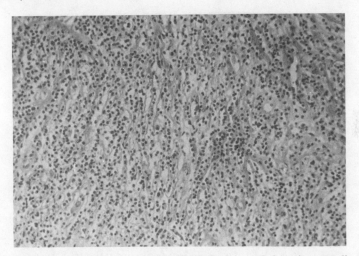

Fig. 8. Case 2. After 4 injections of IFN. Note that tumor cells have been totally replaced by a multitude of lymphocytes.

Histopathologic Findings

Tumor response to the intralesional HuIFN-β therapy was followed histopathologically in 6 of the 8 cases treated. The microscopic findings suggested that, as a general trend, a prominent lymphocyte mobilization that occurs in response to the I.T. injection of IFN might play an important role in the anti-cancer effect of the preparation. Sequentially obtained specimens of resected tissues were observed by light and electron microscopy.

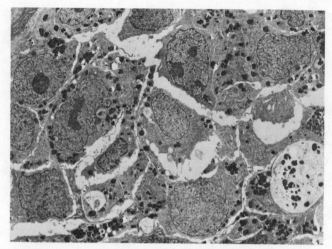

Fig. 9.   Case 1. Electron microscopic view of tumor cells before therapy.

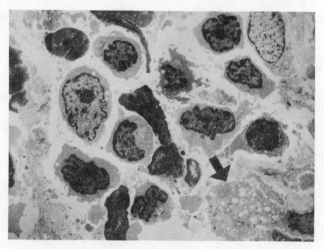

Fig. 10.   Case 1. After a single I.T. injection of 60×10^4 IU of IFN. Periphery of tumor lesion. Numerous lymphocytes and tumor cells (arrow) are seen.

Light Microscopic Observation

Lymphocytic cytotoxic reactions appeared to be a principal histopathologic change evoked by the local injection of the IFN. In contrast to the tumor tissue prior to treatment in which the entire lesion is occupied by malignant cells (Fig. 5), numerous lymphocytes are seen around the tumor tissue and infiltrating among the tumor cells 48 hours after the initial I.T. injection of 6×10^5 U of IFN (Fig. 6). After the second local dose, disintegration of the

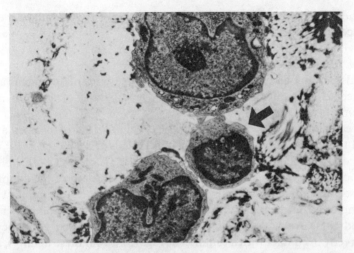

Fig. 11. Case 1. After a single I.T. injection dose of IFN. A small lymphocyte (arrow) is seen coming into contact with a tumor cell.

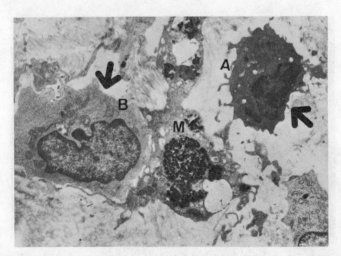

Fig. 12. Case 1. After 2 I.T. injections of IFN. A tumor cell (M) brought into contact with 2 lymphocytes (arrows) has undergone marked degenerative changes. One (A) of the lymphocytes has a long process with a dense cell membrane, while the other (B), whose cytoplasm is light, is in direct contact with the malignant cell.

tumor architecture was evident, with lymphocytic infiltration among tumor cells which, in some areas, where seen immediately adjoining the lymphocytes (Fig. 7). Malignant cells were no longer demonstrable and were replaced with numerous lymphocytes in small lesions after 4 injections of IFN (Fig. 8).

These findings seem to suggest that the mobilization of lymphocytes represents the principal means by which I.T. injections of IFN-β induce the disappearance of tumor cells.

Electron Microscopic Observations

We also examined preparations from the same series of specimens as those subjected to light microscopy. An electron micrograph of a tumor prior to initiation of treatment is shown in Fig. 9.

A great number of lymphocytes with a wide variety of profiles are seen around the tumor 48 hours after the initial HuIFN-β dose of 6×10^5 U (Fig. 10). Occasional tumor cells are observed to be in contact with infiltrating lymphocytes (Fig. 11). After the second local dose, some of the lymphocytes are closely adjoining tumor cells, which are apparently degenerating (Fig. 12). Scanning electron micrographic examination of the same specimens as those for used these transmission electron micrographs revealed lymphocyte-like cells directly in contact with a tumor cell (Fig. 13). From these findings, a direct cytotoxic effect of lymphocytes on tumor cells may be inferred.

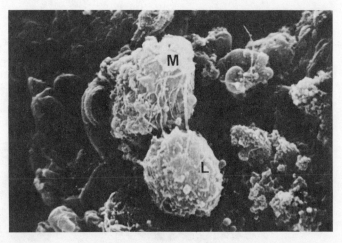

Fig. 13. Case 1. Two cells (probably lymphocyte (L) and tumor cell (M)) are kept in contact with each other.

CONCLUSION

Eight patients with malignant melanoma were treated with intratumoral injections of HuIFN-β. The therapeutic response to the treatment was excellent in 4 cases, good in 2, fair in 1, and unknown in 1. It was our impression that an antitumor effect of the medication usually became apparent after a relatively few I.T. doses. Microscopic observation of treated lesions suggested that the antitumor effect of I.T. injection of HuIFN-β could be largely ascribed to a local mobilization of lymphocytes evoked by the medication. That is, the injections may give rise to a migration of numerous lymphocytes around and into the lesion and thereby induce cytotoxic reactions in the tumor cells. The patients experienced virtually no adverse reactions except pain and reddening at the injection sites. No significant findings of characteristic changes were noted in any of the immunologic parameters studied.

Discussion

Dr. HANAOKA: I know that you have been using BCG for melanoma. Could you kindly explain the indications of BCG therapy and interferon therapy for malignant melanoma?

Dr. ISHIHARA: I have been using BCG for the past 7 or 8 years. I have employed it for the melanoma metastasis of systemic or other forms. To give some of my impressions concerning metastasis melanoma, it is more difficult to use BCG than interferon, because BCG has many side effects. For example, when we inject it in amounts of 0.2 mg or more, we see a strong fever reaction in most of the cases. Repeated injections may cause loss of appetite, fatigue and general malaise. Depending on the use of BCG, it has a very strong effect on skin metasthesis. But the problem is that we cannot generalize its use. Also, as for the histological change, I have observed changes with time from 28 hours to 3 weeks and I have found many neutrophiles in BCG, while many lymphocytes were observed in interferon. With BCG injection, local flare and ulcer appear as well as fever. In terms of efficacy BCG alone is more effective than interferon; however, flare and swelling persist, and the ulcer persists for a long time. BCG is more painful for patients. But pain can be mitigated depending on how BCG is used. Anyhow, because of the side effects of BCG, interferon has a slightly wider range of applications. But as for the clinical efficacy, BCG would probably make a skin metastasis of less than 1 cm disappear after one or two injections, while in the case of interferon we would need about 3 to 4 injections for smaller tumors and 7 to 10 injections for larger tumors. But I have an impression that interferon is easier to use clinically with fewer side effects on patients.

Dr. FURUE: Is there any case where a tumor located at a distant site disappeared after local injection?

Dr. ISHIHARA: When I enlarged the slide of the 4 mm small skin tumor, I noticed many small subcutaneous metastatic lesions, and they disappeared after local injection. Within one week 4 to 5 metastatic lesions appeared. But at the time of 67 injections, metastasis almost completely stopped. In the beginning I was slightly afraid of the doses so I started with 300,000. But recently I have come to conclude that the initial dose can be 1.2 or 1.5 million or even 3 million in a single dose. When it amounts to a record high of more than 100 million in terms of local injection, certain systemic effects seem to occur. This patient continued to have a normal immunological ability and did not have any relapse or recurrence.

Dr. STRANDER: I would like to ask just one question. It is pertinent to all the work with intratumoral injection. In earlier studies with BCG, have you injected any other things into tumors like protein preparation, controlled saline solution, etc.? If so, did you see any infiltration of lymphocyte when you injected any other substances?

Dr. ISHIHARA: I have tried the local injection of saline solution and other agents such as picibanil, bestatin and vincristine. And we saw many neutroplicles. Consequently I was very surprised when I first injected interferon and saw lymphocytes. There was no other agent which produced such a great amount of lymphocyte.

Interferon Therapy for Malignant Brain Tumors

Masakatsu NAGAI,* Toshimoto ARAI,* Seiya KOHNO,[2]* and Masayoshi KOHASE[2]*

*Department of Neurosurgery, Dokkyo University School of Medicine, Mibu, Tochigi-Pref.,
[2]* Department of Measles Virus, National Institute of Health of Japan, 3260 Nakato, Musashi-murayama, Tokyo, Japan

INTRODUCTION

About 10 years have passed since interferon (IFN) was first put to clinical use for the treatment of malignant tumors.[1,2] Many of the clinical studies reported so far have employed leukocytic IFN (α-type), primarily for the control of malignant lymphoma, leukemias, and osteosarcoma. Few reports are as yet available on the therapeutic use of fibroblast IFN (β-type) and, to our knowledge, there are no reported cases of brain tumors treated with either type of IFN. Since September 1979 we have conducted phase I and phase II clinical studies of human fibroblast interferon (HuIFN-β) in malignant brain tumors. This preliminary report documents the results thus far obtained on this new antitumor agent, along with some pertinent basic experimental data.

MATERIALS AND METHODS

Seven patients with malignant brain tumors were treated in this study. Histopathologic diagnoses in this series were medulloblastoma in 2 cases and glioblastoma in 5 cases.

The HuIFN-β preparation used had a specific activity of 10^7 IU/mg protein (Toray Industries, Inc.). The drug was administered in doses ranging from 0.3 to 3.0×10^6 IU and was either dissolved in 100 ml saline and administered by I.V. drip infusion over 1 hour or injected locally or intrathecally in 1–2 ml of saline solution. The dosages were given daily or 2 to 3 times a week for as long as possible, 2 months was the shortest period.

The efficacy of the IFN therapy was assessed by the clinical improvements,

257

changes in Karnofsky's performance status (P.S.), and computerized tomographic (CT) findings. In a follow-up CT study, the volume of the tumor as visualized by CT scan (contrast-enhanced area) was measured and integrated for all slices by the ROI method, and this computed volume was then compared with the pretreatment value to calculate the percent reduction of tumor.

In order to investigate the toxicity of IFN, each patient was serially checked for vital signs, clinical symptoms (e.g., chills, nausea, vomiting, headache, and dizziness), hepatic and renal function, as well as for changes in immunologic parameters.

In the pharmacokinetic study, serial measurements were made of IFN levels in the blood and cerebrospinal fluid following administration, in addition to *in vivo* experiments which will be described later. The quantitative assays were performed by the CP inhibition method using FL cells and Sindbis virus. (For details of this procedure refer to the article by Kohase *et al.* in this volume.)

In Vitro Study

In an attempt to evaluate the effectiveness of IFN for inhibiting the growth of tumor cells, we established a primary culture of tumor tissue specimens taken at surgery from one case each of medulloblastoma and glioblastoma. A study was also made of the antitumor efficacy of a combined treatment with IFN and autologous lymphocytes in these tumors.

The specimens were dissociated by dispase, spread on Falcon dishes for monolayer culture, and incubated at 37°C in a CO_2 incubator. The medium employed was Dulbecco's modification of Eagle's MEM plus 20% fetal bovine serum. HuIFN-β was added to the medium for 2 weeks, starting at 1 week of cultivation, and cells were then enumerated by means of a Coulter counter or the area of a colony was measured to determine the percent inhibition of growth.

In Vivo Study

In order to evaluate the safety of intrathecally or locally administered IFN the following two experiments were carried out:

(1) An adult mongrel dog received 1×10^6 IU of HuIFN-β injected into the cisterna magna as 0.2 ml of solution in distilled water through a cisternal tap done under general anesthesia. Subsequently, IFN titers of serial samples taken from cerebrospinal fluid (CSF) and juglar venous blood were measured with a simultaneous check of vital signs.

(2) Another adult mongrel dog was craniectomized under general anesthesia. After immobilizing and awakening the animal, 10^5 IU of a crystalline preparation of HuIFN-β was applied to the cerebral cortical surface, and EEGs were taken to follow eventual changes in the pattern.

CASE REPORTS

Case 1 (Y.T.): A 6-year-old boy with medulloblastoma

In September 1979 this patient underwent suboccipital craniectomy and biopsy of the tumor. On the 10th postoperative day he was started on HuIFN-β, which was given for 2 months as the single therapy (total dose, 10.5 × 10⁶ IU). The percent reduction of tumor (as estimated from the computed volume) attained during this treatment was 45.7%. After an additional dose of 6.3 × 10⁶ IU of IFN combined with radiotherapy (LINAC; total dose, 6,800 rads), the percent tumor reduction amounted to 62.6%. IFN was continued further without concomitant irradiation, and in June 1980 (after 10 months of the IFN regimen, a total dose of 43.6 × 10⁶ IU) the volume of the tumor was estimated to be 6.5 cm³, which was 85.2% smaller than the pretreatment volume (Fig. 1). The patient has since been receiving IFN in 1.5 × 10⁶ IU injections once a week on an outpatient basis. In a CT done in December 1980, after 15 months of IFN therapy, the tumor was no longer demonstrable. Figure 2 gives a comparison of the CT scans made before and after 15 months of IFN therapy. In this case IFN was administered by I.V. injection. The patient's current clinical symptoms are markedly improved and he is in complete remission without any signs of spinal dissemination.

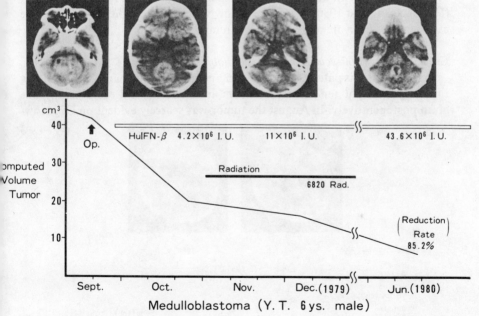

Fig. 1. Reduction curve of computed volume of the tumor on CT (contrast enhanced) corresponding to each period (Case 1).

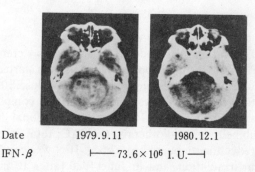

Date   1979.9.11   1980.12.1

IFN-β ⊢——— 73.6×10⁶ I. U.——⊣

Medulloblastoma（Y. T. 6ys. male)

Fig. 2. Comparison of CT (contrast enhanced) findings pre- and posttreatment in Case 1.

Case 2 (H.I.): A 1-year-old boy with medulloblastoma with onset at age 7 months (September 1979)

The patient had the tumor partially removed by suboccipital craniectomy and received radiotherapy (LINAC; 4,000 rads) postoperatively. Three and a half months later IFN therapy was initiated for the control of the remaining tumor. The drug was administered I.V. for 2.5 months in a total dose of 15.62×10^6 IU. With this regimen the size of the tumor was reduced by 79.6% (Fig. 3). In August 1980 no tumor shadow was noticeable on CT (Fig. 4). The case can thus be evaluated as complete remission.

Case 3 (K.I.): A 60-year-old man with glioblastoma

In May 1979 this patient underwent an operation for the partial removal of a tumor in his right temporal lobe. Combined chemo- and radiotherapy was given postoperatively. In August the tumor was scarcely evident on CT. How-

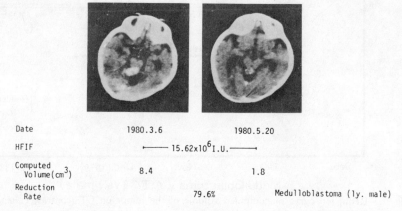

Date   1980.3.6   1980.5.20

HFIF   ⊢——— 15.62x10⁶I.U.———⊣

Computed
Volume(cm³)   8.4   1.8

Reduction
Rate   79.6%   Medulloblastoma (1y. male)

Fig. 3. Comparison of CT (contrast enhanced) findings pre- and posttreatment and the reduction rate in Case 2.

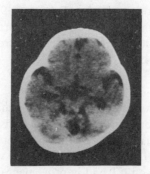

1980.8.5.
(8 months after operation)
Medulloblastoma (1y. male)

Fig. 4.   CT pictures (contrast enhanced) of Case 2, 8 months after surgery.

ever, when a recurrence of the tumor was discovered in December of the same year, the tumor had already encroached upon the lateral ventricle. Treatment with intravenous IFN was begun. Although the tumor appeared to have been reduced in size on CT scan 1.5 months later, at the end of January 1980 (Fig. 5), the patient died the following month. An autopsy revealed widespread dissemination in the intracranial subarachnoid space, including the optochiasmatic and quadrigeminal cisterns, as well as in the spinal cord.

Glioblastoma (60y. male)

| 79.5.24. | 79.8.9. | 79.12.17. | 80.1.29. |

Pretreatment - Operation - Radiation --- MeCCNU ------------ HFIF -------------- HFIF 1.05×10^7 I.U.

Fig. 5.   CT pictures (contrast enhanced) of Case 3 corresponding to the period of each treatment.

Case 4 (T.K.): A 30-year-old man with glioblastoma

   This patient had a tumor in his right frontal lobe which had been removed partially in December 1978; he received radiotherapy and chemotherapy postoperatively. The tumor recurred in February 1980; his general condition was poor, and he again underwent surgery on February 27. Therapy with intravenous IFN was instituted on March 4, but it proved to be ineffective and the patient died on April 4.

Case 5 (K.O.): A 14-year-old girl with glioblastoma

This patient suffered from a brain stem tumor that was first recognized in September 1979. Radiation therapy produced transient remission. A relapse occurred in March 1980 and therapy with I.V. interferon was started. After a total dose of 82.9×10^6 IU over 3.5 months, there was partial remission with a reduction of tumor size on CT and improvement of clinical symptoms. Unfortunately, however, her condition deteriorated and she died 3 months later (September 1980). An autopsy revealed an extension of the tumor from the brain stem to the thalamus and cerebellum.

Case 6 (M.K.): A 30-year-old man with glioblastoma

In February 1980 this patient underwent a partial removal of a right parietal glioblastoma with external decompression. Chemo- and radiotherapy were given postoperatively but proved to be of little benefit. CT done in May of the same year demonstrated a large tumor mass (Fig. 6). The patient was started

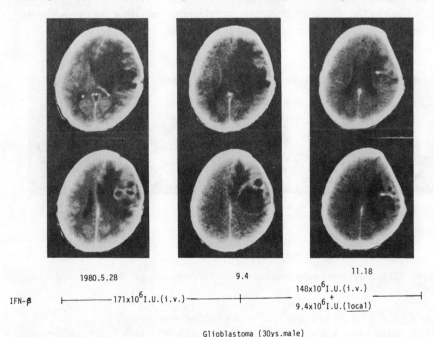

IFN-β   ├──────171x10⁶I.U.(i.v.)──────┤

1980.5.28   9.4

11.18
148x10⁶I.U.(i.v.)
+
9.4x10⁶I.U.(local)

Glioblastoma (30ys.male)

Fig. 6.   CT pictures (contrast enhanced) of Case 6 corresponding to the IFN therapy.

on daily intravenous IFN, and a total dose of 171×10^6 IU was given over a 3-month period. At the end of that time CT disclosed a large cyst formation, indicating that the therapeutic regimen had produced a fairly good result. At this juncture it was felt to be worthwhile to administer IFN locally into the cyst via Ommaya's reservoir,[3] and treatment with IFN by two routes, intralesional and intravenous, was thus initiated. After 2.5 months of this regimen the tumor had almost disappeared on CT and the patient was in complete remission. His clinical improvement was also marked; he now was free from the convulsive seizures which previously had occurred frequently and was able to walk as a result of recovery from left hemiparesis.

Case 7 (T.N.): A 60-year-old woman with glioblastoma

The patient had a bulky tumor extending from the right frontal lobe to the basal ganglia. In September 1980 the tumor was removed partially. Residual tumor tissues around the site of resection and extending to the opposite hemisphere via the corpus callosum were evident on CT (Fig. 7). For half a month from the end of October she received IFN intravenously, but the tumor appeared to grow rapidly, so IFN was locally administered of using Ommaya's reservoir and a catheter inserted into the dead space formed after tumor resection. A CT scan performed after half a month of this regimen demonstrated

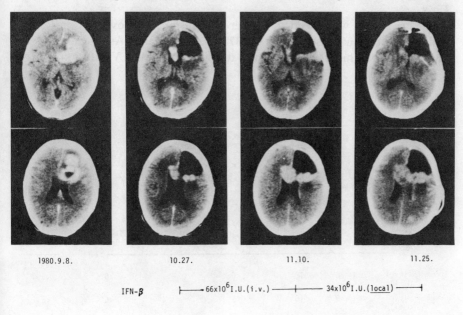

1980.9.8.   10.27.   11.10.   11.25.

IFN-β |——— 66x10⁶I.U.(i.v.) ———|——— 34x10⁶I.U.(local) ———|

Glioblastoma (T.N.) 60 ys. female

Fig. 7. Sequential CT (contrast enhanced) of Case 7.

Table 1. IFN therapy for malignant brain tumors (Phase I-II study).

Case	Age/sex	Diagnosis	Dose (× 10⁶ IU)	Route	Duration (mos)	Response	P.S. (Karnofsky %)
1. Y.T.	6, M	Medulloblastoma	43.6+	I.V.	15	CR	20 → 80
2. H.I.	1, M	Medulloblastoma	15.6	I.V.	9	CR	20 → 80
3. K.I.	60, M	Glioblastoma	10.5	I.V.	2	PG	40 → 0
4. T.K.	30, M	Glioblastoma	12.3	I.V.	1.5	PG	20 → 0
5. K.O.	14, F	Glioblastoma	82.9	I.V.	3.5	PR	50 → 0
6. M.K.	30, M	Glioblastoma	171.0+	I.V.	6	CR	30 → 70
			9.4+	local	2		
7. T.N.	60, F	Glioblastoma	66.0+	I.V.	0.5	PR	20 → 40
				local	0.7		

CR: Complete remission, PR: Partial remission, PG: Progression, +: ongoing.

partial disappearance and necrotization of malignant tissue, and the disease was considered to be in partial remission. The patient has not as yet received radiation therapy or chemotherapy.

A brief summary of these 7 cases is given in Table 1, together with the change in Karnofsky's performance status in each case.

Side-Effect
Fever

The use of IFN was attended by fever in all instances: above 38°C in 1 case, at the 38°C level in 4 cases, and at the 37°C level in 2 cases. As shown in Fig. 8, the body temperature reached a peak 4 to 5 hours after the I.V. infusion of IFN

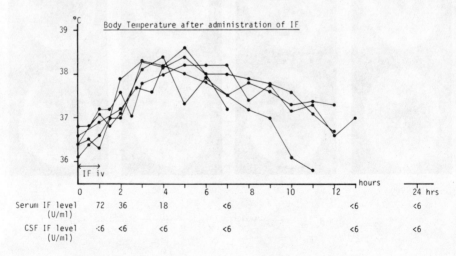

Fig. 8. Fever type after I.V. drip infusion of 0.7 × 10⁶ IU of HuIFN-β (Case 1). IFN levels in serum and in CSF are noted at each point.

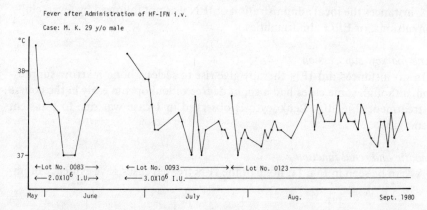

Fig. 9. Declining curve of the peak of body temperature in Case 6. (See text.)

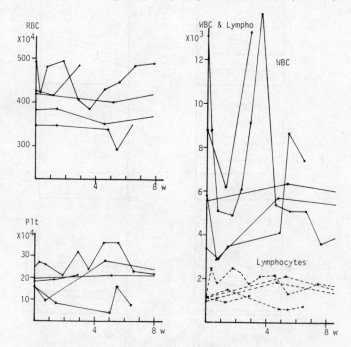

Fig. 10. Blood cell count during IFN therapy in 5 cases.

and returned to normal by 8 to 10 hours after treatment. As the medication was repeated, however, a tolerance phenomenon developed; thus the temperature peak tended to decline gradually as the treatment proceeded (Fig. 9). The fervescence was accompanied by chills in 2 cases, by headache in 1 case, but by symptoms of gastrointestinal upset (nausea, vomiting, anorexia, etc.) in none.

In 2 instances the local administration of IFN was not followed by fever, chills, convulsions, or EEG abnormalities.

Bone marrow suppression

In no instances did IFN therapy give rise to serious bone marrow suppression, although some cases had a slight degree of leukopenia early in the course of treatment (Fig. 10). Leukocytosis observed in 1 case was due to transient meningitis.

Hepatic and renal function

As can be seen in Fig. 11, none of the IFN treated cases gave evidence of im-

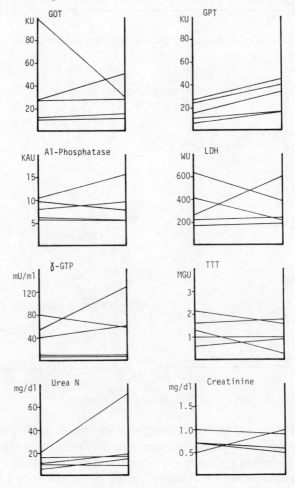

Fig. 11.   Laboratory findings of hepatic and renal function pre- and post-interferon therapy.

paired liver and renal function. An elevated urea-N level was noted in 1 case shortly before the patient's death.

Immunologic parameters

As showed in Fig. 12, there were no significant changes in any of the cases in the parameters of humoral and cellular immunity recorded before and after IFN therapy. It should be noted that a PPD skin test was converted to negative in a patient unsuccessfully treated with IFN just before his death (Case 4).

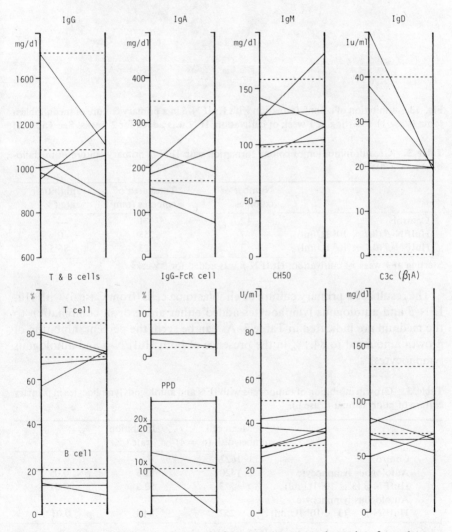

Fig. 12. Laboratory findings on immunologic parameters pre- and post-interferon therapy.

RESULTS *IN VITRO* STUDY

The percent inhibition of growth as calculated from the planimetry of the tumor cell colony formed in primary culture of a medulloblastoma specimen (Case 1) was 86.5% at an IFN concentration of 10^3 IU/ml (Fig. 13 and Table 2).

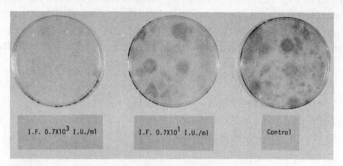

I.F. 0.7X10³ I.U./ml   I.F. 0.7X10¹ I.U./ml   Control

Fig. 13. Inhibition of colony formation with HuIFN-β in a primary culture of medulloblastoma (Case 1). (Starting at 1 week of cultivation, IFN was added for 2 weeks. See Table 2.)

Table 2. Growth inhibition of colony formation with IFN in primary culture of medulloblastoma (Case 1).

	Number of colonies	Total area of colonies (mm²)	Inhibition rate (%)
Control	12	171	—
HuIFN-β (0.7×10^1 IU/ml)	7	258	0
HuIFN-β (0.7×10^3 IU/ml)	3	23	86.5

Starting at 1 week of cultivation, HuIFN-β was added for 2 weeks.

The results of a primary culture of glioblastoma cells (from Case 6) with HuIFN-β and autologous lymphocytes added either alone or in combination to the medium are indicated in Table 3. As can be seen, the percent inhibition of growth amounted to 84.1% in the presence of both HuIFN-β and autologous lymphocytes.

Table 3. Growth inhibition of tumor cells with IFN and autologous lymphocytes in primary culture of glioblastoma (Case 6).

	Mean cell number/dish (n = 4)	Inhibition rate (%)	
Control	1622	—	
Autologous lymphocyte	1420	12.5	$p < 0.05$
HuIFN-β (3×10^3 IU/ml)	773	52.3	$p < 0.01$
Autologous lymphocyte HuIFN-β + (3×10^3 IU/ml)	257	84.1	$p < 0.01$

Starting at 1 week of cultivation, HuIFN-β and/or lymphocytes were added for 2 weeks.

Pharmacokinetics of IFN in Clinical Cases and Results of In Vivo Study

Clearance curves of IFN in blood and CSF following the I.V. administration of IFN in Case 1 are shown in Fig. 14. Immediately after termination of drip infusion the IFN titer in blood was 72 IU/ml, which cleared within 6 hours. The IFN titer in CSF was undetectably low.

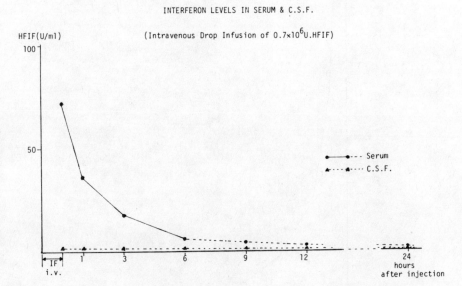

Fig. 14. Clearance curves of IFN in serum and CSF following I.V. administration in Case 1.

The clearance curve of IFN in CSF following injection into the cisterna magna of a mongrel dog is represented in Fig. 15. The IFN titer peaked at 11,000 IU/ml 30 minutes after administration and was detectable for 12 hours. Blood samples taken simultaneously were not found to contain IFN at any recognizable level. During and after IFN administration vital signs remained entirely unaffected.

After application of IFN (10^5 IU) onto the cerebral cortical surface of a mongrel dog, electrocorticograms (waking) were recorded from nearby cerebral structures for 30 minutes. No abnormal patterns were observed (Fig. 16) nor did any convulsive seizures occur.

DISCUSSION AND SUMMARY

A total of 7 patients with malignant brain tumors were treated with HuIFN-β for more than 2 months in a study undertaken to assess the antitumor efficacy of this agent. In 2 medulloblastoma cases in this series the systemic administra-

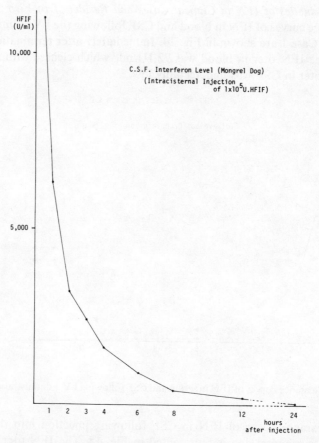

Fig. 15.   Clearance curve of IFN in CSF following the intracisternal injection in a mongrel dog. IFN titer in the serum was not detectable at any time.

tion (I.V.) of the drug proved to be markedly effective. In 2 glioblastoma cases, on the other hand, local administration of the drug was attempted after I.V. infusion failed to produce a favorable effect in 3 other cases. In these 2 cases IFN was thus administered intralesionally via Ommaya's reservoir after animal experiments confirmed the safety of the drug applied by this route. This therapeutic regimen produced complete remission in one case and partial remission in the other.

The pharmacokinetic study of IFN-β in clinical cases demonstrated that the drug, when injected I.V., is not transferred to the CSF, a finding which suggests the desirability of intrathecal or local use in the management of brain tumors. Although some pertinent animal experiments have been reported,[4-6] questions of whether IFN will pass through the blood-brain barrier, and

UNDER ANESTHESIA

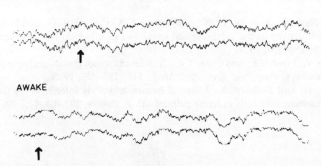

AWAKE

Fig. 16. Electrocorticograms after the application of 10^5 IU of HuIFN-β onto the cerebral surface of a mongrel dog. (Arrows indicate the time of application.)

whether it diffuses into tissues remain to be answered by further in-depth studies.

Tumor tissue specimens taken from one case each of medulloblastoma and glioblastoma were subjected to primary culture in the presence of HuIFN-β to determine the percent inhibition of tumor growth *in vitro*. The figures thus obtained correlated well with actual therapeutic results. As already pointed out by Strander,[7] this procedure is considered one of the most important screening tests in the evaluation of IFN therapy.

Aside from a transient fever, IFN therapy was free from major side-effects, and, accordingly, seems to be easier to use than conventional anticancer drugs. Future studies will be necessary to elucidate its immunologic influence, particularly on natural killer cell activity.

Before an appropriate regimen of IFN therapy can be established, studies will have to be conducted with larger groups of cases to determine the optimal dosage and the time, frequency, and duration of administration. The anticancer efficacy of IFN therapy used in combination with radiotherapy and/or chemotherapy should also be investigated. IFN seems to offer a very promising means for controlling malignant brain tumors and hence deserves intensive study for future development.

REFERENCES

1. Gresser, I.: Antitumor effects of interferon. *Adv. Cancer Res.*, **16**: 97–140, 1972.
2. Strander, H., Cantell, K., Carlström, G., and Jakobsson, P. A.: Clinical and laboratory investigations on man: Systemic administration of potent interferon to man. *J. Natl. Cancer Inst.*, **51**: 733–742, 1973.
3. Ommaya, A. K., Okon, M. A., and Punjab, M. B.: Subcutaneous reservoir and pump for sterile access to ventricular cerebrospinal fluid. *Lancet* Nov. **9**: 983–984, 1963.

4. Cathala, F. and Baron, S.: Interferon in rabbit brain, cerebrospinal fluid and serum following administration of polyinosinic-polycytidylic acid. *J. Immunol.*, **104**: 1355–1358, 1970.

5. Ho, M., Nash, C., Morgan, C. W., Armstrong, J. A., Carroll, R. G., and Postic, B.: Interferon administered in the cerebrospinal space and its effect on rabies in rabbits. *Infect. Immun.*, **9**: 286–293, 1974.

6. Habif, D. V., Lipton, R., and Cantell, K.: Interferon crosses blood-cerebrospinal fluid barrier in monkeys. *Proc. Soc. Exp. Biol. Med.*, **149**: 287–289, 1975.

7. Strander, H. and Einhorn, S.: Effect of human leukocyte interferon on the growth of human osteosarcoma cells in tissue culture. *Int. J. Cancer*, **19**: 468–473, 1977.

Discussion

Dr. YAMAMOTO: You have conducted the primary culture using a colony of glioblastoma. Is this the continuous exposure? If not, what method is used for the primary culture?

Dr. NAGAI: It is the continuous exposure.

Dr. YAMAMOTO: What are the units?

Dr. NAGAI: 10^3, which were effective.

Dr. YAMAMOTO: Did you use common media? Or was it soft agar or something?

Dr. NAGAI: We used the common medium. It was a monolayer culture.

Dr. BORDEN: These are important observations for a very difficult clinical problem. I just want to make sure I understand the results in terms of response. In terms of patients who did not receive other forms of therapy while they were receiving interferon, if I understood your report correctly, there was one of the medulloblastoma patients who showed clear evidence of partial response without receiving any radiation and one of the glioblastoma patients who did not receive any other therapy who also showed a very good partial response. In that patient you were also administering interferon by the reservoir in addition on the systemic administration. Is that correct? Are there other patients from this series who did not receive other therapies while they were receiving the interferon?

Dr. NAGAI: In the first case of medulloblastoma, which I showed you, we gave only interferon and we achieved a reduction rate of over 45 %. The last case, case No. 7, showed a glioblastoma in which local injection resulted in partial remission. The patient is still in this phase now. Because of many cases of relapse and recurrence, most cases underwent chemotherapy and radiotherapy. Radiotherapy is commonly conducted in all the patients with primary cerebral tumors. In the future we would like to try the treatment with pure interferon only.

Dr. BORDEN: Interferon alone then produced no responses? The first patient you mentioned had 45 % reduction in volume, then received radiation. In the glioblastoma patients, how many received interferon alone and showed a substantial reduction in measurable tumor?

Dr. NAGAI: In case No. 1 with medulloblastoma, the patient did receive radiation as well, thus producing complete remission. In the case with glioblastoma, I cannot give a conclusive evaluation as it is only six weeks since we started this study.

Dr. YOKOTA: I would like to ask you a question concerning local application. You have obtained a drastic effect by local application. Is it due to a high local concentration or is it due to T cell or NK cell response to tumor-specific antigen? Because the effect appears to be very tumor-specific and peripheral normal cells do not seem to receive any side effect.

Dr. NAGAI: I think you made two very valuable suggestion. Cyst fluid and cerebral spinal fluid have been collected to look at the interferon level and NK activity, but I did not get the results in time for this conference. As for the localized concentration, we cannot carry out biopsy as often as dermatologists can; when there is a chance, we would like to try more biopsy. In case No. 6 of glioblastoma where complete remission was observed, we did conduct a biopsy. And in this case, we did not see any effect of local administration, but during the previous 6 months we had given interferon intravenously. Consequently we saw a big cyst formation on CT, and histologically we observed so-called gemistocytic astrocytes with reduced capacity for proliferation. Unlike the case of skin, lymphocytes do not tend to accumulate in the brain, but we succeeded in observing some histological change. We would like to study it in the future as well.

Dr. REVEL: I'd like to ask a question of Dr. Ishihara on the work with the melanoma. You presented very interesting data on regression of metastatis. How is interferon affecting the prognosis of melanoma? Can you give any indication on survival of patients and on how you expect to improve their survival? Do you think that the metastases that you can treat locally are most important? Or do you think it is more necessary to treat profound metastasis?

Dr. ISHIHARA: There are two different cases—metastasis seen only in skin and metastasis in organs and skin. In the case where metastasis is only seen in skin, the prognosis is very favorable and there has been no recurrent metastasis observed in most cases. However, when metastasis occurs in organs, such as liver and lung, and skin at the same time, prolongation of life is not expected. Also, a large dose may be conducive to many side effects. However, I give repeated injections, because I believe it has some effect in prolonging life. I think I have not answered some part of your question concerning peripheral injection. We conduct injection on the periphery of the tumor because direct intratumor injection is not likely to produce many lymphocytes. As for the life prolongation effect, I started this treatment in April this year. So presently we are considering how we can continuously use interferons in patients after lesions have disappeared. I am a dermatologist, so I cannot keep the patients in the hospital when the skin lesions are gone. And naturally patients prefer to leave the hospital. I am trying to find a way to follow up these patients on an ambulatory basis. Of course patients are reluctant to come back for an injection every other day. Therefore, in the future, we may try to give subcutaneous injections to those patients once a week to study various parameters and to see whether there is a recurrence of metastasis. I would like to study those cases over a longer time span.

Conference on Clinical Potentials of Interferons in Viral Diseases and Malignant Tumors

Explanation of Contents of Film

Yasuiti NAGANO

National Hospital of Sagamihara, Kanagawa

We have previously reported that the activity of IFN on mouse Ehrlich ascites carcinoma cells is cytostatic rather than cytocidal (C. R. Soc. Biol., 173. 20 & 960, 1979).

The following film shows, through phase contrast microscopy, how mouse myeloid leukemic cells (myeloblasts) differentiate to become phagocytes and cease to divide and grow when treated with IFN.

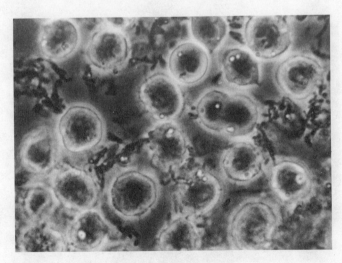

Fig. 1. Culture of myeloblastic cell line originated from a case of spontaneous myelogenous leukemia in mice. No active movement, no phagocytosis.

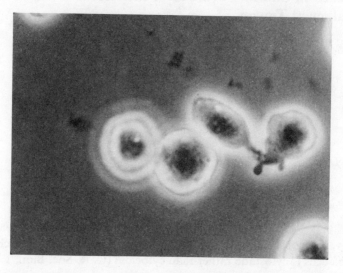

Fig. 2.　A few hours following addition of IFN. Note the abnormal divisions.

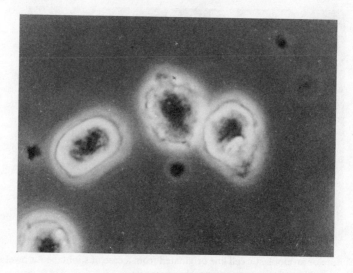

Fig. 3.　42 hours after addition of IFN. Small pseudopods begin to appear.

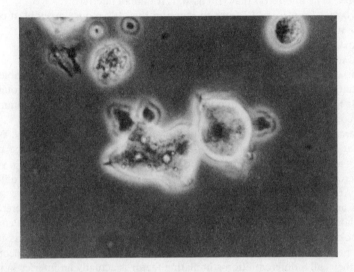

Fig. 4. After 3 days. Pseudopods are prominent. Cells migrate activity and do not divide any more.

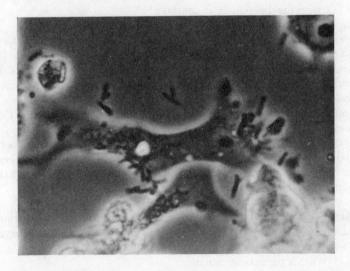

Fig. 5. After 5 days. Amoeboid movement is characteristic in some cells, which are also phagocytic and stop to divide.

Discussion

Dr. Ishida: The interferon that you used, is it human interferon?

Dr. Nagano: I am sorry I forgot to mention this. It's mouse myeloblast cells and mouse interferon.

Dr. Ishida: Is the mouse interferon very pure?

Dr. Nagano: No, it's not so pure. It's about 10^6 units per mg protein.

Dr. Ishida: I am concerned, because a colony-stimulating factor is capable of differentiating myeloblasts into macrophage and microphage. The glycoprotein has a similar molecular weight to interferon, so I thought there might be contamination of glycoprotein.

Dr. Nagano: That's one possibility. But I think there is another possibility. When we look at the list of differentiation-stimulating factors, some percentage of these factors are interferon inducers. When we treated the cells that I've shown you with interferon inducers such as poly I.C., endotoxin and myxovirus, we see differentiation. At this time, the cells themselves produce interferon, which, we suppose, exerts an effect upon them. However, if you ask me whether a differentiation-stimulating factor was also present or not, the answer is still not known. People who are looking at differentiation-stimulating factors say that contaminants in interferon preparation are the contributing factor. I always say to those people that what they call a differentiation-stimulating factor is actually an interferon inducer, and that it is interferon that stimulates differentiation directly. And I further ask them if they can give me the counter proof. So we have a very congenial argument going on.

Dr. Machida: I believe that in your film, interferon was kept for 72 hours. If interferon is removed during the differentiation, does so-called "disdifferentiation" occurs? Or does the differentiation continue?

Dr. Nagano: We have not done this yet.

Dr. Ebina: I am also working on a film of macrophages and interferon. The problem which concerns me most is that it is only after 72 hours following interferon administration that macrophage-like cells appear. So how do you define differentiation? When bacteria is given, phagocytosis is seen even in normal cells. I believe the large cell seen in the center of the film is the macrophage. When we look at other parts on the screen, there are dead cells and many other things in the film which makes macrophages unclear.

Dr. Nagano: In the beginning, you saw the round lymphocyte-like cell producing pseudopods, and it started to move around. As it grows larger, it beings to eat foreign objects. So this constitutes the criterion. And the control cells that are not given interferon do not show these changes when they are cultured.

Dr. Ebina: What percentage of cells became large cells?

Dr. Nagano: It's difficult to say in this film, but according to other experiments unfortunately only 50 or 60 % of cells become large cells. Unless we have 100 % transformation, complete cancer treatment cannot be expected.

Dr. Ebina: What is the magnification?

Dr. Nagano: 400 times magnification.

III.

SAFETY CONTROL

Comparative Kinetics of Circulating Interferon and Physiological Response in Cynomolgus Monkeys Given Intramuscular and Intravenous Injections of α and β Interferons

Shudo Yamazaki, Masayoshi Kohase, Masashi Tatsumi, Eiko Onishi, Chiharu Morita, Sachi Otaki, Seiya Kohno, and Reisaku Kono

National Institute of Health of Japan, Murayama Annex, Gakuen, Musashimurayama, Tokyo, Japan

INTRODUCTION

For clinical trials of human interferon (IFN) it is important to have an established system which will permit both *in vivo* quantitative studies of pharmacologic actions and safety tests of the IFN. The difficulty in selecting appropriate experimental animals is related to the "species specificity" of IFN action, a distinct nature possessed by all IFNs, although various degrees of cross-reactivity between different species have been noticed. Furthermore, it has also been suggested that the 3 distinct types of human interferon, α, β, and γ, may behave differently from each other *in vivo* just as they are distinguished *in vitro* in antigenic, physicochemical, and some biological properties. Therefore, an experimental animal susceptible to the distinct types of human IFN is required to study the comparative pharmacokinetics and pharmacodynamics *in vivo*. It has been shown that human IFN is highly active in monkey cells *in vitro*,[1] so comparative experiments between IFN-α and IFN-β were designed to determine whether cynomolgus monkeys could be used to investigate the pharmacologic actions and safety of human IFN preparations.

METHODS AND RESULTS

Fibroblast (F)-IFN was provided by Toray Industries, Inc., and lymphoblastoid (Lb)-IFN and leukocyte (Le)-IFN were supplied by the Green Cross Corp.

Fourteen cynomolgus monkeys, female and over 5 years old, were used after

281

a 3-month period of health care and stabilization at the National Institute of Health in Tokyo.

Prior to performing the animal experiments, baseline experiments were carried out *in vitro* to obtain information necessary for the subsequent animal experiments. The first experiment examined the cross-reactivity of IFN in the cynomolgus monkey cells by comparing IFN-α and IFN-β with simultaneous titrations in human and monkey cells. As shown in Table 1, Le-IFN-α was found to be equally as active on the primary cultures of cynomolgus monkey kidney (MK) as on human-derived FL cell cultures; the MK to FL ratio was about 2 when titration was done by the plaque inhibition method. In contrast, F-IFN-β revealed a much higher titer in the human cells than in the monkey cells, giving a MK to FL ratio lower than one. Similar results were obtained when IFN titers were compared in MK cells and human embryonic lung cells by the CPE-inhibition method.

Table 1. Comparative titers of human IFN assayed in monkey and human cells.

Human IFN	Plaque inhibition[a]		MK/FL
	MK[b]	FL[c]	
Leukocyte			
Sample 1	1,700	800	2.1
Sample 2	50	20	2.5
Fibroblast			
Sample 1	130	560	0.23
Sample 2	16	125	0.13
	CPE-inhibition[a]		MK/HEL
	MK	HEL[d]	
Leukocyte			
Sample 1	840	480	1.8
Sample 2	96	48	2.0
Fibroblast			
Sample 1	113	1,680	0.067
Sample 2	10	144	0.069

a) Challenge virus = vesicular stomatitis virus.
b) MK = primary cultures of monkey kidney cells.
c) FL = a cell line derived from human amnion.
d) HEL = human embryonic lung cells (9th passage).

These results indicate that both types of human IFN are active in cynomolgus monkey- cells, although there was a difference between IFN-α and IFN-β in the level of cross-reactivity. This difference may vary depending on the cells, viruses, and other conditions used in the assay system. Under the experimental conditions we used, the MK cells were more sensitive to IFN-α than to IFN-β. The result is not inconsistent with the general idea that the α type of IFN is more cross-reactive than the β type.[2]

Another baseline experiment was done to test the stability of IFN-α and IFN-β in the blood of cynomolgus monkey. If either type of IFN was particularly unstable in the blood or was taken up preferentially by the blood cells as soon as it entered the circulation, then the resultant loss of serum IFN might influence the clearance rate of circulating IFN. As seen in Fig. 1, IFN-α was quite stable in the whole blood as well as in the plasma, while IFN-β was slowly degraded to a level of 25% of the initial IFN activity by 5 hours. It should be noted that there was no significant difference in the amount of IFN recovered from either plasma or whole blood, suggesting that a significant loss of either type of IFN due to adsorption of free IFN molecules to blood cells may not occur in blood flow. Even if some loss by adsorption occurs, it may not have a significant influence on the clearance rate of circulating IFN.

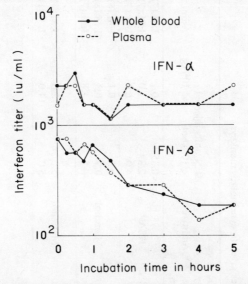

Fig. 1. Comparative stability of human Le-IFN-α and F-IFN-β in monkey blood or plasma. Interferon was mixed with either plasma or whole blood, and the mixtures were shaken continuously and incubated in a 37°C water bath for various periods of time, as shown. Samples were centrifuged and the supernatants assayed for IFN activity.

Using these data, we carried out *in vivo* experiments to study the comparative pharmacokinetics of IFN-α and IFN-β administered to monkeys. The nature and doses of the human IFN preparations used for these experiments are described in Table 2. Although Lb-IFN is generally considered to be a source of IFN-α, the Lb-IFN preparation provided to us by Green Cross Inc. was found to consist soley of IFN-β, which was completely neutralized by anti-F-IFN serum but not by anti-Le-IFN serum. For each IFN administered monkey, one control monkey was injected with the placebo material, which contained

Table 2.　IFN preparations and doses given to cynomolgus monkeys.

IFN production system	Type of purified IFN	Specific activity IU/mg protein	Additive	IFN units injected ×10⁶/shot	×10⁶/kg	Administration	Total IFN units injected ×10⁶/body	Placebo (HSA) mg/shot
Fibroblast cells + poly 1:C	β	$> 10^7$	HSA[a]	0.35 2.8 14.0	0.1 1.0 6.0	I.M.(7), I.V.(7) I.M.(7), I.V.(7) I.M.(7), I.V.(7)	5 39 196	0.7 5.6 28.0
Lymphoblastoid cells + HVJ	β	1×10^6	Mannitol	0.3 0.9 4.5	0.1 0.3 1.8	I.M.(8), I.V.(6) I.M.(8), I.V.(6) I.M.(7), I.V.(6)	4 13 63	1.0 3.0 15.0
Leukocytes (buffy coat) + HVJ	α	3×10^6	Mannitol	35.0 35.0	12.0 14.0	I.M.(1) I.V.(1)	35 35	— —

a) HSA: human serum albumin.

human serum albumin in the same concentration as the respective IFN preparation.

The experimental procedure over a period of one month and laboratory test items are summarized in Table 3. In the group for testing F-IFN and its placebo, 6 monkeys were inoculated on the days marked with triangles; they received 7 intramuscular (I.M.) injections followed by 7 intravenous (I.V.) injections in the thigh. Samples were taken by bleeding for various laboratory tests at the points shown by arrows. In the Lb-IFN group, 6 monkeys were injected with either IFN or placebo, 7 times I.M. then 6 times I.V., followed by one I.M. shot. All 12 monkeys were autopsied at the end of one month and subjected to histopathologic examinations. The 2 monkeys given Le-IFN were not sacrificed.

Table 3. Experimental procedure and laboratory tests.

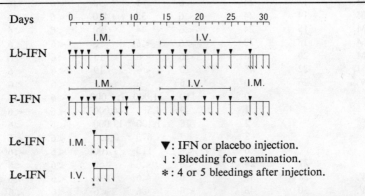

Test items	F/Placebo		Lb/Placebo		Le/Placebo
Body weight	●	●	●	●	●
Body temperature	●	●	●	●	●
White cell count	●	●	●	●	●
Red cell count	●	●	●	●	●
Platelet count			●	●	●
T-cell count			●	●	●
Hemogram	●	●	●	●	●
Blastogenesis			●	●	●
Transaminase	●	●	●	●	●
Serum IFN assay	●	●	●	●	●
Inhibitor to IFN	●	●	●	●	●
Autopsy	●	●	●	●	
Histopathol, exam.	●	●	●	●	

Kinetics of Serum IFN

Table 4 shows the circulating IFN titers in monkeys which were given 3 different doses of F-IFN-β. With I.M. administration, the highest titer was demonstrated one to 3 hours after injection in all monkeys. In monkey no. 3, which received 6 mega international units (IU) of IFN/kg, antiviral activity was detectable even at 48 hours after administration. Interestingly, accumula-

Table 4.   Serum IFN titers in monkeys given 3 different doses of F-IFN-β and its placebo by I.M. and I.V. injections.

Injection route	Day of bleeding[c]	Time of bleeding[d]	Interferon group[a]			Placebo group[b]		
			Monkey 1	Monkey 2	Monkey 3	Monkey 4	Monkey 5	Monkey 6
I.M.	6/12	0	<6	<6	<6	<6	<6	<6
		1	24	90	6,000	<6	<6	<6
		3	20	120	4,500	<6	<6	<6
		6	15	60	3,000	<6	<6	<6
		12	<6	20	2,300	<6	<5	<6
I.M.	13	24	<6	5	90	<6	<6	<6
I.M.	14	24	<6	33	410	<6	<6	<6
I.M.	15	24	<6	44	390	<6	<6	<6
I.M.	18	72	<6	<6	<6	<6	<6	<6
I.M.	20	48	<6	<6	15	<6	<6	<6
I.M.	22	48	<6	<6	19	<6	<6	<6
I.V.	26	0	<6	<6	<6	<6	<6	<6
		0.5	110	11,000	152,000	<6	<6	<6
		1	49	4,560	46,000	<6	<6	<6
		2	18	1,100	13,000	<6	<6	<6
		3	7	670	7,600	<6	<6	<6
		6	<6	110	1,100	<6	<6	<6
	27	24	<6	<6	60	<6	<6	<6
I.V.	28	48	<6	<6	9	<6	<6	<6
I.V.	30	48	<6	<6	<6	<6	<6	<6
I.V.	7/3	72	<6	<6	<6	<6	<6	<6
	4	24	<6	<6	1,300	<6	<6	<6
I.V.	5	48	<6	<6	<6	<6	<6	<6
I.V.	7	48	<6	<6	<6	<6	<6	<6
I.V.	10	72	<6	<6	<6	<6	<6	<6
		0.5	260	1,400	15,000	<6	<6	<6
	11	24	<6	<6	<6	<6	<6	<6
	12	48	<6	<6	<6	<6	<6	<6
	13	72	<6	<6	<6	<6	<6	<6

a) Monkeys no. 1, 2, and 3 were injected with 0.35×10^6 IU, 2.8×10^6 IU, and 14.0×10^6 IU of IFN, respectively, by a single shot on each day of bleeding.

b) Monkeys no. 4, 5, and 6 were injected similarly with the placebo material which contained as much human serum albumin as had been added as stabilizer to the IFN preparations given to monkeys no. 1, 2, and 3, respectively (see Table 2).

c) Serum samples were harvested by bleeding at 10 A.M. just before administration, except on days 6/12 and 6/26 when monkeys were bled at the indicated time intervals after administration.

d) Time of bleeding in terms of hours after previous administration.

tion was observed when high doses of IFN were administered daily (compare the titers on day 6/13 and 6/14). With I.V. administration, 100% of the injected IFN was demonstrated at 30 min, but the titer fell rapidly and no antiviral activity was detected at 48 hours. Circulating IFN titers were dose-dependent in both cases. No antiviral activity was demonstrable in the sera from placebo monkeys.

Similar results were obtained with the monkeys which received Lb-IFN-β or Le-IFN-α (data not shown).

Clearance Rate

To compare the clearance rate of IFN by the two injection routes (I.M. and I.V.), a total amount of circulating IFN was calculated from each serum IFN titer and plasma volume (approximately 5% of body weight) and expressed as the percent fraction of a total IFN amount given by a single shot (Figs. 2 and 3).

The following results were obtained:

1) A significant difference was seen in the clearance rate of IFN by the two administration routes.

2) The clearance rate varied according to dose: with a lower dose there was a more rapid clearance (Fig. 2).

3) The maximum serum titer obtained at one hour after I. M. administration

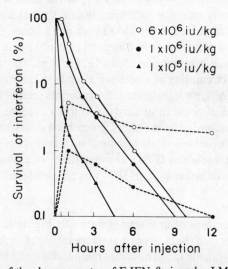

Fig. 2. Comparison of the clearance rates of F-IFN-β given by I.M. and I.V. injections. Monkeys were injected with 3 different doses of F-IFN-β as described in the legend to Table 4. Circulating IFN units were calculated from the serum IFN titers shown in Table 4 and the plasma volume obtained from the body weight of each monkey. Survivals of serum IFN are expressed as percentages of total IFN units injected either I.M. (-----) or I.V. (——).

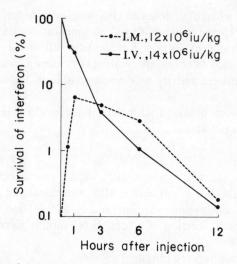

Fig. 3. Comparison of clearance rates of Le-IFN-α given by I.M. and I.V. injections. Monkeys were injected with 35 × 10⁶ IU of Le-IFN-α either I. M. or I. U. Blood samples were taken at indicated intervals after injection, and the sera were separated and assayed for IFN activity. Survivals of circulating IFN are expressed as percentages of total IFN units injected by a single shot.

of the highest dose of F-IFN-β was only 5% of the total IFN injected, but the titer decreased slowly over the following hours, so that a relatively high concentration of IFN remained in the blood even at 12 hours. This compares with the rapid clearance of serum IFN observed in monkeys injected I.V.

4) A similar result was obtained with IFN-α (Fig. 3); only 6% of the total IFN injected was circulating at one hour after I.M. administration of a high dose of Le-IFN. Thus, no significant difference was seen between the two types of IFN in the level of circulating antiviral activity obtained by I.M. injection when they were compared in monkeys given high doses of IFN. This finding differs from that observed with humans, in whom IFN-α appeared in the circulation at high levels and IFN-β at much lower or undetectable levels when an equivalent dose of either type of IFN was administered I.M.[3,4]

Body Temperature

The body temperature of monkeys is normally higher than that of humans, and it has been reported that the normal temperature at 10 A.M. of cynomolgus monkeys is 38.32 ± 0.40 °C.[5] The rectal temperature was measured at 10 A.M. before every injection. The temperatures fluctuated over a wide range, and although the temperatures of some monkeys rose after the first injection, a fever specifically caused by F-IFN-β administration was not observed.

However, early transient changes in body temperature were observed in monkeys given Lb-IFN-β (Figs. 4 and 5). High fever exceeding 40°C was recorded at 6 hours after I.M. administration and at one hour after I. V. administration of Lb-IFN-β. The fever response seemed to be dose-dependent; temperatures

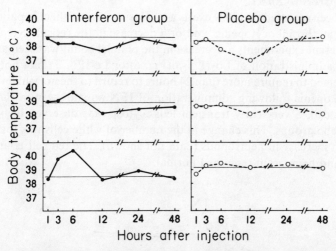

Fig. 4. Fever response of monkeys to I.M. administration of human Lb-IFN-β or placebo. Monkeys were injected I.M. with 0.3×10^6 IU of IFN or its placebo (top panel), 0.9×10^6 of IFN or its placebo (middle panel), or 4.5×10^6 IU of IFN or its placebo (bottom panel). Rectal temperatures were measured at indicated intervals after injection. A straight line in each panel indicates the pre-injection temperature.

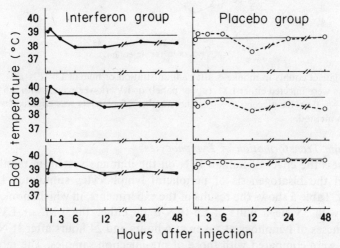

Fig. 5. Fever response of monkeys to I.V. administration of human Lb-IFN-β or its placebo.

Monkeys were treated in the same way as described in the legend to Fig. 4 except that administration was by I.V. injection.

in the placebo group did not exceed the pre-injection level. A similar but less signicant response was observed with Le-IFN-α (data not shown).

Myelosuppressive Effect

It has been reported that IFN exerts a myelosuppressive effect in patients, e.g., leukopenia, thrombocytopenia, and/or a decrease in the reticulocyte count.[6,7] In the present experiments a decrease in the platelet count was seen at 6 hours after the administration of Lb-IFN-β (Fig. 6) or Le-IFN-α (data not shown), and it seemed to require more than 24 hours to return to the normal level. However, leukopenia following administration of IFN was not seen in those monkeys. Instead, a very early transient leukocytosis was observed in both IFN and placebo groups. This change in the number of white cells was found to be due to an increase in neutrophils (data not shown). The red cell count, T-cell counts, and hemogram remained normal.

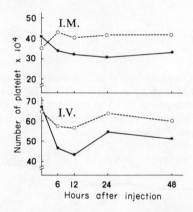

Fig. 6. Platelet counts in monkeys after administration of human Lb-IFN-β.
Monkeys were injected either I.M. (upper panel) or I.V. (lower panel) with 4.5×10^6 IU of IFN (——) or its placebo (······). The number of platelets was counted by Brecher-Cronkite's method.

Blastogenic Transformation of Lymphocytes

To assess the effect of human IFN on the immune system in monkeys, we examined the blsatogenesis of peripheral lymphocytes stimulated by PHA or ConA. Table 5 shows the results of the experiments, in which monkeys were injected with 35 mega units of Le-IFN-α by either the I.M. or I.V. route. Blastogeneses of lymphocytes taken at 6 hours and 24 hours after IFN administration were compared with those of pre-injection samples. The most significant inhibitory effect on blastogenesis was demonstrated with the lymphocytes harvested at 6 hours after I.M. administration of IFN. At 24 hours, a partial recovery of blastogenic reaction was seen. Interestingly, the effect was correlated with concentrations of circulating IFN, e.g., the higher concentration of IFN was detected in the serum taken at 6 hours from the monkey injected I.M. A suppressive effect on blastogenesis was also seen with IFN-β.

Table 5. Effect of human IFN-α on blastogenesis of monkey lymphocytes.

Injection	Time	Control	PHA	S.I.[a]	ConA	S.I.
I.M.	Pre-injection	455 ± 42[b]	1,907 ± 163(4.2)		5,499 ± 47(12.1)	
	Post 6 hours	271 ± 9	322 ± 33(1.2)		297 ± 10(1.1)	
	Post 24 hours	381 ± 10	1,231 ± 107(3.2)		1,569 ± 231 (4.1)	
I.V.	Pre-injection	691 ± 189	1,411 ± 570(2.0)		2,180 ± 228 (3.2)	
	Post 6 hours	273 ± 23	521 ± 28(1.9)		410 ± 12 (1.5)	
	Post 24 hours	397 ± 13	731 ± 201(1.8)		1,407 ± 178 (3.5)	

a) Stimulation index.
b) Mean ± SD cpm.
  2×10^5 cells/120 μl/well; PHA: 50 μg/ml; ConA: 50 μg/ml.
  Incubation time: 72 hours; ^{3}H-TdR labelling time: 18 hours.

Other Laboratory Tests

Serum samples were tested for transaminase, antimeasles virus HI titer, and anti-IFN activity. A transient elevation of serum transaminase was seen in the monkeys injected with Lb-IFN-β or Le-IFN-α, but not in the monkeys that received F-IFN-β. The F-IFN-β was purer and the specific activity was 10 to 100 times higher than that of Lb-IFN-β or Le-IFN-α.

All the monkeys had an HI titer to measles virus ranging from 32–512 before IFN was administered. At the end of one month, the HI activity in the samples taken from treated monkeys had dropped 2- to 4–fold.

A low level of IFN-neutralizing activity was detected in the sera taken from the IFN-treated monkeys, but no such activity was detected either in the pre-injection sera or in the sera obtained from the placebo group. This anti-IFN activity was probably due to neutralizing antibody formed by repeated injections of IFN.

Twelve monkeys were sacrificed for autopsy 3 days after the last administration of either IFN or placebo. Gross autopsy findings were normal, and no histologic changes obviously related to the IFN treatment were noted in any of the organs and tissues except for the lymphocytic organs, namely the thymus, spleen, and lymph nodes. A marked change was found in the T-cell zone of these organs by a histochemical examination for acid α-naphthyl acetate esterase (ANAE) activity. ANAE activity has been found to be a useful T-cell marker, and T-lymphocytes display a solitary red brown nodule of reaction product (T-pattern) which can be readily distinguished from the diffuse, cytoplasmic staining of monocytes (M-pattern).[8]

T-cell zones present in the paracortical and interfollicular regions of the lymph nodes from the placebo monkey clearly demonstrated ANAE (+) activity, as shown in Fig. 7A. In contrast, almost all the lymphocytes present in the T-cell zone of the monkeys injected with Lb-IFN were replaced with many small lymphocytes lacking ANAE activity (Fig. 7B). The same findings were seen in the medullar region of the thymus and the periarteriolar region of the spleen. The nature and significance of these ANAE (—) small lymphocytes are not known at present.

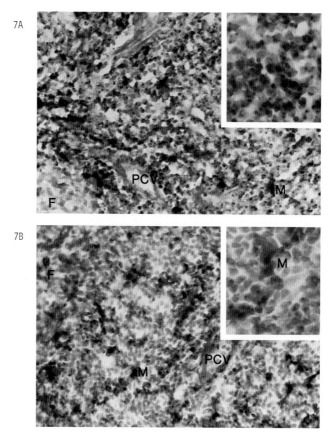

Fig. 7. ANAE reactivity of the cells in the paracortical area of the lymph nodes of the monkeys treated with Lb-IFN (B) or with a placebo (A).

The monkeys were autopsied and examined on the 31st experiment day, 3 days after the last injection of multiple I.V. and I.M. doses (see Table 3). Note: almost all the cells in the paracortical T-cell area of the placebo-treated animal showed a typical T-pattern reaction product (A). The same cells had aggregated densely in this area of the Lb-IFN-treated animal and were ANAE-negative under the same staining condition, remaining a normal reactivity of monocytes. (B). Inserts in both A and B are high magnification views.

F: cortical lymph follicle; PCV: postcapillary venule; M: monocytes.

In this report, we have presented some data from animal experiments which were designed to determine whether human IFN preparations would have the same effects in cynomolgus monkeys as in humans. The experiments showed that, although the pharmacokinetic behavior of IFN-β after I. M. injection was somewhat different from that in humans, the biological effects and many physiological responses of the monkeys to human IFN preparations seemed to be comparable to those clinically observed in patients. These results indicate that cynomolgus monkeys would be a useful experimental animal for studying the pharmacologic actions of human IFN preparations.

REFERENCES

1. Bucknall, R. A.: "Species specificity" of interferons: A misnomer? *Nature*, **216**: 1022, 1967.
2. Gresser, I., Bandu, M. T., Brouty-Boye, D., and Tovey, M.: Pronounced antiviral activity of human interferon on bovine and porcine cells. *Nature*, **251**: 543–545, 1974.
3. Edy, V. G., Billiau, A., and De Somer, P.: Non-appearance of injected fibroblast interferon in the circulation. *Lancet*, **i**: 451–452, 1978.
4. Billiau, A., De Somer, P., Edy, V. G., De Clercq, E., and Heremans, H.: Human fibroblast interferon for clinical trials: Pharmacokinetics and tolerability in experimental animals and humans. *Antimicrob. Agents Chemother.*, **16**: 56–63, 1979.
5. Honjo, S., Fujiwara, T., Takasaka, M., Suzuki, Y., and Imaizumi, K.: Observations on the diurnal temperature variation of cynomolgus monkeys (*Macaca irus*) and on the effect of changes in the routine lighting upon this variation. *Jap. J. M. Sc. & Biol.*, **16**: 189–198, 1963.
6. Greenberg, H. B., Pollard, R. B., Lutwick, L. I., Gregory, P. B., Robinson, W. S., and Merigan, T.C.: Effect of human leukocyte interferon on hepatitis B virus infection in patients with chronic active hepatitis. *New Engl. J. Med.*, **295**: 517–522, 1976.
7. Cheesman, S. H., Rubin, R. H., Stewart, J. A., Tokoff-Rubin, N. E., Cosimi, A. B., Cantell, K., Gilbert, J., Winkle, S., Herrin, J. T., Black, P. H., Russell, P. S., and Hirsch, M. S.: Controlled clinical trial of prophylactic human-leukocyte interferon in renal transplantation. *New Engl. J. Med.*, **300**: 1345–1349, 1979.
8. Knowles, D. M. and Holck, S.: Tissue localization of T-lymphocytes by the histochemical demonstration of acid α-naphthyl acetate esterase. *Lab. Invest.*, **39**: 70–76, 1978.

Discussion

Dr. REVEL: What is the possible function of the enzyme in LT lymphocytes that you found being decreased by interferon treatment?

Dr. YAMAZAKI: The method of examining ANAE activity is used generally as a very simple and convenient T-cell marker method.

Dr. REVEL: Is it a decrease in total T-cell population or . . . ?

Dr. YAMAZAKI: I don't know. I cannot answer exactly yet, but we found that all the cells inTDA were replaced by a number of small lymphocytes lacking this enzyme activity, as you saw in the slide, and we have not yet done the characterization of those cells. We'd like to do that.

Interferon Standards: Current Status and Future Needs

George J. GALASSO

Development and Applications Branch Microbiology and Infectious Diseases Program National Institute of Allergy and Infectious Diseases, Bethesda, Maryland 20205, U.S.A.

Since its discovery in 1957 and until recently, interferon (IFN) has been studied as an antiviral agent. With its demonstrated potential as an anticancer agent and its effects on the immune system, interest in IFN has multiplied manyfold. In one respect this publicity is working to the deteriment of IFN. The public is expecting a miracle drug. There is no question that IFN is not the cure for cancer or the penicillin of viral diseases. There is also no question in my mind that it will indeed prove to be of some clinical value in both infectious diseases and cancer patients. However, a few years from now when this has been proven, the public will be disappointed because they have been led to believe it is a miracle drug instead of being impressed with its actual potential. On the other hand, this publicity has led to increased work and a fierce competition to be the first to purify or to clone IFN. The progress that has been made in the past year has been truly remarkable. It is expected that IFN produced in bacteria will be available within a few months for clinical studies.

This recent flurry of activity and availability of material emphasizes the need for accurate comparisons among laboratories of the materials tested and the results obtained. Toward this end, International Reference Preparations of Interferon are made available by the National Institute for Biological Standards and Control, London, and the National Institute of Allergy and Infectious Diseases (NIAID), Bethesda. These reference preparations have been officially recognized by the World Health Organization (WHO) and consist of human leukocyte, human fibroblast, rabbit, mouse, and chick IFNs.[1,2]

Since the only means of quantitating IFN is by measuring its biological activity and since various assays were developed soon after its discovery, it became apparent that some mechanism had to be developed so that results from

295

different laboratories could be compared. The need for research reference reagents was clear. Working standards became available and after some experience with them, a meeting was held in London in 1969 (Table 1). The data were reviewed and the participants agreed that since there were so many different kinds of bioassays and since each laboratory seemed to have a favorite, interim reference preparations should be adopted to permit comparison of results obtained by use of the various methods. It was agreed that human leukocyte, rabbit, mouse, and chick preparations would be provided by the Medical Research Council (MRC) and the NIAID. In 1978 the WHO, having recognized the general acceptance, need, and usage of these preparations adopted them and a human fibroblast IFN reagent as international reference preparations.

Table 1. Preferred expression of IFN unitage.

1. An International Unit, as defined by an appropriate international IFN standard preparation, if one exists;
2. A research unit, as defined by a research standard preparation, if available from a national agency;
3. If no research standard preparation exists, as the minimal amount of IFN producing an arbitrarily defined degree of activity in a given test system; in essence, a laboratory unit.

The importance of these materials is attested to by their use at an increasingly rapid rate, the absence of controversy regarding their unitage, and the results reported in the literature in terms of reference units (Table 2).

Table 2. NIAID distribution of international reference preparations of human and mouse IFNs.

	Human leukocyte	Human fibroblast Number of ampoules	Mouse
Distributed prior to 1979	191	61	518
Distributed in 1979	128	104	140
Distributed in 1980	163	107	80

The primary purpose of these standards is to compare the observed titrations in one's own preferred assay to the unitage of the standard. Once the standard is received, it should be diluted, divided into separate tubes, and stored at $-70°$C. A large lot of an internal laboratory standard of a similar type should also be produced and stored in a similar fashion. The standard material should be assayed in a given laboratory repeatedly (more than 4 times) in order to obtain a valid estimate of the mean titer and the variation that is observed within the particular assay performed. In performing these assays, an attempt should be made to obtain the greatest precision, such as by using small dilution steps, e.g., 2-fold, and many replicate cultures to test each dilution. The dose-response curves for the international reference preparation and the comparable internal laboratory standard must be parallel and the ratios between the observed titers of the external and internal standards should be reproducible. The geometric mean titer of the internal standard can then be determined in relations to the titers of the external standard. The laboratory preparation, then calibrated, can be used in each experimental titration to provide the basis, by the same ratio method, for reporting titiers of test samples in international reference units. The laboratory standard should be included in all subsequent assays in which unknown samples are run.

Other reagents distributed by the NIAID which have proven to be of immense value have been antisera to mouse, human leukocyte, and human fibroblast IFNs. These materials were prepared by repeated injection of rabbits from which sera were collected when significant anti-IFN levels were obtained. Greater than 95 % of the antibodies to known contaminants present in the IFN preparations used for immunization were removed by immunoabsorption techniques utilizing antigens bound to Sepharose 4B. This material was distributed sparingly to all investigators who requested it. It has contributed to a great variety of important data and was responsible for the first recognition of the antigenic differences between leukocyte and fibroblast IFNs. This led to the realization that a separate reference preparation for fibroblast IFN was needed, and it was subsequently developed by the NIAID.

More recently, the discovery of immune or γ IFN has again indicated a need for new reference preparations. We are currently supporting the development of the appropriate reagents for both human and mouse IFN-γ. It is hoped that these will be available within the year.

DNA recombinant technology resulting in the cloning of IFN has yielded unprecedented rapid discoveries about the structure of IFN. These findings have in turn, led to the realization that there may be at least ten different leukocyte IFNs and perhaps more. There are also multiple forms of fibroblast IFN. Utilizing monoclonal antibody techniques, it may be possible to develop specific antibodies to each of these IFNs. Whether they will cross-react remains to be proven. It may eventually be necessary to make such serologic reagents available, but for the time being it would seem that the group-reactive antisera currently available through the NIAID would be the most useful.

Since there is considerable interest in the antitumor effect of IFN and its immunomodulatory effects, such as increases in T-cell cytotoxicity, natural killer cell activity, antibody-dependent cell cytotoxicity, and macrophage phagocytosis, it will be necessary to develop new standard assay systems to quantitate these properties of the various new IFN preparations in progress and to define the reference preparations in these terms as well as antiviral titer.

Finally, it will eventually be necessary to do comparative studies of the various IFNs. Just as we have found that fibroblast and leukocyte IFN behave differently in patients, we are sure to find other differences between the various cloned products. It is too early to predict which of the various materials will prove most efficacious, but at a future period in time it will be necessary for an independent sponsor, such as a government agency, to support comparative studies.

It appears that new questions develop faster than we can provide answers. This is an exciting time for IFN and antivirals in general, but if we are to continue to make useful progress, we must assure that the proper controls and standards are used.

REFERENCES

1. Interferon standards: a memorandum. *J. Biol. Stand*, 7: 383–395, 1979.
2. WHO Technical Report Series, 638: 1979.

Discussion

Dr. KUWATA: You said that besides standardizing the antiviral action of interferon, tests are going on to standardize the anticellular action of interferon, that is, the effects of interferon for the suppression of cell growth or the enhancement of NK activity. Would you please tell us what kinds of tests are now going on at NIH to evaluate such actions of human interferons?

Dr. GALASSO: What I meant to indicate was that up until now we quantitated interferon on the basis of its antiviral activity. Those who are interested in the antitumor effect and other effects of interferon are not satisfied with just an antiviral titer. So it is important that we develop new ways of measuring interferon, and I suggested that these ways are being developed but not that any specific test is currently being done.

Dr. KAWADE: As one of the few survivors in the field of mouse interferon, I must say that it is highly desirable to have separate mouse α and β interferons and, especially, separate anti-α and anti-β antibody references. In contrast to human cells, various mouse cells usually produce both α and β species, but, for instance, people tend to consider mouse interferon produced by fibroblasts to be β in analogy to human interferon, but this is often wrong. So I wonder how you consider the mouse reference preparations.

Dr. GALASSO: My slide indicated that there aren't less people interested in mouse research, because that is approximately at the same level as it always was. We do feel that work in the mouse is terribly important, and when we develop new standards such as we are doing now for α interferon we include α for mouse as well as human. The need for the two, for α and β, is taken under advisement, and this will be considered. There is no attempt on our part at the present time to do anything about it, but perhaps you are correct and this should be done.

Potency Standardization of Human Interferon Preparations for Clinical Trials

Masayoshi Kohase, Seiya Kohno, Shudo Yamazaki, Akira Shishido, and Reisaku Kono

National Institute of Health of Japan, Murayama Annex, Gakuen, Musashimurayama, Tokyo, Japan

SUMMARY

A procedure for determining human interferon (IFN) potency is described in this paper. Severalyears' experience with the procedure demonstrated that it offers several advantages for evaluating both α and β types of IFN: (1) it gives a reproducible titer with moderate sensitivity, and (2) most of the manipulations can be automated so that (3) subjective elements inherent in conventional assays can be eliminated. An additional feature of this method, due in large part to the use of sindbis virus, is its poor sensitivity to the naturally occurring virus-inhibitor (s) frequently found in human sera.

INTRODUCTION

Determination of potency is one of the essential elements involved in the control of human IFN preparations intended for clinical studies. Each assay procedure for IFN now in use in various laboratories has certain advantages over others for particular experimental purposes. When it is necessary to titrate a large number of samples either singly or in batches simplicity of the procedure and reproducibility of the results are of prime importance.

The method originally described by Finter[1] was our first choice for titrating IFN samples. This method, based on the suppression of the viral cytopathic effect (CPE), measures the amount of a dye taken up by viable cells rather than grading the CPE microscopically. The benefits of introducing photometry are twofold. First, it eliminates subjective factors and/or deviations in the scores assigned by individual observers, and second, the automated measurements can be processed by a microcomputer. We had previously used a system consisting of FS-7 cells and vesicular stomatitis virus (VSV).[2] Although it was satisfactory for assaying a small number of IFN samples, certain shortcomings became evident when frequent, large-scale titrations were necessary; these included a long generation time, the high nutritional requirements of the cells, and the sensitivity of VSV against naturally occurring inhibitor(s) in human sera.[3]

MATERIALS AND METHODS

Cell Cultures

FL cells were grown in Eagle's minimum essential medium (MEM) containing 100 units/ml of penicillin and 100 μg/ml of streptomycin and supplemented with 5% heated calf serum (CS). The cells, which were adjusted to 1×10^5 cells/ml, were cultured in 700 ml glass roux bottles (50 ml/bottles). Three- or 4-day-old cells were then seeded on 96-well plastic microplates (5.5×10^4 cells/0.1 ml/well) with MEM containing 10% CS. They were incubated at 37° C for 4 hours or overnight in humidified air containing 5% CO_2 before use. FS-7 cells grown in MEM containing 5% fetal bovine serum (FBS) were incubated for several days at 37° C in a CO_2 incubator after seeding. Piror to use in IFN titration, the medium was replaced with MEM containing 5% CS.

Viruses

Vesicular stomatitis (VSV), semiliki forest (SFV), and sindbis viruses were grown and titrated by plaque formation in primary chick embryo cell cultures. They were stored at −80° C.

IFN Assay

IFNs (0.05 ml) were serially ($2 \times$) diluted with MEM on transfer plates with a multimanifold pipetter and added to the cell seeds in the 96-well microplates. The cells, after an overnight exposure to IFN, were challenged with sindbis virus in serum-free MEM whose buffer capacity had been strengthened by the addition of HEPES (N-2-hydroxylethylpiperazine-N'2'-ethanesulfonic acid, 10 mM)-NaOH (pH 7.4). The cells were incubated for 1–2 days until complete CPE was observed in the control cells which had received no IFN, and were then exposed for 30 min to 0.05 ml/well of 0.02% neutral red solution in MEM containing 5% CS. After a thorough washing with phosphate-buffered saline (PBS), the cell-bound dye was extracted by the addition of 0.1 ml/well of 30% ethanol, 0.01 N HCl. The optical densities of the extracts were measured *in situ* by a Titertech Multiscan photometer.

One unit was defined to be the reciprocal of the IFN dilution at the point where the incorporation of dye was 50% in uninfected control cells. Internal reference IFN-α and IFN-β, which had been frequently calibrated by the international references, MRC B, 69/29 and WHO G023 902–527, respectively, were included in every run to express the resulting titers in terms of international units.

RESULTS

Challenge Virus

Figures 1, 2, and 3 represent the results of experiments in which IFN-α- and IFN-β- treated FL cells were challenged with different doses of VSV, semiliki forest (SFV), and sindbis viruses. The cells were stained at 20 hours (Figs. 1 and 2) and at 48 hours (Fig. 3) after infection. The 50% end point of the uptake of the dye (Materials and Methods) decreased as the dose of VSV (Fig. 1) or SFV (Fig. 2) increased. The dose dependency usually became more evident when the cultures were incubated longer. These findings indicate the necessity of holding the multiplicity of infection and the incubation time constant to obtain reproducible titers.

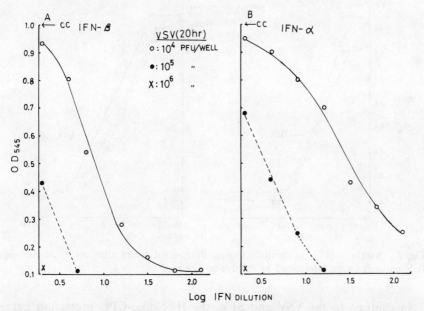

Fig. 1. Assays of IFN-α and IFN-β using VSV as a challenge virus. FL cell monolayers were treated with IFN overnight and then inoculated with the indicated doses of VSV after removal of the IFN. Twenty hour after the virus challenge, grades of CPE were determined by the dye-uptake method. Two rows of microplate were used for each sample, and eluates from 2 wells at each IFN dilution were pooled for measuring the optical density.

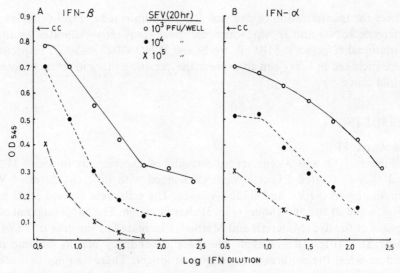

Fig. 2. Assays of IFNs using SFV. All procedures were similar to those described in the legend to Fig. 1 except that SFV was used as the challenge virus.

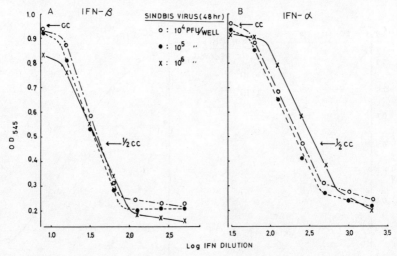

Fig. 3. Assays of IFNs using sindbis virus. Forty-eight hours after the virus challenge, IFN potencies were determined by the dye-uptake method.

In contrast to the VSV and SFV, the IFN dose-CPE protection curves observed with sindbis virus (Fig. 3) were hardly affected by the challenge dose within a wide range of 10^4–10^6 PFU/ml. Therefore, it can be anticipated that the use of this virus will reduce the amount of effort needed to obtain reproducibility.

Incubation Time with IFN

To determine the appropriate time period for exposure of the cells to IFN, the experiments shown in Figs. 4A and B were performed. FL and FS-7 cells were treated with serially diluted IFN-α or IFN-β for the periods indicated on the abscissa before the challenge with 10^5 PFU/well of sindbis virus. The antiviral state in these cells was expressed as the titer of the IFN (ordinate).

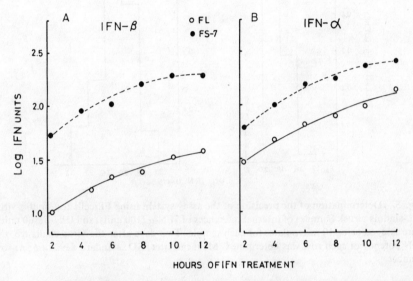

Fig. 4. Effect of incubation time on the kinetics of developing an antiviral state. Monolayers of FL cells and FS-7 cells were treated with IFN-α (30 units) and IFN-β (30 units) at 37°C. At the times indicated in the figure, the monolayers were washed twice with fresh medium and challenged with sindbis virus (10^5 PFU/well). Two days after the virus challenge, IFN titers were determined. Two rows of a microplate were used for each determination.

The antiviral state in these cells continued to increase during the exposure to IFN up to 12 hours. Although it does not reach a plateau, we routinely use overnight (12 hours) incubation with IFN for convenience.

Precision, Sensitivity, and Reproducibility

The IFN-α and IFN-β samples were titrated by multiple simultaneous runs. The results are summarized in Figs. 5A and B, in which titiers are expressed as exponents of 10. The IFN-β sample, which had an expected titer of 1.90 international units (IU), gave a titer of 1.92 with a standard deviation (SD) of 0.06. A slightly broader distribution of the titer was seen in IFN-α assays (Fig. 5B), the SD of which was 0.09. Another characteristic of our assay was that the observed titers of IFN-α were always higher than the international reference.

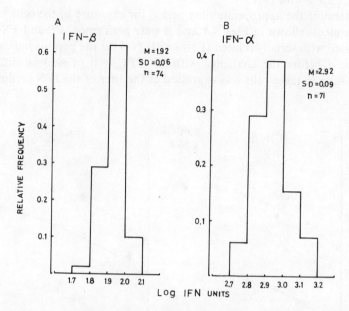

Fig. 5. Determination of the precision of the assay system using FL cells and sindbis virus (FL-sindbis virus). Samples of internal references of IFN-α (100 units) and IFN-β (160 units) were assayed using 10 microplates for each sample. Two days after the virus challange, the IFN potency of each row was determined. M: mean titer; SD: standard deviation; n: row number.

The mean titer of 2.92 calculated from the results in Fig. 5B is 8 times greater than the reference.

When a preparation of IFN is repeatedly assayed on different days, the distribution of its titer is expected to be much broader. Figures 6 and 7 show that this was indeed the case. In experiments summarized in Fig. 6, we carried out 24 independent assays on a sample of IFN-β, the expected titer of which was 2.20 IU. Although the mean titer (2.19) was very close to the expected value, the SD increased 2-fold (0.12) compared to simultaneous assays (0.06, Fig. 5A). The SD of the distribution of titers of an IFN-α sample in 40 independent titrations was almost tripled (0.29, Fig. 7; 0.09, Fig. 5B).

Considering the variety of factors which influence the bioassay of a biologically active substance like IFN, we think the fluctuation reported here falls in an acceptable range. In addition, most of the day-to-day variations, such as small changes in the cellular sensitivity to IFNs, may be cancelled by correcting observed titers with internal or international references assayed at the same time.

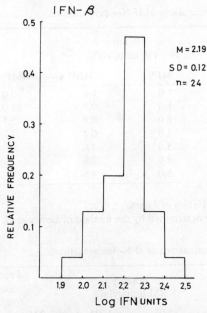

Fig. 6. Determination of reproducibility and sensitivity of FL-sindbis virus system in the assays of IFN-β. Reference IFN-β samples (160 units) were assayed on 24 different days. The challenge dose of the virus was 10^5 PFU/well. The resulting potencies obtained independently on different days were from 2 rows of the microplate.

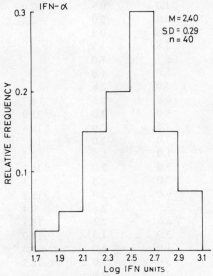

Fig. 7. Determination of reproducibility and sensitivity of FL-sindbis virus system in the assays of IFN-α. Samples of international reference IFN-α (100 units) were assayed on 40 different days. The procedures were the same as those used in Fig. 6.

Table 1.   Potency determinations of IFN-α preparations.

Lot No.	Potency (M units/vial)		Protein content (mg/vial)[c]	
	MF[a]	NIH[b]	MF	NIH
021	1.0	1.0	10.0	19.0
022	1.0	0.9	21.0	22.5
026	1.0	0.8	2.5	2.5
028–2	1.0	0.4		1.7
028–3	5.0	4.0		11.0
029–2GS	8.0	7.0		8.3
030–3	5.0	4.6		8.2

a) Manufacturer.
b) National Institute of Health of Japan.
c) Protein contents were determined by the method of Lowry *et al.*

Table 2.   Potency determinations of IFN-β preparations.

Lot No.	Potency (M units/vial)		Protein content (mg/vial)	
	MF	NIH	MF	NIH
78002	1.0	0.8	1.2	1.5
78004	1.0	1.1	1.2	1.0
78005	1.0	0.9	1.0	1.2
78006	1.0	0.9	2.0	1.9
78007	8.0	5.0	2.2	2.1
L001	0.8	0.7		
L002	2.8	3.2		
L004	5.5	7.0		
L0051	1.0	1.0		12.0
L0053	3.0	2.8		38.0
L0061	0.8	0.5	8.7	9.0
L0063	3.0	2.0	21.9	18.0
L0073	3.0	2.6	18.4	13.4
L0083	3.0	2.0	10.7	15.0
L0091	1.0	0.5	4.7	5.4
L0093	3.0	2.0	16.7	17.0
L0103	3.0	2.5	9.3	9.8
L0113	6.0	5.0	15.8	15.8
L0123	3.0	2.6	9.4	9.8
L0133	3.0	2.2	12.3	12.5
L0143	3.0	1.5	14.0	13.5
L0151	1.0	1.0	3.0	3.0
L0163	3.0	3.0	12.5	11.9
L0173	3.0	2.0	9.0	7.5
L0183	3.0	2.0	12.0	11.0

Testing IFNs in the Final Containers

Tables 1 and 2 summarize our potency tests on the IFN-α and IFN-β preparations, respectively. Most had been used in clinical studies under the supervision of the IFN Project Team, the Ministry of Health and Welfare. A small number of earlier lots were assayed by the direct reading of CPE of FS-7 cells challenged with VSV. These tables also indicate the amount of protein contained in the preparations. Analysis by gel electrophoresis revealed that the majority of protein is human serum albumine added as a stabilizer.

Considering the fluctuation which is inevitably associated in any bioassay, we can conclude that titers reported by manufactures and those obtained by us are in good agreement.

DISCUSSION

Progress in clinical studies and in the techniques of large-scale production has brought a growing need for a reliable method of titrating a large number of human IFN preparations. The method should give reproducible titers with a minimum of subjective steps, such as reading and grading CPE under a microscope. Automation in read-out and in computation of results is another requirement, because it not only saves time and labor but also removes subjective factors from the assay. It has been pointed out frequently that IFN-induced reduction of yields of viral components or infectivity is theoretically the best measure of the antiviral state. We decided, however, that we could sacrifice the theoretical advantage or even the sensitivity of the assay to some extent to meet the requirements for reliability and objectivity.

As noted earlier, we found the principles of the IFN assay described by Finter[1] best suited to our purposes. This method has been successfully used in many laboratories[4-6] for titrating various species of IFNs. We modified the original method slightly by using FL cells and sindbis virus. This cell line showed certain advantages, over others, i.e., a shorter generation time and lower nutritional requirements. We deliberately avoided the use of VSV, the most widely used challenge virus, for following reasons: (1) the growth and consequently the virus-induced CPE are extremely sensitive to the shift to an acid pH in the culture medium,[7] (2) it is labile to naturally occurring inhibitor (s) in human serum,[3] and (3) its use is discouraged or prohibited in many countries, including Japan.

In addition to the advantage that the use of sindbis virus offers (Figs. 3–7), the virus has other attractive characteristics which contrast with those of VSV. Sindbis virus is much less sensitive to a change of pH during its growth and to the presence of serum inhibitor (s) (data not shown). In addition, it belongs to the least hazardous group of animal viruses that can be handled in ordinarily equipped laboratories. These characteristics were particularly useful when levels of circulating IFN-α or IFN-β were determined after injections into patients. In our laboratory, none of the sera from more than 80 individuals showed any virus inhibitory activity (data not shown). In some preliminary studies, it was shown that this system worked well for titrating IFN-γ produced by the treatment of bufiy coat cells with a phytohemagglutinin.

Finally, it must be pointed out that an adequate supply and distribution of reference IFNs are prerequisites for the control of IFN preparations. In Japan, freeze-dried provisional references of IFN-α and IFN-β are available in large quantities so that we can include them in every run.

REFERENCES

1. Finter, N. B.: Dye uptake methods for assessing viral cytopathogenicity and their application to interferon assays. *J. Gen. Virol.*, **5**: 419–427, 1969.
2. Havell, E. A. and Vilček, J.: Production of high-titered interferon in cultures of human diploid cells. *Antimicrob. Agents Chemother.*, **2**: 476–484, 1972.
3. Thiry, L., Clerc, J.C.-L., Content, J., and Tack, L.: Factors which influence inactivation of vesicular stomatitis virus by fresh human serum. *Virology*, **87**: 384–393, 1978.
4. McManus, N. H.: Microassay for interferon: Microspectrophotometric quantitation of cytopathic effect. *Appl. Environ. Microbiol.*, **31**: 35–38, 1976.
5. Borden, E. C. and Leonhart, P. H.: A quantitative semimicro, semiautomated colorimetric assay for interferon. *J. Lab. Clin. Med.*, **89**: 1036–1042, 1977.
6. Armstrong, J. A.: Semi-micro, dye-binding assay for rabbit interferon. *Appl. Microbiol.*, **21**: 723–725, 1971.
7. Fiszman, M., Leaute, J. B., Chany, C., and Girard, M.: Mode of action of acid pH values on the development of vesicular stomatitis virus. *J. Virol.*, **13**: 801–808, 1974.
8. Lowry, O. H., Rosebrough, N. J., Farr, A. L., and Randall, R. J.: Protein measurement with the Folin phenol reagent. *J. Biol. Chem.*, **193**: 265–275, 1951.

Discussion

Dr. EBINA: I wish to ask you three questions. First, what is the sensitivity of this assay; second, have you ever used or carried out a comparison with WISH cells, which is a popular cell line; and third, what is the reason for not using plaque reduction? We are using the plaque reduction method and have obtained good sensitivity with WISH cells and the VSV line.

Dr. KOHASE: To answer your last question first, we do not use the plaque reduction method because the method I have shown has the advantage of easily obtaining a large amount of samples. With regard to WISH cells, we did not compare their sensitivity with FL cells. With regard to the sensitivity, the sensitivity of the β interferon was the expected level, and that of the α was two- to five-fold higher.

Dr. EBINA: So the sensitivity does not seem to be so good. I think it might be better to use a method in which each unit could be measured.

Dr. KOHASE: We can measure each unit with this method. I would not say that the sensitivity is extremely good, but it is not so bad, either.

Dr. MACHIDA: I reported in a previous interferon symposium that the IF titer changes according to the inoculum size regardless of the number of hours after infection in the EL-VSV line. You showed that the challenge virus at 3 doses from 10^4 to 10^6 showed almost the same titer at 48 hours, and I was impressed with your results, but have you looked at the results at different intervals?

Dr. KOHASE: I used 2 days because the results were not dose-dependent. If we measure on the first day, the results were dose-dependent. In this system, if we try to measure on the first day, using 10^6 or 10^5 PFU/well, we get an almost identical titer on the first day at either 10^6 or 10^7.

Interferon-Induced Disease in Mice and Rats

Michael G. Tovey and Ion Gresser

Laboratory of Viral Oncology Institut de Recherches Scientifiques sur le Cancer, Villejuif, France

INTRODUCTION

Treatment of newborn mice with potent mouse interferon (IFN) preparations resulted in an acute "early" syndrome characterized by inhibition of growth, delay in the maturation of several organs, diffuse liver cell necrosis, and death. When IFN treatment was discontinued at 1 week of life, mice appeared to recover, but subsequently developed a progressive glomerulonephritis ("late syndrome"). Treatment of newborn mice with electrophoretically pure mouse IFN also induced both the early and late disease syndromes, whereas preparations without IFN activity but containing the major contaminants collected during the purification procedures were inactive.

Treatment of newborn rats with potent IFN preparations also resulted in inhibition of growth, dealy in maturation, and the subsequent development of glomerulonephritis.

After infection at birth with lymphocytic choriomeningitis (LCM) virus, most strains of mice developed a similar acute early syndrome and surviving mice subsequently developed glomerulonephritis. We postulated that the endogenous IFN induced by LCM virus early in life was partly responsible for these syndromes. Administration of a potent antimouse IFN serum to LCM virus infected mice neutralized the circulating endogenous IFN and inhibited the development of both the early and late syndromes.

These results suggest that large amounts of exogenous or endogenous IFN at a crucial stage in the rapid growth or development of mice and rats can induce lesions in several different organs. Some lesions (i.e., in the kidney) only become apparent weeks or even months after exposure to IFN.

Interferon is a potent antiviral protein. There are abundant experimental data indicating that the production of IFN in the course of viral infections is an integral part of the host response, and IFN treatment of animals and (recently) humans is associated with prophylactic and therapeutic antiviral effects. For many years, most investigators believed that IFN inhibited viral multiplication within the cell without affecting host cell metabolism or function. It is now widely accepted, however, that IFN can also affect cell division and function both in cell culture and in the animal. If this is so, we might expect to find instances in which too much IFN instead of being beneficial, might even prove inimical to the host. This is the subject of our presentation.

When newborn mice were inoculated daily from birth subcutaneously or intraperitoneally with potent mouse IFN preparations (.05 ml of IFN with a titer of 8×10^{-5} reference units), there was a progressive inhibition of growth in the first week of life. The mean weight of IFN treated mice was 60 to 80% of the weight of control-inoculated litter mates. When IFN treatment was continued for the next few days, *all* of the mice died (Table 1A).[1] At autopsy, the most striking abnormality was a pale gray liver. Light microscopic examination revealed a marked steatosis, large areas of cell degeneration, and necrosis without any inflammatory reaction. The only other abnormalities on light microscopic examination were some diminution of the cortical region of the thymus in some mice, and poorly differentiated germinal follicles in the spleens of most mice. No renal lesions were present. Examination of liver sections under the electron microscope showed a marked accumulation of fat in hepatocytes. No viral particles were observed.

In these experiments, IFN treatment proved lethal only when begun on the day of birth and continued daily for the first week of life. When treatment was initiated on day 6 and continued daily for 14 days, mice grew normally and liver lesions were not observed. The effect of IFN on newborn mice depended, therefore, not only on the amount of IFN administered but also on the immaturity of the host.

What happened to these mice when IFN treatment, begun at birth, was stopped on the 7th day of life (a time when steatosis and discrete foci of liver cell necrosis were present)? The majority of these mice appeared to recover and they gained weight. However, in the ensuing months a number of these mice died. At autopsy, although the liver and other organs appeared normal, the kidneys were pale and the surface was granular. Histologic examination revealed a severe glomerulonephritis (Table 1B).[2] The kidney pathology can be summarized as follows: in "early" lesions (30th day) the glomeruli appeared moderately enlarged with some thickening of the mesangium, some segmental foci of measangial proliferation, and some thickening of capillary loops. By immunofluorescence there were focal and segmental granular deposits of IgG, IgM, and C3 in the mesangial spaces and along some glomerular basement membranes (GBM). Subsequently (> 45 days), the lesions were more conspicuous with hyalinization of glomerular tufts (with epithelial crescents and

Table 1. Effects of treatment of suckling mice with mouse IFN.

	Mouse strain	No. experiments[a]	Mouse IFN[b]	Injected with			
				Control preparation	Inactivated mouse IFN	Human IFN	Uninoculated
A) Lethality of mouse IFN preparations (Daily IFN treatment continued)	Swiss	5	107/107[c]	0/52	0/15	0/23	0/142
	C₃H	1	15/15	0/30	0/15	NT	0/18
B) Development of glomerulo-nephritis[d] (Daily IFN treatment stopped at day 6 to 8)	Swiss	9	60/60[e]	0/50	0/18	1/18	2/65
	C₃H	1	13/17	—	—	—	0/13

a) For experimental details see references 1 and 2.
b) Mice injected daily subcutaneously with 0.05 ml of a C-243 cell IFN preparation (titer 3.2×10^{-6} reference units).
c) Number of mice dead/total number of mice injected. Mean day of death = 11 days.
d) Results pooled; mice sacrificed between 20 and 274 days of life.
e) Number of mice with histologic confirmation of glomerulonephritis per total number of mice killed.

voluminous subendothelial deposits). In well-advanced disease, virtually all glomeruli were sclerotic and there was extensive sclerosis and diffuse atrophy of tubules. By immunofluorescence there were coarse granular deposits of IgG, IgM, and C3 along the GBM.

Although glomerular lesions were first seen by light microscopy towards the 3rd week of life, electron microscopic examination of the kidneys of IFN treated mice at 8 days of life showed a marked delay in the maturation of glomeruli. Furthermore, there was a marked thickening of the glomerular basement membrane, involving mainly the lamina rara interna and characterized by lacunae containing coarse granules, fibrillary material, and finely granular electron-dense deposits.[3]

We should emphasize at this point that, under our experimental conditions, *all* Swiss and C3H mice treated with potent IFN preparations have shown the liver lesions described above, and *all* Swiss mice treated for the first week of life developed glomerulonephritis (Table 1). These syndromes have been seen in *all* strains of mice tested, and also in axenic and nude mice.

These experiments were carried out with partially purified mouse IFN preparations having a specific activity of 10^7 reference units per mg protein. Mice were injected with approximately 50 μg of protein per day. Control preparations consisting of mock mouse IFN preparations, heated or periodate-inactivated mouse IFN preparations, or human IFN preparations did not induce disease in mice. All these preparations contained comparable amounts of protein.

Nevertheless, we wanted to determine the effect of even more purified mouse IFN preparations. Recently, we have tested electrophoretically pure mouse IFN prepared by Dr. Michel Aguet in our laboratory based on methods developed by De Maeyer- Guignard *et al.*[4,5] This material had a specific activity of 0.5 to 1.0 $\times$ 10^9 units/mg protein. After electrophoresis in polyacrylamide gels in SDS, and staining with Coomassie Blue, only 3 bands corresponding to molecular weights of 35,000, 28,000, and 22,000 were observed. Biological activity of IFN was found only in eluates of gel slices corresponding to these bands. We injected newborn mice with 25 μl of IFN (containing 500 nanograms of protein). We also tested the original partially purified IFN (having a comparable titer) and preparations containing the major contaminants collected during the purification procedures. Only partially and highly purified IFNs inhibited mouse growth, delayed maturation of different organs, induced liver lesions, caused death, and induced glomerulonephritis. It was concluded, therefore, that IFN itself was the responsible factor in inducing these lesions.

Furthermore, this phenomenon was not confined to mice. When newborn rats were injected with rat IFN preparations (but not mouse or human IFN preparations), there was also a clear-cut inhibition of growth, delay in the maturation of several different organs, and the late development of glomerulo-nephritis.[6] Liver lesions were not observed, however.

The experiments discussed so far have concerned the use of exogenous IFN-let us now turn to some of the effects of endogenous IFN induced in newborn mice by lymphocytic choriomeningitis virus. When newborn mice of most strains were injected at birth with this virus, they grew poorly and after the 8th day began to die. The only histologic lesions observed were in the liver, which showed steatosis and focal or diffuse necrosis. Mice surviving this acute episode, subsequently developed glomerulonephritis. In other words, the syndromes induced in mice with LCM virus were identical to those induced by treatment of mice with IFN (Table 2). To explain this similarity of syndromes we proposed two hypotheses:[8] (1) IFN was lethal for suckling mice because it activated a latent virus (such as LCM virus), or (2) some of the manifestations of LCM virus disease in suckling mice were in fact due to endogenous IFN induced by the virus. We found no evidence to support hypothesis (1) because neither LCM virus nor mouse hepatitis virus nor any other infectious agent was re-covered from the liver and kidneys of IFN treated suckling mice.[1]

Table 2. Similarity in syndromes induced in suckling mice by IFN and LCM virus.

| Time | Clinical findings | Injected with | | Comments |
		Mouse IFN	LCM virus	
Early 2–3 weeks	Decreased weight gain	+	+	Similar curves of weight gain
	Delay in maturation of several organs	+	+	
	Liver cell steatosis leading to necrosis	+	+	Similar histology
	Mortality	+	+	
Late 1 month	Glomerulonephritis	+	+	Similar histology Deposits of C3 and IgG along GBM

We therefore turned our attention to the second hypothesis. First, we found that, despite previous reports to the contrary, LCM virus induced large amounts of IFN in suckling and adult mice.[7, 8] We then injected newborn mice with LCM virus and a potent sheep antiglobulin to mouse IFN.[8] Injection of this immunoglobuline neutralized the endogenous IFN and resulted in a 100-fold increase in the serum LCM virus titer. Despite this marked increase in circulating virus, anti-IFN globulin-treated mice grew normally, showed no liver lesions, and the incidence of death was much decreased.[8] Furthermore, injection of this anti-IFN antibody also markedly inhibited the appearance of the glomerulonephritis characteristic of late LCM virus disease.[9] LCM virus was present in the blood and kidneys of these mice in amounts comparable to control virus-infected mice developing glomerulonephritis.[9]

The lethality of LCM virus for suckling mice varies markedly with the mouse strain. Thus, virus-infected BALB/c mice exhibit minimal liver lesions and none die, whereas C3H mice have extensive liver lesions and all mice die. An intermediate pattern is observed with Swiss mice (36% mortality). The results of our experiments suggest that the genetic control of susceptibility or resistance is determined not by the extent of virus multiplication but by the amount of IFN produced. Thus, although there were no differences in the titers of LCM virus in the plasma or liver among the three strains of mice, there was a marked difference in the amount of IFN produced and the duration of inter-feronemia: BALB/c mice produced small amounts of IFN detectable in the plasma mostly on the 3rd day, Swiss mice produced more IFN detectable on the 3rd and 4th day, whereas C3H mice produced larger amounts of IFN and interferonemia lasted between the 3rd and 6th days.[10] Our results suggest, therefore, that the amplitude of the IFN response in C3H mice is in large part responsible for the severity of LCM disease. This interpretation is further supported by experiments showing a marked decrease in the incidence of mortality in virus-infected C3H mice when they were injected with a potent antimouse IFN globulin.[10] Furthermore, the relative resistance of BALB/c mice was not caused by insensitivity to IFN action because exogenous IFN did inhibit their growth and did induce comparable liver lesions. We suggest, therefore, that the minimal disease occurring in BALB/c mice was related to their minimal IFN response.

We believe this ensemble of results shows that the presence of both exogenous or endogenous IFN in large quantities in an immature animal can be harmful. Furthermore, a brief exposure to IFN at a critical period of rapid growth and maturation can be an important factor in the development of disease that only becomes manifest later in life. Space is too limited for me to discuss the possible mechanisms of action of IFN in inducing disease. Discussion of the various possibilities may be found in the references cited.[1-3,6,8,9] Instead let us emphasize several important points and consider why our results may be of relevance to human pathology. First, we may ask whether there are other instances in which IFN may be in part responsible for disease. Virelizier et al. have shown that C3H and A2G strain mice can become carriers of mouse hepatitis virus (MHV-3) and develop a progressive neurologic disease lasting for weeks or months.[11] These virus carrier mice also showed a chronic inter-feronemia,[12] and thus the possibility exists that IFN may be exerting untoward effects in some of these mice.

IFN does not cross the placental barrier in mice,[13] probably for a very good reason. Pregnant animals can contract virus infections and produce circulating IFN. If IFN crossed the placenta, it might well affect the developing embryo. But what about a virus that crosses the placenta and infects the embryo? Is it possible that the embryo-toxic effects ascribed to rubella virus, for example, may be related to IFN induced in the embryo itself? In other words, is it possible that cellular lesions considered heretofore as being caused by the virus are in fact caused by host substances (such as IFN) induced by the infectious agent? Recently, Hooks, and coworkers found immune IFN in the sera of patients with systemic lupus erythematosus, rheumatoid arthritis, scleroderma, and Sjögren's syndrome.[14] Serial serum samples showed a good correlation between IFN titers and disease activity, and these investigators suggested that the production of IFN might contribute to immunologic aberrations in autoimmune disease.[14]

In case these speculations might be misunderstood, it should be emphasized, however, that we do not feel that the results presented here constitute an argument against the use of IFN in patients. Over the years, we have pleaded long and hard the potential clinical usefulness of exogenous IFN.[15] We have been too often witness in the past 15 years to IFN's therapeutic efficacy in viral and neoplasic diseases of mice not to believe that comparable results would be obtained in man, were it properly used. We have also been witness to its extraordinary activity and to the varied effects IFN exerts on cells.[16] In some instances, IFN inhibits specialized cellular functions and in other instances it enhances cellular functions.[16,17] Factors such as the amount of IFN and the time of treatment determine the biological effects observed. Aside from the theoretical interest, these considerations are of utmost importance in determining how to use IFN in patients. Our results emphasize that we are dealing with a most potent substance, and as with hormones, use of IFN must be based on knowledge of its effects and, if possible, of its mode of action.

REFERENCES

1. Gresser, I., Tovey, M. G., Maury, C., and Chouroulinkov, I.: Lethality of interferon preparations for newborn mice. *Nature*, **258**: 76–78, 1975.
2. Gresser, I., Morel-Maroger, L., Maury, C., Tovey, M. G., and Pontillon, F.: Progressive glomerulonephritis in mice treated with interferon preparations at birth. *Nature*, **263**: 420–422, 1976.
3. Morel-Maroger, L., Sloper, J. C., Vinter, J., Woodrow, D., and Gresser, I.: *Lab. Invest.*, **39**: 513–522, 1978.
4. Sipe, J. D., De Maeyer-Guignard, J., Fauconnier, B., and De Maeyer, E.: Purification of mouse interferon by affinity chromatography on a solid-phase immunoadsorbent. *Proc. Natl. Acad. Sci. USA*, **70**: 1037–1040, 1973.
5. De Maeyer-Guignard, J., Tovey, M. G., Gresser, I., and De Maeyer, E.: Purification of mouse interferon by sequential affinity chromatography on poly (U) and antibody-agarose columns. *Nature*, **271**: 622–625, 1978.
6. Gresser, I., Morel-Maroger, L., Châtelet, F., Maury, C., Tovey, M. G., Bandu, M-T.,

Buywid, J., and Delauche, M.: Delay in growth and the development of nephritis in rats treated with interferon preparations in the neonatal period. *Am. J. Pathol.*, **95**: 329–333, 1979.

7. Rivière, Y. and Bandu, M.-T.: Induction d'interferon par le virus de la choriuméningite lymphocytaire chez la souris. *Ann. Microbiol. (Institut Pasteur)*, **128A**: 323–329, 1977.

8. Rivière, Y., Gresser, I., Guillon, J.-C., and Tovey, M. G.: Inhibition by anti-interferon serum of lymphocytic choriomeningitis virus disease in suckling mice. *Proc. Natl. Acad. Sci. USA*, **74**: 2135–2139, 1977.

9. Gresser, I., Morel-Maroger, L., Verroust, P., Riviere, Y., and Guillon, J.-C.: Anti-interferon globulin inhibits the development of glomerulonephritis in mice infected at birth with lymphocytic choriomeningitis virus. *Proc. Natl. Acad. Sci. USA*, **75**: 3413–3416, 1978.

10. Rivière, Y., Gresser, I., Guillon, J.-C., Bandu, M.-T., Ronco, P., Morel-Maroger, L., and Verroust, P.: Severity of lymphocytic choriomeningitis virus disease in different strains of suckling mice correlates with increasing amounts of endogenous interferon. *J. Exp. Med.*, **152**: 633–640, 1980.

11. Virelizier, J.-L., Dayan, A. D., and Allison, A. C.: Neuropathological effects of persistent infection of the mouse by mouse hepatitis virus (MHV-3). *Infect. Immun.*, **12**: 1127–1140, 1975.

12. Virelizier, J.-L., Virelizier, A.-M., and Allison, A. C.: The role of circulating interferon in the modifications of immune responsiveness by mouse hepatitis virus (MHV-3). *J. Immunol.*, **117**: 748–753, 1976.

13. Gresser, I.: Unpublished observations.

14. Hooks, J. J., Moutsopoulos, H. M., Geis, S. A., Stahl, N. I., Decker, J.L., and Notkins, A. L.: Immune interferon in the circulation of patients with autoimmune disease. *New Engl. J. Med.*, **301**: 5–8, 1979.

15. Gresser, I.: Clinical use of exogenous interferon. In: 3rd Int. Symp. Medical and Applied Virology. Reprinted from: M. Sanders and M. Schaeffer (eds.), Viruses Affecting Man and Animals. W. H. Green, St. Louis, Mo. USA, 1971 pp. 416–429.

16. Gresser, I.: On the varied biologic effects of interferon. *Cell. Immunol.*, **34**: 406–415, 1977.

17. Gresser, I. and Tovey, M. G.: Antitumor effects of interferon. *Biochem. Biophys. Acta*, **516**: 231–247, 1978.

Discussion

Dr. Niethammer: I have a question for Dr. Tovey. I would like to hear your ideas about whether the same thing could happen in humans. When you think about suckling mice and the state of development they are in, then they are certainly comparable to humans in some age of intrauterine life, say, 3–4–5 months of intrauterine life. so the problem might be that we get some similar results, for example, in intrauterine infection of rubella. Do you have any ideas about that?

Dr. Tovey: I agree with your suggestion. I think rubella might indeed be a candidate. We have found that most interferon does not cross the placenta, and this may be for a very good reason.

Dr. Beladi: Have you any comparative data concerning the effect of interferon α and interferon β on the newborn mice?

Dr. Tovey: As yet, we don't. But we have isolated the different sorts. We have them, and if we ever manage to get sufficient quantities, we would very much like to do this.

Dr. Bektimorov: I have two questions for Dr. Tovey. The first is whether there is any critical age in mice when interferon stops inhibiting the growth of the mice and developing glomerulonephritis. There is a critical age of mice in relation to some viruses such as Coxackie virus and arboviruses. The next question is, did you check the distribution of interferon in newborn mice in comparative studies with adult mice? Maybe this interferon in newborn mice just passes to the kidney and other cells. What do you think about these suggestions?

Dr. Tovey: With regard to the second part, it's very difficult to do those sorts of studies in newborn mice on where the interferon goes, for obvious reasons. For the first point, yes, there is a critical period. If you start treatment at 6 days with the same amount of IFN and continue for the same period of time, then you do not see these lesions.

Histopathological and Physiological Studies on Suckling Mice Treated with High Doses of Purified Mouse Interferon

Yoshihiro Kiuchi,* Takane Matsui,* Shizuko Taguchi,* Jiro Suzuki,* Kiyoshi Okada,[2]* Jun Utsumi,[3]* and Shigeyasu Kobayashi[3]*

*Tokyo Metoropolitan Institute of Medical Science, 3–18, Honkomagome, Bunkyo-ku, Tokyo,
[2]*Tokyo Metropolitan Ohkubo General Hospital, 2–44–1, Kabukicho, Shinjuku-ku, Tokyo,
[3]*Basic Research Laboratories, Toray Industries, Inc., 1111, Tebiro, Kamakura, Japan

INTRODUCTION

It has been well established that interferon (IFN) has a variety of biological activities. It was originally discovered as an antiviral agent, but later its anti-tumor action was clearly demonstrated in many laboratories. Clinical application of IFN are now making rapid progress because of recent innovations in techniques for mass production and purification. There are three types of IFN, α, β, and γ, which are produced in different kind of cells and which differ in some of their biological and physicochemical properties.

Safety tests of IFN as a drug should be designed from various points of view. One of the most striking properties of IFN is species specificity. The best way to check the safety of human IFN preparations is to test them in humans, but this is, of course, impossible in practice. Accordingly, model experiments such as those with mice and mouse IFN will provide a reliable source of information which is useful in clinical applications of human IFN.

Since IFN is one of the physiological mediators produced in the body after stimulation with foreign substances, toxicity is hardly to be expected. However, in most clinical situations a very high dose of IFN is needed in order to obtain some effect. Therefore, the pharmacologic action of IFN should be surveyed thoroughly and even minimal side-effects should not be neglected. All of the clinical trials so far have been carried out with preparations which have a specific activity of less than 10^6–10^7 IU/mg protein (a purity of less than 1 %). Toxic responses caused by contaminating proteins or additives in the IFN preparations should be strictly distinguished from those of IFN itself. It is clear that more data on the safety of IFN should be accumulated to facilitate further clinical applications.

Several attempts have been made by Gresser's group using animal models to reveal possible adverse effects of IFN. They reported that IFN inhibits liver regeneration in partially hepatectomized mice and that administration of IFN to suckling mice results in a retardation of their growth.[1,2] They also reported recently that daily administration of IFN to newborn mice caused death or glomerulonephritis, depending on the protocol.[3-5]

Safety tests with suckling or fetal mice have significance beyond their relevance to general sensitivity. Infection with certain kinds of virus, especially hepatitis B and herpes simplex viruses, is known to take place between mothers and their infants at the time of delivery. This maternal transmission may be prevented by the administration of IFN to pregnant women, but first it is necessary to study carefully the adverse effect of IFN on the development of infants. We thus decided to administer purified mouse IFN to suckling and pregnant mice. The present paper will describe our findings on the effect of IFN given in a single shot or by repeated injections on the growth and the histopathology of infant mice.

MATERIALS AND METHODS

Mouse IFN was produced in mouse L-MS cells induced with Newcastle disease virus (NDV), Miyadera strain, as described by Sano et al.[6] Purification was carried out by a combination of zinc acetate precipitation, SP-Sephadex, and copper-chelate chromatography as follows. NDV in the harvested medium was inactivated by maintaining the pH at 2 with HCl for 4 days at 4°C. Zinc acetate was added to the harvested medium to a concentration of 20 mM (pH 6.0–6.5), and the zinc acetate precipitate was dialyzed against 0.01 M HCl (pH 2.0). The crude IFN solution obtained was applied to a SP-Sephadex column and the activity was eluted with 0.1 M phosphate buffer (pH 8.2). The eluted IFN activity was adsorbed to a copper-chelate Sepharose column and eluted with a pH gradient from pH 3 to pH 9 formed in 0.1 M acetate buffer containing 0.5 M NaCl. Fractions of high IFN activity were collected and desalted by gel filtration with Sephadex G-25. Consequently, the final preparation has a specific activity of $3–10 \times 10^7$ international reference units (IU)/mg protein. The zinc acetate precipitate was also employed as a crude IFN preparation after lyophilization (1×10^6 IU/mg protein). Mouse serum albumin (MSA) was added to the final preparation as a stabilizing agent and the mixture was lyophilized. The ratio of IFN to MSA in the preparation employed in the experiments was 10^6 IU/0.2 mg MSA. IFN activity was determined according to the method based on inhibition of viral RNA synthesis and converted into IU. Two strains of mice, C57BL/6 and BALB/c, were chosen, the former as a high responder to IFN inducers and the latter as a low responder, as described by De Maeyer et al.[8] Both strains were obtained from the Institute of Medical Science, University of Tokyo, as SPF mice and were bred in an Isorack using a Filtercap. A Co^{60}1 MR-irradiated diet was given. Cages, bedding, and water were sterilized by autoclaving and the Filtercap by ethylene oxide.

Newborn mice were injected I.P. with 0.05–0.1 ml of IFN or MSA preparations within 24 hrs after birth. In the experiments with repeated administration, mice were injected I.P. once every day except Sunday.

To determine spontaneous motor activity, the amount of horizontal movement by the mice was measured with a Varimex II (Tokai Medical Instruments Co.). Three mice taken from each of the 3 groups were put into 3 separate cages, and the groups were compared in pairs: IFN-treated mice vs. MSA-treated mice; MSA-treated mice vs. untreated mice; IFN-treated mice vs. untreated mice. Each comparison was carried out for at least 2 hrs in a dark room with a light on in the cage. The amount of movement of the 3 mice in one hour was calculated.

To determine the weight of organs, mice were bled by cardiac puncture after anesthesia by chloroform. The liver, spleen, kidney, heart, lung, thymus, and brain were removed from each mouse and weighed by PDA-100 electronic balance (Cho Measuring Instruments Co.). The body weight of each mouse was determined daily by a PN-200 Mettler scale.

For histopathologic examination each organ was fixed with PBS-formalin, embedded in paraffin, stained with hematoxilin-eosin, and examined under a light microscope.

RESULTS

Administration of a Large Amount of IFN in a Single Shot
Newborn mice of the two strains were injected I.P. on the day of birth with IFN or MSA (10^5, 10^4, 10^3, 10^2 IU of mouse IFN or 0.02 mg of MSA per mouse). Separate litters were employed for each group. They were killed on day 1, 3, 5, 7, 14, or 21 and examined histopathologically. They were weighed daily until the day of sacrifice. The growth curves for 7, 14, and 21 days are shown only for mice injected with 10^5 IU of IFN and with MSA and for untreated mice (Figs. 1–5). No significant differences in the growth curves were detected among the IFN-treated, MSA-treated, and untreated mice. Some of IFN-treated mice even showed better growth than untreated mice. Histopathologic examinations also revealed no differences between the IFN-treated and MSA-treated mice.

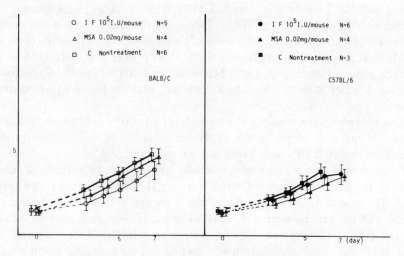

Fig. 1. Growth curve of mice (IF, MSA were injected at 0-day-old).

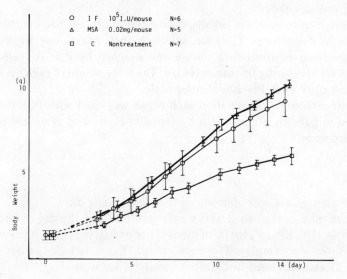

Fig. 2. Growth curve of BALB/c mice (IF, MSA were injected at 0-day-old).

Repeated Administration of IFN

Newborn mice of the two strains were injected I.P. with 10^4 IU of mouse IFN daily from birth for 30 days, and the amount of spontaneous motor activity was determined on day 30. Immediately afterwards they were killed and various organs were weighed and examined histopathologically. The body weight of the mice was followed daily during the 30 days, and the growth curves are

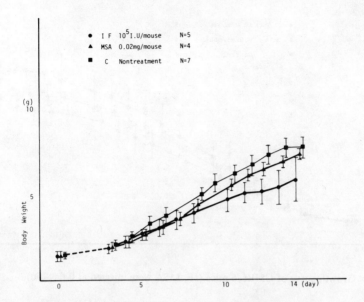

Fig. 3. Growth curve of C57BL/6 mice (IF, MSA were injected at 0-day-old).

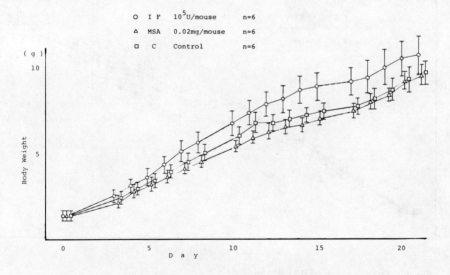

Fig. 4 Growth curve of BALB/c mice (IF, MSA were injected at 0-day-old).

shown in Figs. 6 and 7. No differences were found among the three groups. Table 1 shows the weight of various organs from the mice. Again, there were no

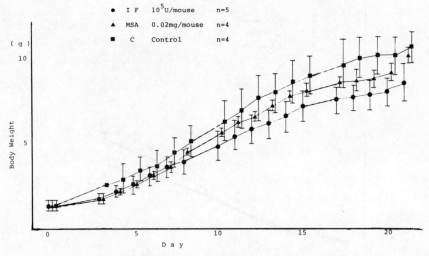

Fig. 5. Growth curve of C57BL/6 mice (IF, MSA were injected at 0-day-old).

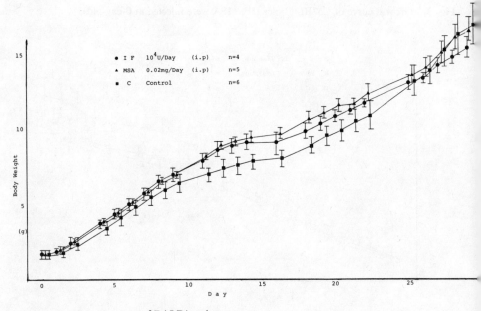

Fig. 6. Growth curve of BALB/c mice.

differences in the weight of whole body, liver, spleen, kindney, heart, lung, brain, and thymus. Determination of spontaneous motor activity with Varimex II did not reveal any significant differences, as shown in Table 2.

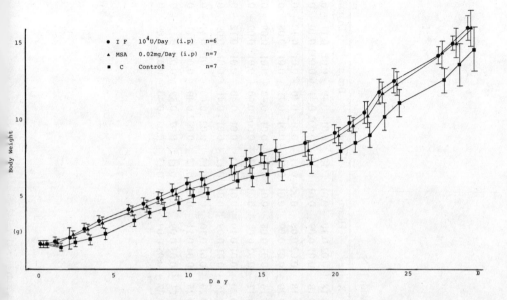

Fig. 7.   Growth curve of C57BL/6 mice.

On histopathologic examination, focal necrosis with calcification was observed in about half of mice from both the IFN- and MSA-treated groups without regard to the strain. Most of the lesions were considered to be due to technical error at the time of injection judging from the location of the lesions, and they seemed to be unrelated to the presence of the IFN or MSA. Peritonitis was also observed in a few mice from both groups but it was also considered to be due to technical error.

Administration of a Large Amount of IFN to Pregnant Mice
Pregnant mice were injected I.P. with 2×10^5 IU of IFN 6 times at intervals of 3 days in the 20 days from fertilization to delivery. As shown in Table 3, the growth rate varied depending on litter size but no effect from the IFN administration was observed.

Comparison of Purified and Crude IFN Preparations
Newborn mice from two strains, C57BL/6 and BALB/c, were injected I.P. with 10^4 IU of purified (10^8 IU/mg protein) or crude (10^6 IU/mg protein) IFN preparation daily from birth to the 8th day. As shown in Figs. 8 and 9, there was a significant difference between the growth curve of mice injected with the

Table 1.　Weight of organs from 30-day-old mice serially injected with IFN.

Strain	Treatment	Sex	No.	B.W	Liver	Spleen	Kidney	Heart	Lung	Brain	Thymus
C57BL/6	I F	♀	3	15.29 ± 0.53	0.86 ± 0.07	0.07 ± 0.02	0.18 ± 0.02	0.10 ± 0.01	0.13 ± 0.01	0.40 ± 0.01	0.11 ± 0.03
		♂	3	15.43 ± 0.90	0.87 ± 0.10	0.07 ± 0.01	0.18 ± 0.01	0.09 ± 0.01	0.12 ± 0.002	0.41 ± 0.002	0.10 ± 0.01
	MSA	♀	3	14.75 ± 1.35	0.81 ± 0.12	0.07 ± 0.01	0.18 ± 0.02	0.08 ± 0.004	0.11 ± 0.01	0.40 ± 0.01	0.10 ± 0.02
		♂	4	16.74 ± 0.62	0.97 ± 0.06	0.09 ± 0.01	0.20 ± 0.01	0.09 ± 0.01	0.12 ± 0.01	0.41 ± 0.01	0.08 ± 0.01
	C	♀	4	13.40 ± 0.75	0.60 ± 0.03	0.05 ± 0.01	0.16 ± 0.03	0.08 ± 0.01	0.10 ± 0.01	0.40 ± 0.01	0.09 ± 0.02
		♂	3	15.71 ± 0.95	0.94 ± 0.10	0.07 ± 0.01	0.17 ± 0.02	0.08 ± 0.01	0.11 ± 0.004	0.40 ± 0.01	0.09 ± 0.02
BALB/c	I F	♀	2	14.60 ± 0.66	0.71 ± 0.12	0.10 ± 0.01	0.20 ± 0.01	0.10 ± 0.01	0.12 ± 0.01	0.40 ± 0.01	0.12 ± 0.02
		♂	2	15.53 ± 0.30	0.85 ± 0.05	0.11 ± 0.01	0.25 ± 0.01	0.09 ± 0.01	0.12 ± 0.01	0.41 ± 0.01	0.09 ± 0.02
	MSA	♀	4	15.28 ± 1.08	0.84 ± 0.10	0.10 ± 0.01	0.20 ± 0.01	0.10 ± 0.01	0.13 ± 0.02	0.40 ± 0.01	0.11 ± 0.01
		♂	2	17.32 ± 0.71	1.09 ± 0.04	0.11 ± 0.01	0.25 ± 0.04	0.11 ± 0.02	0.12 ± 0.002	0.40 ± 0.004	0.11 ± 0.02
	C	♀	3	15.27 ± 1.77	0.86 ± 0.11	0.10 ± 0.01	0.21 ± 0.03	0.09 ± 0.02	0.11 ± 0.02	0.39 ± 0.02	0.12 ± 0.01
		♂	3	18.08 ± 2.57	1.04 ± 0.16	0.11 ± 0.01	0.27 ± 0.05	0.09 ± 0.01	0.13 ± 0.03	0.40 ± 0.03	0.09 ± 0.02

IFN: 10^4 IU/day (I.P.).
MSA: 0.002 mg/day (I.P.).
C: Nontreatment.

Table 2. Total number of spontaneous motor movements.

C57BL/6	⌈IFN	2,074/hr[a]	
	⌊C	1,928/hr	
	⌈IFN	3,130/hr	
	⌊MSA	2,966/hr	
	⌈MSA	3,231/hr	
	⌊C	3,729/hr	
BALB/c	⌈IFN	2,592/hr	
	⌊C	2,674/hr	
	⌈IFN	2,235/hr	
	⌊MSA	1,764/hr	
	⌈MSA	3,608/hr	
	⌊C	3,308/hr	

Mice received serial injections of IFN.
a) Total number of 3 mice.

Table 3. Growth curves of offspring from mice injected with IFN during pregnancy.

	Litter size	1-week	2-week	3-week
IFN	8	5.01±0.20	7.90±0.26	10.51±0.46
	10	2.96±0.52	4.73±0.85	6.51±1.36
	5	5.80±0.26	9.01±0.48	11.75±0.24
	6	5.31±0.30	8.52±0.35	11.18±0.44
C	5	5.51±0.53	9.18±0.38	11.61±0.75
	7	5.63±0.30	8.43±0.42	11.39±0.55
	9	4.80±0.66	8.07±0.67	10.84±1.04
	9	4.12±0.20	6.27±0.40	8.88±0.38

Pregnant mice were injected with IFN 6 times in 20 days.
IFN dose: 2×10^5 IU/ one injection.
Strain: BALB/c.

crude preparation and that of mice injected with the purified preparation or with MSA. Upon histopathologic examination, no difference was observed except that there were some necrotic lesions in the livers of mice injected with the crude preparation. Although there is a possibility that the lesions were induced by technical error, they are more likely to be due to contaminants in the crude preparation rather than IFN itself. No abnormality was observed in the brain, kidney, spleen, lung, heart, or thymus.

DISCUSSION

Adult animals are usually employed in general safety tests. In the present investigation IFN was administered to suckling or pregnant mice. The experiments are relevant to two considerations. Suckling mice are at a very early stage of development and are very sensitve to adverse effects from various

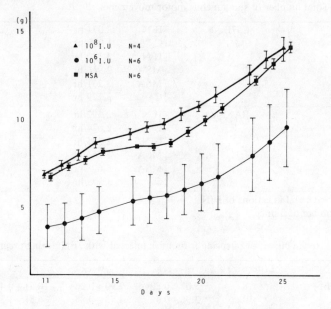

Fig. 8. Growth curve of BALB/c mice (Serial administration of crude mouse IFN).

kinds of substances. As a result, these mice provide a useful tool for safety tests of IFN preparations, despite the difficulty in handling them. Furthermore, since IFN may be given in the near future to pregnant women to prevent maternal transmission of certain viruses, safety tests should be carried out using newborn animals.

Interferon is a new type of biologic, and as such it will be very difficult to assess its toxicity correctly. In addition, IFN is a physiological mediator and this makes evaluation of its safety even more complex.

As shown in experiments 1, 2, and 3, purified preparations of mouse IFN did not induce histopathologic changes in the treated mice. The growth rate of newborn animals is very sensitive to toxic factors in general, but the present study found no differences in the growth rate or in the weight of various organs among the mice treated with IFN and those given MSA or no treatment. It is reasonable to assume that any toxicity against the central nervous system will develop first as a change in spontaneous motor activity rather than as a histopathologic abnormality. However, no change was observed in the amount of movement, and no abnormality was observed in the brain upon histopathologic examination. In experiment 4, the administration of an IFN preparation with a specific activity of 10^6 IU/mg protein resulted in a marked inhibition of the growth rate and a development of lesions in the liver, but these effects were caused by contaminant proteins in the preparation.

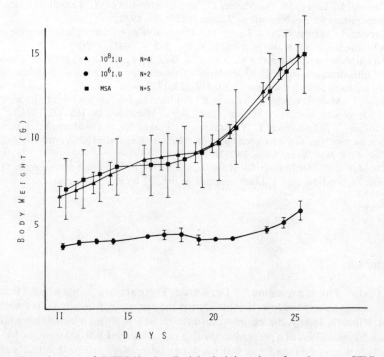

Fig. 9. Growth curve of C57BL/6 mice (Serial administration of crude mouse IFN).

In conclusion, the administration of highly purified mouse IFN did not cause any delay in the growth or any histopathologic abnormality in suckling mice. Death due to necrosis of the liver or glomerulonephritis, as reported by Gresser's group in IFN-treated suckling mice, was not observed in the present investigation. It is not clear whether the discrepancy can be explained by differences in the methods of IFN purification or in the strains of mice employed. In our study, even repeated administration of the purified IFN preparation did not exert any adverse effect on the suckling mice. This at least suggests that some potential adverse effects of IFN administration can be minimized by refining the IFN preparation to a certain level of purity.

REFERENCES

1. Frayssinet, C., Gresser, T., Tovey, M., and Lindahl, P.: Inhibitory effect of potent interferon preparations on the regeneration of mouse liver after partial hepatectomy. *Nature*, **245**: 146–147, 1973.
2. Gresser, I. and Bourali, C.: Development of newborn mice during prolonged treatment with interferon. *Eur. J. Cancer*, **6**: 553–556, 1970.

3. Gresser, I., Tovey, M. G., Maury, C., and Chouroulinkov, I.: Lethality of interferon preparations for newborn mice. *Nature*, **258**: 76–78, 1975.
4. Gresser, I., Maury, C., and Tovey, M.: Progressive glomerulonephritis in mice treated with interferon preparations at birth. *Nature*, **263**: 420–422, 1976.
5. Molel-Maroger, L., Sloper, J. C., Vinter, J., Biol, M. I., Woodrow, D., and Gresser, I.: An ultrastructural study of the development of nephritis in mice treated with interferon in the neonatal period. *Lab. Invest.*, **39**: 513–522, 1978.
6. Sano, E., Matsui, Y., and Kobayashi, S.: Production of mouse interferon with high titers in a large-scale suspension culture system, *Jap. J. Microbiol.*, **18**: 165–172, 1974.
7. Kawade, Y., Matsuzawa, T., Yamamoto, Y., Tsukui, K., and Iwakura, Y.: A rapid and precise microassay of interferon based on the inhibition of viral RNA synthesis *Ann. Rep. Inst. Virus Res., Kyoto Univ.*, **19**: 52–58, 1976.
8. De Maeyer, E., De Maeyer-Guignard, J., and Bailey, D. W.: Effect of mouse genotype on interferon production. I. Lines congenic at the If-1 locus. *Immunogenetics*, **1**: 438–443, 1975.

Discussion

Dr. TOVEY: This is a question for Dr. Kiuchi. There are two points which I think are important to emphasize when considering the discrepancy between our results and Dr. Kiuchi's. Firstly, the lesions were observed only when we injected neonatal mice with 50 microliters of a preparation with a titer of at least 800,000 u/ml, or 10^6 μ/ml, and not when we injected mice with the same volume of only 100,000 units. The second point is, we used only 2 types of interferon preparations: the first was partially purified interferon with a specific activity of 2×10^7 μ/mg protein, comparable to the preparations used by Dr. Kiuchi, and the second was electrophoretically pure interferon, if not of absolute chemical purity then certainly 90% pure; and I should emphasize that we observed exactly the same type and extent of lesions with the 2 types of preparations and absolutely no effect whatsoever with the major contaminants isolated during the purification process. And I think this is convincing evidence that the lesions we observed are indeed due to interferon when administered under the conditions that we have described.

Testing and Control of Interferon

Hope E. HOPPS, John C. PETRICCIANI, Paul D. PARKMAN, and Harry M. MEYER

Bureau of Biologics, Food and Drug Administration, Bethesda, Maryland, U.S.A.

The development of a philosophy and rationale for the testing and control of human interferon (IFN) began in the late 1960s, concomitant with the clinical testing of IFN as an antiviral agent. As possibilities for the clinical use of IFN developed, the decision was made that regulatory control of IFN and IFN inducers would come under the purview of the Division of Biologics Standards, the predecessor organization of the current Bureau of Biologics.

Some background information about our organization may help in understanding the Bureau's operation. In the latter part of the 19th century, following the medical discoveries of Pasteur, Ehrlich, and others, a number of vaccines and serums were developed that were useful for the prevention or treatment of certain infectious diseases, such as rabies, diphtheria, and tetanus. These, together with smallpox vaccine, which had already been in use for about a century by that time, were the first biological products.

Although the need for special care in the preparation and testing of vaccine and antitoxins was foreseen early in their development, it was not until 1902 that the "Biologics Control Act" gave official recognition to the U.S. Public Health Service for its broad health responsibility.

This legislation would not have been enacted even then except for an accident in St. Louis. Since 1894, the city of St. Louis had employed a bacteriologist to prepare diphtheria antitoxin for free distribution to physicians. During 1901, 10 children to whom antitoxin had been administered died from tetanus. These deaths were due to tetanus organisms in the serum derived from the horse used to produce the antitoxin. This unfortunate occurrence shocked Congress into passing the Biologics Control Act. The act established a new Biological Control Service to regulate the sale of viruses, serums, and similar products. This was the beginning of what is now known as the Bureau of Biologics.

333

The Biological Control Service was a division of the Public Health Service Hygienic Laboratory located in Washington, D.C. In 1930 the Hygienic Laboratory was reorganized and expanded and its name was changed to the National Institute of Health. In 1937 the Laboratory of Biologics Control was created within the Institute. By the early 1940s the laboratories for biologics control were situated on the present grounds of the NIH.

In 1948 the Laboratory became part of the National Microbiological Institute (later renamed the National Institute for Allergy and Infectious Diseases). The need for strengthening and expanding biologics control became clear in 1955 when many cases of poliomyelitis occurred in persons who had received killed polio vaccine. Some batches of the vaccine contained residual poliovirus which was undetected by the safety tests used at that time.

In June of 1955, the Secretary of HEW authorized the establishment of a separate division within the NIH to be called the Division of Biologics Standards. In 1972, the Division was transferred to the Food and Drug Administration to become the now-existing Bureau of Biologics, still located on the NIH campus. As a result of investigational new drug (IND) legislation enacted in the 1960s, the Bureau of Biologics has the authority to oversee human experimentation relating to biological product development. In standard practice, a potential manufacturer will contact the Bureau and indicate his interest is developing a certain product, for example, IFN.

On many occasions he will sit down with Bureau scientists to discuss what we might view as problems in terms of human use. We feel it is extremely important that this kind of dialogue be established very early in the development process. Once the basic laboratory work is completed the manufacturer can then submit an IND (Investigational New Drug) application to initiate clinical trials.

The IND contains a minutely detailed description of the production process, along with a description of all of the tests and the results of such tests which have been performed to prove that the product is potent and safe.

In addition, the IND contains a detailed clinical trial proposal describing how the material will be inoculated, including the volume, route, and number of doses, as well as the kinds of clinical observations that will be made.

In attempting to recommend test procedures for assessing the safety of the various types of IFN we have been guided by our earlier experience in dealing with viral and bacterial vaccines.

In Table 1 are summarized some of the recommendations developed at the Interferon Workshop held at the National Institutes of Health, Bethesda, Maryland, in 1979. These procedures, which include tests for sterility, pyrogenicity, and general safety, have been modified from tests now published in the U.S. Code of Federal Regulations (CFR); modifications have been made largely to alleviate the problem of the limited amounts of IFN available for testing.

Table 1. Suggestions for sterility, pyrogenicity, and general safety tests for IFN preparations in final containers to be used in human clinical studies.

Test system	Volume and route	No. units to be tested or animals used	Observation period	Comment
1. Bacterial and fungal sterility[a]	Total contents of 1 vial/ tube of each medium (up to a maximum of 1 ml/tube)	10% of vials in a lot or a maximum of 20 vials	14 days	21 CER 610.12 except for number of samples (d)(2), (5),(6)
2. Rabbit pyrogenicity[b]	1.5×10^6 U/kg or 0.1 ml, whichever is greater; I.V.	3 rabbits	3 hrs	21 CFR 610.13(b)
3. General safety[b]	1.5×10^6 U/kg or 0.1 ml, whichever is greater; I.P.	2 guinea pigs (400 gm each)	7 days	21 CFR 610.11
	0.1 ml; I.P.	2 mice (22 gm each)	7 days	

a) The number of containers to be tested (10% of the lot or a maximum of 20 containers) should be divided equally between the two culture media, (e.g., 10 final containers for bacterial sterility and 10 final containers for fungal sterility), but the contents of only one container should be inoculated into a tube even if the volume is less than 1 ml. If the volume of a container is greater than 1 ml, only 1 ml need be inoculated into a tube; the excess should not be used to inoculate additional tubes of either culture medium. The possibility of using membrane filtration as an alternate method should be discussed with the Bureau on a case-by-case basis.

b) The rabbit pyrogen and general safety test volumes are based on three times the maximum single human dose ($3 \times [30 \times 10^6$ U$] = 9 \times 10^7$ U), assuming a 60 kg human patient (9×10^7 U/60 kg $= 1.5 \times 10^6$ U(kg)). To obtain the dose per rabbit or guinea pig 1.5 $\times 10^6$ U is multiplied by the weight of the individual animal in kilograms or fraction of a kilogram. Because this calculation for mice results in a dose of less than 0.1 ml and the minimum acceptable dosage volume is 0.1 ml, the test in mice should be done with 0.1 ml per mouse.

In regard to the test for bacterial sterility, we have suggested that the sample size for testing of the bulk should be 1% of the bulk container, but need not exceed 10 ml. This reduced volume for testing is intended to conserve material needed for clinical investigation because of the current short supply. For the final container test we have recommended 10% of the vials in a lot, or a maximum of 20 vials.

In addition, we have suggested that tests for mycoplasmas be performed on bulk material; the point for testing of materal would depend on the process used. If manufacturers wish to consider alternate tests for mycoplasmas, then the Bureau should be contacted for discussion of the proposed test.

For the rabbit pyrogenicity test, we have suggested that one use three times a single human dose of 30×10^6 units. Pyrogenicity represents a particular problem since it may be an inherent property of some types of IFN. In assessing the result of pyrogenicity testing one must consider the patient population and the route of administration in relation to the degree of pyrogenicity. Thus, much greater caution would be exercised if the preparation were to be given by other than the subcutaneous or intramuscular route, that is, an intraspinal, intravenous, intra-arterial, or intrathecal route.

The general safety test can be performed according to our current regulations. Again, we have suggested that the inoculum be based on three times the human dose.

During the past 5 years we have seen a burgeoning interest in IFN for use in experimental trials for therapy in malignant disease. Many potential producers of leukocyte, fibroblast, lymphoblastoid, and more recently, recombinant DNA-derived IFNs have come to the Bureau seeking guidance in the kinds of tests which should be performed to make the product acceptable for use in clinical trials. While all aspects of testing have been discussed, the question which most concerns the IFN producer is that of safety. What will the Bureau of Biologics require? How safe is safe? The question of safety is one which cannot be answered in absolute terms.

One of the major safety issues in IFN production concerns the choice of cell substrate used for production. Early adverse experience with SV_{40} virus contamination of primary rhesus monkey kidney cells and also the contamination of primary chick embryo cells with avian leukosis viruses aroused grave concerns generally of the possible presence of viruses or viral genome material which might be oncogenic for humans. Piror to 1978 there was particular concern regarding the use of lymphoblastoid IFN since it was feared that the final product might be contaminated with host nucleic acid. Our assessment of current technology suggest that a manufactorer may now employ purification procedures which can exclude any measurable nucleic acid from the final product.

Questions have recently been raised with respect to toxicologic testing of IFN. Early IFN preparations received from Finland and prepared by Cantell and already been administered to humans and, hence, animal testing was not required. With the advent of many new manufacturers of experimental materials and with the development of new production techniques, the Bureau of Biologics is reconsidering the issue of animal tests. We are recommending that any new product, not yet administered to humans and for which an IND is being sought, be tested for a period of time (perhaps several weeks) in one or two species of animals (guinea pigs, mics, primates, etc.). It is suggested that plans for animal testing be discussed with the Bureau prior to their implementation. It is believed that the use of abbreviated toxicity tests do provide some assurance of product safety prior to use in humans.

My final comments concern the kinds of supplementary guidelines which are being considered for testing human IFN derived from recombinant DNA technology. While no final decisions as to specific testing requirements by the

Bureau have been made, one can presume certain basic recommendations:

(1) IFN production should be performed in accordance with current NIH guidelines for human IFNs produced by recombinant DNA techniques in bacteria.

(2) With regard to purity, potency, and safety, the guidelines sued for IFN derived from human cells should be followed.

(3) The specific activity of the purified IFN should be comparable to the specific activity of the analogous homogeneous IFN derived from human-cells.

(4) The amino acid compositions should be analyzed and compared to the appropriate native IFN species.

(5) Other studies might include the determination of the amino-terminal and carboxy-terminal amino acid sequences, fractionation of peptides following cyanogen bromide or trypsin cleavage, and determination of amino acid composition of the fragments.

Potency assays should be performed on both homologous and heterologous cells, and studies of other biological activities would be encouraged, e.g., natural killer cell activation and antiproliferative activity. Neutralization of the antiviral activity of the IFN could be achieved by an appropriate antiserum and would provide a further test of identity.

In addition, one should carry out a periodic quality control test on the plasmid itself by determining the nucleotide sequence of the cloned IFN gene and assessing the absence of other human gene sequences in the plasmid.

In conclusion, it should be emphasized that the test procedures recommended by the Bureau are not immutably fixed. In view of the rapid technological developments of the past several years, we wish to maintain flexibility in terms of appropriate testing. It is extremely important for us to recognize that we carefully balance our concerns for safety with the need for clinical investigation.

Discussion

Dr. KAUPPINEN: I would like to ask a question about pyrogenicity testing of human interferons in rabbits. This dose of 0.5 million units/kg per rabbit weight is far above that dose which always gives a pyrogenic reaction even though the limulus test gives a negative. So I wonder, does the result tell anything in that case?

Dr. HOPPS: I think that was initiated as a kind of safety factor. What we plan to do at the present time is to study the pyrogenicity of interferon in humans and rabbits. We are all getting some data on this. Then we'll be able to make a better test, whether it will be with rabbits or with limulus. But I agree that this is a kind of over-safety factor which we're using right now.

Dr. KONO: I have a question for Dr. Hopps. In Japanese interferon trials a minute amount of bovine albumin coming from the medium is contained in the preparation, so some of the patients who were treated have antibody to bovine serum. Clinicians are concerned that there may be some danger, especially to pregnant women. What are the thoughts about this in the United States?

Dr. HOPPS: I think that at the present time we are interested in the presence of small amounts of fetal bovine serum in the final product. Fortunately it may become less of a problem because now it is beginning to be possible to purify interferon to such an extent that we will not have fetal bovine serum fragments or small amounts in the final product. I agree that if we continue to use impure preparations that could be a problem. We haven't had any reports of adverse reactions at the present time in terms of numerous administrations. However, we are concerned about it; we have done some guinea pig testing and are looking at that question.

Dr. KOHNO (S.): I would like to show a slide on the tentative guidelines we are using in our country. These are restrictions carried out by the Research Group on Clinical Applications of Interferon of the Ministry of Health and Welfare. These guidelines are similar to those shown by Dr. Hopps. The second column will give you an idea how we are controlling extraneous protein quantitatively. The rest is as shown on the slide. By small amounts of bovine serum albumin, this is the level that we have, and this is the limit, according to our present understanding, of the state of the art of purification.

IV.

FUTURE PROBLEM AND GENERAL DISCUSSIONS

Studies on a Human Interferon-β Gene

Tadatsugu TANIGUCHI, Shigeo OHNO, Yoshiaki FUJII-KURIYAMA, and
Chikako TAKAOKA

*Department of Biochemistry, Cancer Institute, Japanese Foundation for Cancer Research,
Toshima-ku, Tokyo, Japan*

INTRODUCTION

Interferons (IFNs) are species-specific glycoproteins produced by almost
all vertebrates upon induction by viruses and numerous other compounds.[1,2]
The best characterized biological activity of IFNs is their capacity to elicit antiviral activity in taget cells, in conjunction with the *de novo* synthesis of several
proteins, such as oligoisoadenylate synthetase, protein kinase, and phospho-
diesterase.[3-6] In addition to their antiviral effects IFNs appear to be involved
in the regulation of immune responses[7] and in inhibition of tumor growth.[8]

At least three different types of IFNs, classified as α (leukocyte), β (fibroblast), and γ (immune) on the basis of antigenic differences, are produced in
humans.[9] Earlier studies also showed that separate structural genes code for
HuIFN-α and HuIFN-β.[10]

A number of efforts have been made to characterize the biological and
physicochemical properties of the IFNs and to assess their clinical uses, but it has
been difficult ot obtain sufficient quantities of purified IFN for further studies.

We have made use of recombinant DNA technology in order to elucidate
the structure of the IFN-β gene and to study the mechanism of IFN gene induction. In addition, it is hoped that the cloned gene will be useful in the mass
production of IFN in xenogenic hosts such as *E. coli*.

Synthesis and Cloning of HuIFN-β cDNA

Total cytoplasmic RNA was extracted from human fibroblast DIP-2 cells
(provided by Dr. S. Kobayashi, Toray Industries, Inc.) after 4 hours of
induction by poly I : C poly in the presence of cycloheximide, and poly
A-containing mRNA was isolated by oligo(dT)-cellulose affinity chromato-

graphy. Starting from 1.5×10^9 cells, 250 μg of poly A-containing mRNA was obtained. After fractionation of the mRNA into 20 fractions with 5–25% sucrose gradient centrifugation, a small portion of the mRNA from the fractions in the 12S region was injected into *Xenopus* oocytes and IFN activity was determined. The peak fraction contained about 5 μg of mRNA (termed "IFN mRNA" here), and this was used as the template for cDNA synthesis. About 1.5 μg of double-stranded cDNA was synthesized, elongated with dAMP residues, then hybridized with EcoRI-cleaved, dTMP-elongated pBR322. This hybrid DNA was used to transform *E. coli* strain χ 1776, and colonies containing the hybrid plasmid DNA were selected on agar plates containing ampicillin (20 μg/ml). The efficiency of the transformation was about 1.5×10^5 colonies/μg cDNA. For the first screening, 3,600 colonies were picked up and transferred on grid-meshed nitrocellulose filters in triplicate. After the colonies had grown on the filters, DNA from duplicate filters was fixed for *in situ* colony hybridization.[11] Colonies grown on the third filter were kept at 4°C.

"Plus-minus" Method

For colony hybridization, two kinds of ^{32}P-labeled cDNA probes were prepared as follows. First, partially purified IFN mRNA (6 μg) was prepared as described above and ^{32}P-labeled cDNA was synthesized (0.45 μg; specific radioactivity, 6×10^8 cpm/μg). After removing the template RNA by alkali treatment, cDNA was hybridized with about 50-fold excess of mRNA prepared from mock-induced cells, incubated for 4 hours in the presence of cycloheximide. Nonhybridized cDNA with about 10% of the total radioactivity was separated from the mRNA-cDNA hybrid by hydroxyapatite column chromatography, and this cDNA was used as probe A. After alkali treatment to remove mRNA, the cDNA which had hybridized with mRNA was used as probe B. Both probe A and probe B were separately hybridized with colony DNA fixed on nitrocellulose filters.[11] The colonies which hybridized with probe A but failed to hybridize or hybridized much less with probe B were screened by autoradiogram. Four colonies, nos. 319, 644, 746, and 3,548, were in this category (Table 1).

Table 1. Hybridization of colonies of cDNA clones with cDNA probes.

Ampicillin-resistant colony	Extent of hybridization	
	Probe A	Probe B
No. 319	++++	++
No. 644	+++	+
No. 746	++	−
No. 3578	+++++	+

Colony hybridization was done following the procedure of Grunstein and Hogness.[11] Extent of hybridization was determined by visual inspection of the autoradiogram.

Hybridization-translation Assay

For the second screening, these 4 colonies were grown in liquid media and each recombinant plasmid DNA was Prepared, Five μg of each recombinant plasmid or pBR322 DNA was linealized by Hind III digestion, denatured, and then hybridized with the IFN mRNA (2.5 μg) under the conditions in which a RNA-DNA hybrid could be formed but DNA renaturation was negligible.[12] After 4 hours of hybridization, single-stranded plasmid DNA whose cDNA should have hybridized with complementary mRNA was trapped on nitrocellulose filter,[13] and hybridized mRNA was eluted from the filter.[14] After oligo (dT)-cellulose column chromatography to remove possible contaminants such as DNA, the mRNA was microinjected into frog oocytes to determine the interferon mRNA activity. As shown in Table 2, mRNA hybridized with the recombinant plasmid DNA from clone no. 319 (termed TpIF319) gave rise to IFN synthesis, whereas mRNA hybridized with the other plasmid DNA, including pBR322, failed to synthesize IFN in frog oocytes.[15] Plasmid TpIF319 was used as a probe, and another recombinant plasmid TpIF319–13, whose cDNA insert consists of about 800 base paris, was isolated.[16]

Table 2. Hybridization translation assay with IFN mRNA and various recombinant DNAs.

Plasmid DNA	IFN activity (units/ml)
from no. 319	360
from no. 644	< 10
from no. 746	15
from no. 3578	< 10
pBR 322	< 10

IFN mRNA was hybridized with linealized, denatured plasmid DNA, and the hybrid was trapped on a nitrocellulose filter. RNA was eluted, chromatographed on an oligo(dT)-cellulose column, then injected into frog oocytes for IFN synthesis.

Sequence Analysis of the IFN-β cDNA

The locations of several restricition endonuclease cleavage sites of the cDNA insert from TpIF319–13 were determined[17] (Fig. 1) and a nucleotide sequence analysis was carried out according to the procedure of Maxam and Gilbert.[18] As shown in Fig. 2, the sequence analysis of the TpIF319–13 cDNA revealed that the cDNA codes for the IFN-β whose amino acid sequence was determined by Knight *et al.*[19] We concluded that the matured form of IFN-β, which consists of 166 amino acids, is processed from a precursor containing 21 additional amino acids (signal peptide). The complete amino acid sequence of the HuIFN-β predicted from the cDNA sequence is presented in Fig. 1.

The amino acid composition of IFN reported by Knight *et al.*[19] agrees largely with that deduced from the cDNA sequence. The molecular weight of the human fibroblast IFN polypeptide was calculated to be 20,040; this is to

```
                -20                                            -10
        Met Thr Asn Lys Cys Leu Leu Gln Ile Ala Leu Leu Leu Cys Phe Ser Thr
GTC AAC ATG ACC AAC AAG TGT CTC CTC CAA ATT GCT CTC CTG TTG TGC TTC TCC ACT
                 20                                            40


                1                                             10
Thr Ala Leu Ser Met Ser Tyr Asn Leu Leu Gly Phe Leu Gln Arg Ser Ser Asn Phe
ACA GCT CTT TCC ATG AGC TAC AAC TTG CTT GGA TTC CTA CAA AGA AGC AGC AAT TTT
 60                       80                            100


                20                                            30
Gln Cys Gln Lys Leu Leu Trp Gln Leu Asn Gly Arg Leu Glu Tyr Cys Leu Lys Asp
CAG TGT CAG AAG CTC CTG TGG CAA TTG AAT GGG AGG CTT GAA TAT TGC CTC AAG GAC
     120                       140                       160


                    40                                        50
Arg Met Asn Phe Asp Ile Pro Glu Glu Ile Lys Gln Leu Gln Gln Phe Gln Lys Glu
AGG ATG AAC TTT GAC ATC CCT GAG GAG ATT AAG CAG CTG CAG CAG TTC CAG AAG GAG
         180                       200                       220


                        60                                        70
Asp Ala Ala Leu Thr Ile Tyr Glu Met Leu Gln Asn Ile Phe Ala Ile Phe Arg Gln
GAC GCC GCA TTG ACC ATC TAT GAG ATG TCT CAG AAC ATC TTT GCT ATT TTC AGA CAA
             240                       260                       280


                            30                                        90
Asp Ser Ser Ser Thr Gly Trp Asn Glu Thr Ile Val Glu Asn Leu Leu Ala Asn Val
GAT TCA TCT AGC ACT GGC TGG AAT GAG ACT ATT GTT GAG AAC CTC CTG GCT AAT GTC
                 300                       320                       340


                                100                                       110
Tyr His Gln Ile Asn His Leu Lys Thr Val Leu Glu Glu Lys Leu Glu Lys Glu Asp
TAT CAT CAG ATA AAC CAT CTG AAG ACA GTC CTG GAA GAA AAA CTG GAG AAA GAA GAT
                     360                       380


                                    120
Phe Thr Arg Gly Lys Leu Met Ser Ser Leu His Leu Lys Arg Tyr Tyr Gly Arg Ile
TTC ACC AGG GGA AAA CTC ATG AGC AGT CTG CAC CTG AAA AGA TAT TAT GGG AGG ATT
400                       420                       440


130                                       140
Leu His Tyr Leu Lys Ala Lys Glu Tyr Ser His Cys Ala Trp Thr Ile Val Arg Val
CTG CAT TAC CTG AAG GCC AAG GAG TAC AGT CAC TTG GCC TGG ACC ATA GTC AGA GTG
     460                       480                       500


150                                       160               166
Glu Ile Leu Arg Asn Phe Tyr Phe Ile Asn Arg Leu Thr Gly Tyr Leu Arg Asn
GAA ATC CTA AGG AAC TTT TAC TTC ATT AAC AGA CTT ACA GGT TAC CTC CGA AAC TGA
         520                       540                       560


AGA TCT CCT AGC CTG TGC CTC TGG GAC TGG ACA ATT GCT TCA AGC ATT CTT CAA CCA
         580                       600                       620


GCA GAT GCT GTT TAA GTG ACT GAT GGC TAA TGT ACT GCA TAT GAA AGG ACA CTA GAA
         640                       660                       680
```

Fig. 1.   The nucleotide sequence of the cDNA from TpIF319–13.[17]

be compared with values of 20,000 and 26,000 for glycosylated IFN-β[20,21] and 16,000 for unglycosylated IFN[22] estimated by electrophoretic mobilities in sodium dodecylsulfate polyacrylamide gels.

The protein structure deduced from the DNA sequence agrees with the physicochemical properties of HuIFN-β in the following respects. Hydrophobic amino acids such as leucine,[25] isoleucine,[11] phenylalanine,[9] and valine[5] are abundant, and this findings is consistent with the well-known hydrophobicity of IFN.[23] There are 3 cysteine residues (at positions 17, 31, and 141) in HuIFN-β which is consistent with the notion that S-S bonds may play a role in the maintenance of IFN activity.[23] HuIFN-β is known to be a glycoprotein, and since N-glycosidic linkage occurs on the sequence Asn-X-Ser or Asn-X-Thr (where X could be any amino acid),[24] a possible candidate for this type of glycosylation is the asparagine residue at position 80, which is followed by Glu-Thr.

Comparison of the Sequences of HuIFN-β and HuIFN-α

HuIFN-α and HuIFN-β share almost all the biological properties known to date,[2] and the induction and shut-off of their synthesis seem to be under similar control.[21] Nonetheless, antibodies directed against IFN-α do not neutralize IFN-β and *vice versa*, and the reported 13 N-terminal amino acid sequences of those IFNs show no homology. We therefore decided to compare our cDNA sequence of IFN-β with that of IFN-α, which was cloned and analyzed by Weissmann and his colleagues.[25,26] The coding sequences of the two cDNAs showed homologies of 45% at the nucleotide level and 29% at the amino acid level (Fig. 2).[27]

The longest stretches of contiguous conserved amino acids were Gln-Phe-Gln-Lys (positions 47–50 of IFN-α and 49–52 of IFN-β) and Cys-Ala-Trp (positions 139–141 and 141–143, respectively); the latter sequence is notable because it includes Cys and Trp, which are preferentially conserved in related proteins.[28] The amino acid conservation was highest between the interferon polypeptides (not considering the signal sequences) for Trp, Phe, Arg, Cys, and Tyr residues, in agreement with the general experience that the amino acids most likely to be conserved between related proteins are Trp > Cys > Tyr > Arg > Phe > His.[29] Even where amino acids are conserved, the codons show one or more nucleotide changes in half the instances. The codons of 3 out of 7 conserved Leu residues are unrelated, as are 2 of 4 codons pertaining to conserved Ser residues. This suggests that there is a strong selective pressure favoring the conservation of several amino acids. It is quite likely that at least some of the conserved amino acids are essential for a function common to IFN-α and IFN-β, perhaps the induction of the virus-resistant state in the target cell. On the basis of our findings, we concluded that the two genes were derived from a common ancestor about 500 to 1,000 million years ago.[27]

It has recently been reported that HuIFN-α includes many subspecies (α_1, α_2, . . . and so on)[29,30] and that human fibroblasts produce another β-type IFN, IFN-β_2.[31,32] It will be of interest to determine the evolutionary relationship of these IFNs with a third type of IFN, IFN-γ.

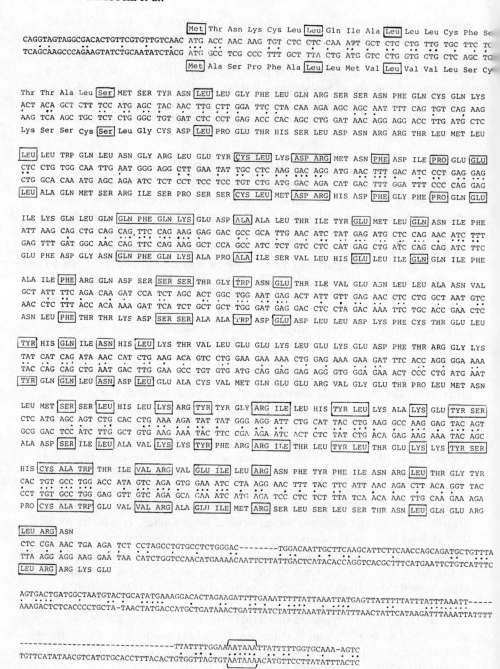

Fig. 2. Comparison of the nucleotide and amino acid sequences of HuIFN-α, and HuIFN-β, cDNA. Identical amino acids are framed and identical nucleotides are marked with a dot.

Analysis of the Chromosomal Gene for IFN-β (IFN-β₁)

In order to study the structural organization and the mechanism of human IFN-β gene expression, it was desirable to obtain a chromosomal DNA segment which contained the IFN-β gene and its regulatory region.

The human gene bank prepared by Lawn *et al.*[33] was screened by an *in situ* procedure using the ^{32}P-labeled TpIF319–13 cDNA insert as probe, and a recombinant phage, λIFN-121, was isolated. The nucleotide sequences of the protein-coding as well as the noncoding regions of the chromosomal gene were identical to the cDNA sequence, indicating that, like IFN-α, the IFN-β (IFN-β₁) gene is devoid of intervening sequences.[29,34–37]

In the region upstream from the putative transcription initiation site, significant nucleotide sequence homology was observed between the IFN-α and -β genes (Fig. 3).[34] Since both genes are derived from a common ancestor and since they are induced by common (or related) inducers, this conserved sequence may play an important role in the regulation of gene expression.

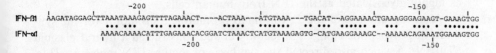

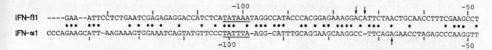

Fig. 3. A comparison of the nucleotide sequences upstream of the putative transcription initiation sites on the IFN-β₁ and IFN-α₁ genes.[34] Dots indicate identical nucleotides. Arrow indicates putative transcription initiation site. TATA box is underlined.

Expression of the IFN-β Gene in E. coli

In order to express the IFN-β gene in *E. coli*, we first made use of a *lac* portable promotor and fused this promotor fragment with IFN-β cDNA as follows.[38] Since the N-terminal amino acid of mature HuIFN-β is methionine, it was possible for *E. coli* to synthesize the mature IFN-β directly by using the ATG sequence for this methionine in the cDNA as the initiator for protein synthesis. The N-terminal portion of the IFN-β cDNA was first fused with a β-galactosidase gene. After exonucleolytic digestion of the cDNA, it was fused again to the 105 base paired *lac* portable promotor which had been previously linked to a bacterial plasmid, and the resulting hybrid plasmids were introduced into *E. coli* strain LG 90.[38] Plasmids which expressed a high level of β-galactosidase activity were screened, and one of them pLG117, was shown to have the sequence which was expected to initiate the protein synthesis (see Fig. 4).

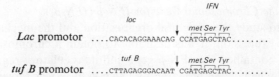

Fig. 4. Nucleotide sequence of the junction between bacterial promotors and HuIFN-β_1 gene. Junction between promotor DNA and IFN-β_1 DNA is indicated by an arrow. Both DNAs should give rise to a mature form of IFN-β.

The β-glactosidase gene was replaced by the c-terminal portion of the IFN-β cDNA to restore the IFN-β gene, and a plasmid 117R was obtained. This plasmid gave rise to a protein whose biological and physicochemical properties were identical to human IFN-β when introduced into various *E. coli* strains. Assuming the specific activity of the IFN-β to be 2×10^8 units/ml, a bacterial clone which contained pLG117R synthesized about 50–100 IFN molecules per cell.[39] This, however, could be a low estimate because bacterial IFN is not as highly glycosylated as the IFN from human cells.

We next made use of the *E. coli tuf B* promotor, a promotor for the synthesis of polypeptide elongation factor Tu, and constructed a hybrid plasmid pTuIFNβ-5 which also directed the synthesis of mature IFN molecules (Fig. 4). An *E. coli* strain HB101 which contained this plasmid produced about 10 time more IFN molecules than the same strain containing pLG117R.[39]

Acknowledgments

The comparison of the nucleotide sequences of IFN-α and -β cDNA was done with Dr. C. Weissmann and his colleagues, and the construction of hybrid plasmids with *lac* promotor was carried out in collaboration with Dr. M. Ptashne and his colleagues at Harvard University.

We wish to express our appreciation to Drs. H. Sugano and M. Muramatsu for their support and interest. We also want to thank Ms. Y. Shimizu for typing this manuscript.

REFERENCES

1. Isaacs, A. and Lindenmann: *J. Proc. Roy, Soc.*, **B147**: 258, 1957.
2. Stewart, W. E., II: The Interferon System. Springer Verlag, Vienna, 1979.
3. Lebleu, B., Sen, G. C., Shaila, S., Cabrer, B. and Lengyel, P.: *Proc. Natl. Acad. Sci. USA*, **73**: 3107, 1976.
4. Hovanessian, A. G., Brown, R. E., and Kerr, I.: *Nature*, **268**: 537, 1977.
5. Hovanessian, A. G. and Kerr, I.: *Eur. J. Biochem.*, **93**: 515, 1979.
6. Schmidt, A., Cherhajovsky, Y., Shulman, L., Federman, P., Berissi, H., and Revel, M.: *Proc. Natl. Acad. Sci., USA*, **76**: 4788, 1979.
7. Johnson, H. M.: *Texas Repts. Biol. Med.*, **35**: 357, 1977.
8. Gresser, I.: *Texas Repts. Biol. Med.*, **35**: 394, 1977.

9. Interferon Nomenclature. *Nature*, **286**: 110, 1980.
10. Cavalieri, R. L., Havell, E. A., Vilček, J., and Pestka, S.: *Proc. Natl. Acad. Sci. USA*, **74**: 3287, 1977.
11. Grunstein, M. and Hogness, D. S.: *Proc. Natl. Acad. Sci. USA*, **72**: 3961, 1975.
12. Casey, J. and Davidson, N.: *Nucleic Acids Res.*, **4**: 1579, 1977.
13. Nygaard, A. O. and Hall, B. D.: *Biochem. Biophys. Res. Commun.*, **12**: 98, 1963.
14. Harpold, M. M., Dobner, P. R., Evans, R. M., and Bancroft, F. C.: *Nucleic Acids Res.*, **5**: 2039, 1978.
15. Taniguchi, T., Sakai, M., Fujii-Kuriyama, Y., Muramatsu, M., Kobayashi, S., and Sudo, T.: *Proc. Japan Acad.*, **55**: 464, 1979.
16. Taniguchi, T., Fujii-Kuriyama, Y., and Muramatsu, M.: *Proc. Natl. Acad. Sci. USA*, **77**: 4003, 1980.
17. Taniguchi, T., Ohno, S., Fujii-Kuriyama, T., and Muramatsu, M.: *Gene*, **10**: 11, 1980.
18. Maxam, A. M. and Gilbert, W.: *Proc. Natl. Acad. Sci. USA*, **74**: 560, 1977.
19. Knight, E., Jr., Hunkapiller, M. W., Korant, B. D., Hardy, R. W. F., and Hood, L. E.: *Science*, **207**: 525, 1980.
20. Knight, E., Jr.: *Proc. Natl. Acad. Sci. USA*, **73**: 520, 1976.
21. Hayes, T. G., Tip, Y. K., and Vilček, J.: *Virology*, **98**: 351, 1979.
22. Havell, E. A., Yamazaki, S., and Vilček, J.: *J. Biol. Chem.*, **252**: 4425, 1977.
23. Tan, Y. H., Barakat, F., Berthold, W., Smith-Johannsen, H., and Tan, C.: *J. Biol. Chem.*, **254**: 8067, 1979.
24. Neuberger, A., Gottschalk, A., Marshall, R. D., and Spiro, R. G.: In: A. Gottschalk (ed.), The Glycoproteins, Their Composition, Structure and Function. Elsevier, N.Y., 1972, p. 450.
25. Nagata, S., Taira, H., Hall, A., Johnsrud, L., Streuli, M., Ecosodi, J., Boll, W., Cantell, K., and Weissmann, C.: *Nature*, **284**: 316, 1980.
26. Mantei, N., Schwarzstein, M., Streuli, M., Panem, S., Nagata, S., and Weissmann, C.: *Gene*, **10**: 1, 1980.
27. Taniguchi, T., Mantei, N., Schwarzstein, M., Nagata, S., Muramatsu, M., and Weissman, C.: *Nature*, **285**: 547, 1980.
28. Dayhoff, M. O.: Atlas of Protein Sequence and Structure, vol. 5. Nat. Biomed. Res. Fdn., Washington, 1972.
29. Nagata, S., Mantei, N., and Weissmann, C.: *Nature*, **287**: 401, 1980.
30. Goeddel, D. V., Leung, D. W., Dull, T. J., Gross, R. M., Lawn, R. M., McCandliss, R., Seeburg, P. H., Ullrich, A., Yelverton, E., and Grag, P. W.: *Nature*, **290**: 20, 1981.
31. Sehgal, P. B. and Sagar, A. D.: *Nature*, **287**: 95–97, 1980.
32. Weissenbach, Shulman, L., Soreq, H., Nir, U., Wallach, D., Perricaudet, M., Tiollais, P. and Ravel, M.: *Proc. Natl. Acad. Sci. USA*, **77**: 7152, 1980.
33. Lawn, R. M., Fritsch, E. F., Parker, R. C., Blake, G., and Maniatis, T.: *Cell*, **15**: 1157–1174, 1978.
34. Ohno, S. and Taniguchi, T.: *Proc. Natl. Acad. Sci.*, *USA*: 1981 (in press).
35. Houghton, M., Jackson, I. J., Porter, A. G., Doel, S. M., Catlin, G. H., Barber, C., and Carey, N. H.: *Nucleic Acids Res.*, **9**: 247, 1981.
36. Tavernier, J., Derynck, R., and Fiers, W.: *Nucleic Acids Res.*, **9**: 461, 1981.
37. Nagata, S., Brank, C., Henco, K., Schambock, A., and Weissmann, C.: *J. Interferon Res.*, **1**: 333, 1981.
38. Taniguchi, T., Guarente, L., Roberts, T. R., Kimelman, R., Douhan, J., III, and Ptashne, M.: *Proc. Natl. Acad. Sci. USA*, **77**: 5230, 1980.
39. Taniguchi, T., Hirose, T., Takaoka, C., and Ohno, S.: unpublished observations.

Discussion

Dr. YAMANE: I wonder whether the secretion of interferon proceeds well or not. Is it extracted from the bacteria itself?

Dr. TANIGUCHI: That is correct.

Dr. YAMANE: I think clinicians will be somewhat concerned because, as you know, *E. coli* is a rich source of pyrogenic substance. Your work is very impressive theoretically, but what do you have in mind for its practical application in the future?

Dr. TANIGUCHI: It is true that there is a high possibility of contamination by the proteins of *E. coli*, but on the other hand, if we take a different standpoint, interferon is the only heterogenous protein that is produced in *E. coli*, because the gene is cloned. Purification with the use of an antibody column, for example, is very difficult in the case of material of human origin, unless a very good antibody is used. But by skillful use of the antibody column, I believe that interferon can be considerably purified. However, we have not yet conducted such experiments. If the general percentage were low that might present a problem, but if the percentage is high, purification will be further simplified.

Dr. YAMANE: I think it is important that secretion proceed well . . .

Dr. TANIGUCHI: Yes, since *E. coli* is a gram-negative bacteria, secretion cannot be occurring in the medium but must be occurring in the periplasm. Our interferon does not appear in the periplasm, so it is probably maintained in the cell.

Dr. YAMANE: So the only way to get it would be to mash the cell?

Dr. TANIGUCHI: Yes, or it may be possible to get it our using bacillus, or maybe a eukaryotic cell could be used to get it out in the medium.

Dr. MATSUO: I would like to ask a question concerning your comment that there is a strong possibility that the HuIFN alphagene does not have a glycosylation site.

Dr. TANIGUCHI: I said that that there is no possible candidate sequence, if glycosylation occurs with the N-glycosidic acid pattern; but there seem to be various glycosylation systems, so there may be glycosylation in another form. This difference in the sequence may be one reason why the leukocyte interferon does not have the glycosylation.

Dr. MATSUO: We are conducting purification of the leukocyte interferon, and studies by Stewart or by Cantell suggest that the high molecular weight interferon of 21,000 is a glycoprotein. In your studies, did the messenger RNA that you needed to obtain the complementary DNA have to be harvested at a particular time to get the leukocyte interferon molecule? In other words, would it be possible to have a gene with a glycosylation site if it were harvested at a different time?

Dr. TANIGUCHI: The example I showed today was the fibroblast interferon, but I have also read, in *Nature* I believe, that some of the leukocyte interferons may have the glycosylation site. I do not know how such genes could be obtained, but I would tend to think that the key is not the timing of harvesting but the selection of special cells or the screening of various interferon genes obtained at different times.

Dr. BARON: Have you had any opportunity to synthesize any of those small common peptide areas to determine whether these sequences have any biological activity?

Dr. TANIGUCHI: That's a very interesting question. The answer is, we have not done anything on that, but I am sure that some other people are working on this in order to make active peptides. I wonder if anybody heard about this at the Washington meeting. In order to exert antiviral function, the molecule has to interact with the cells. Then they will elicit the biological functions. Therefore, even if the part of the sequence is responsible as a whole molecule, I don't know whether this is enough to elicit the biological functions. That is one possible problem that we can foresee.

Dr. BARON: Yes, I think there are many problems, but at least with some polypeptide hormones, partial sequences can give partial activity.

Dr. TANIGUCHI: I see; that's very interesting.

Monitoring of Interferon Therapy, Diagnosis of Viral Diseases, and Detection of Interferon Deficiencies by Assay of an Interferon-Induced Enzyme in Human Peripheral White Blood Cells

M. Revel,* A. Schattner,* D. Wallach,* G. Merlin,* H. Levavi,* T. Hahn,[2*] and S. Levin[2*]

* Department of Virology, Weizmann Institute of Science, Rehovot, and [2*] Department of Pediatric Research, Kaplan Hospital, Rehovot, Israel

INTRODUCTION

With the increasing number of patients undergoing interferon (IFN) therapy for viral diseases and malignancies, it is important to have a method to monitor the response of the patient to IFN. During viral diseases, IFN production in the organism probably plays an important protective function, since injection of anti-IFN serum increases the mortality of virus-infected mice.[1]

Direct assay of IFN activity in the serum is possible,[2-7] but it involves lengthy biological procedures which are often imprecise because of the low levels and short half-life of IFN activity usually observed. As an alternative to IFN assay in the serum, we suggested[8,9] the measurement of the variations in an enzyme, (2'-5') oligo A synthetase, which is induced in the cells exposed to IFNs. Induction of this enzyme, which takes place at the transcriptional level,[10] appears to be clearly related to the antiviral and antimitogenic effects of IFNs.[11,12] We have developed a simple and rapid assay which allows the measurement of the enzyme level in leukocytes from 1-2 ml of blood.[8,9] Differentiated mouse lymphocytes have a relatively high level of the enzyme,[13,14] and the activity can also be detected in several tissues. Moreover, after experimental viral infection of mice, the enzyme level is increased in blood and tissues.[15-17]

In humans, we have used our assay procedure to measure the level of (2'-5') oligo A synthetase in peripheral blood mononuclear (PBM) cells of healthy volunteers, of patients receiving either HuIFN-α or HuIFN-β injections, and of patients with viral, autoimmune, and malignant diseases. The results obtained and the main applications of this enzyme assay will be reviewed here.

THE ASSAY

The procedure is summarized in Fig. 1. Two ml of heparinized venous blood are diluted with 2 ml phosphate-buffered saline (PBS), layered on 3 ml of ficoll-hypaque (Pharmacia Fine Chemicals), and centrifuged for 30 min at 400 g. The interphase cells (mononuclear cells) are collected, washed twice in 5 ml PBS, and counted. An aliquot of 10^6 cells is pelleted in an Eppendorf microtest tube, and 0.1 ml lysis buffer (20 mM Hepes buffer, pH 7.5, 5 mM $MgCl_2$, 120 mM KCl, 7 mM dithiothreitol, 10% glycerol, 0.5% Nonidet-P40) is added at 4° C. After a few minutes, the extract is clarified by centrifugation for 6 min at 8,000 g and can then be frozen at −70° C. Extracts from granulocytes can be prepared from the same sample as described.[9]

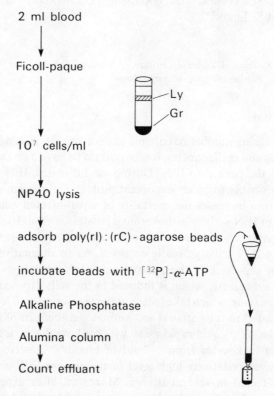

Fig. 1. Flow scheme of the enzyme assay.
(Assay of (2′–5′) oligo A synthetase in human peripheral lymphocytes or granulocytes.)

For enzyme assay, 0.01 ml thawed extract is added to 0.025 ml poly (rI): (rC)-agarose beads (PL biochemicals; the beads have been previously washed with 1 ml of buffer C: 10 mM Hepes buffer, pH 7.5, 50 mM KCl, 5 mM $MgCl_2$,

7 mM dithiothreitol, 20% glycerol). After gentle mixing, the beads suspended in the extract are incubated for 15 min at 30°C; at this step, the (2′–5′) oligo A synthetase binds to the beads. Tubes with cell extracts from 3 healthy donors and tubes without cell extract are routinely included in addition to the extracts to be tested. The beads are pelleted in the Eppendorf microfuge, washed with 1 ml buffer C, and all liquid is carefully removed. A reaction mixture of 0.01 ml is added which contains 10 mM Hepes buffer, pH 7.5, 5 mM $MgCl_2$, 7 mM dithiothreitol, 10% glycerol, 2.5 mM [^{32}P]-α-ATP (0.1–0.3 Ci/mmol), 3 mg/ml creatine kinase, 10 mM creatine phosphate, and 40 μg/ml poly (rI):(rC). Incubation is carried out for 14–20 hours at 30°C. Then, 1 unit of bacterial alkaline phosphatase in 0.01 ml of 140 mM Tris-base is added. After 1 hour at 37°C, 0.02 ml water is added, and the beads are removed by centrifugation. From the supernatant, 0.01 ml is applied to a 0.3 ml column of alumina (acid alumina WAl from Sigma) equilibrated in 1 M glycine-HCl buffer, pH 2. Three ml of the same buffer are applied to the column and directly collected in scintillation vials which are then counted in the ^{3}H-channel of a Tricarb scintillation counter (Packard) by Cerenkov radiation. This procedure measures the $(A2'p)_nA$ nucleotides formed.[8]

The results can be expressed in cpm or pmol ATP incorporated per hour and per μg protein, or per 10^5 cells. The assay itself uses only 2.5×10^4 cells and usually gives 6–8×10^3 cpm. We routinely express the results in percent of the mean enzyme activity found for the samples from healthy donors.

ENZYME LEVEL IN PBM CELLS FROM HEALTHY DONORS

In a group of 63 samples from healthy blood donors, we found that the mean (2′–5′) oligo A synthetase activity was 130 pmoles $(A2'p)_nA$ per hr and 10^5 cells (about 5 μg protein). The standard deviation was $\pm 40\%$, and this is taken as the statistical range of normal values. The (2′–5′) oligo A synthetase level of mononuclear cells in the normal human population appears, therefore, high and constant. We did find, in this group of 63, 3 high values outside the statistical deviation, but these were later diagnosed as pathologic cases. We also found enzyme activity in the granulocytes, but this amounted to only 0.1–0.3 fold the activity of mononuclear cells. Erythrocytes, thrombocytes, and serum had no significant enzyme activity in our assays. Incubation of mononuclear cells and granulocytes for 20 hours *in vitro* with 100 U/ml human HuIFN-α led to at least 5-fold increases in the enzyme level.

ENZYME INCREASES IN PATIENTS RECEIVING IFN THERAPY

IFN-α

The first study was done on a group of patients receiving intramuscular

(I.M.) injections of HuIFN-α prepared from fresh human leukocytes by the method of Cantell and Hirvonen.[18] (This IFN is produced at the Israel Biological Institute, Ness Ziona, by Dr. Hagai Rosenberg and T. Bino). The dose was 1–3 $\times$ 10⁶ units, according to the weight of the patient (0.8–1 $\times$ 10⁵ U/kg).

Figure 2 shows the enzyme activity in the PBM cells of some of these patients relative to the mean enzyme value of the healthy population (solid horizontal line). The standard deviation of the normal value is shown by the two broken lines. Blood samples were taken immediately before the first injection (day 0) and then every 24 hours just prior to the next injection of IFN. For 2 of the patients (curves 1 and 2), there was a rapid 6–8-fold increase in enzyme level during the first 2 days following the onset of therapy. Curve 1 indicates the

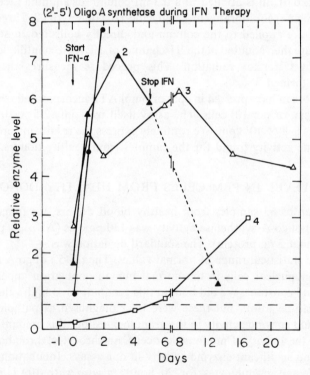

Fig. 2. (2′–5′) Oligo A synthetase levels in peripheral mononuclear white blood cells of patients under IFN therapy.

The mean enzyme activity in the blood cells of healthy donors is shown as 1 (horizontal full line), with the dotted horizontal lines representing the standard deviation of this value in 60 normal blood samples. In 4 patients receiving IFN therapy, IFN injections were started on day 0. The curve represents the enzyme level in these patients relative to the normal value. The dotted line in curve 3 relates to the period after IFN injections were stopped. For details see text.

enzyme changes in a critically ill 2-year-old boy with fulminans hepatitis who received 10^6 U of IFN daily. The enzyme activity increased from 6,800 cpm on day 0, to 33,200 on day 1 and 56,200 cpm on day 2. Despite treatment, however, death occurred. Curve 2 relates to a case of severe viral encephalitis in a 14-month-old infant who received 1.2×10^6 U daily. The symptoms disappeared after 5 days of treatment and IFN injections were discontinued. During treatment the enzyme level was high, but returned to normal one week after the last injection (broken line). Curve 3 represents the case of a young girl with laryngeal papillomatosis. The starting enzyme level on day 0 was higher than normal, as observed in most viral diseases (see below). The injection schedule in this patient was 1.5×10^6 U every second day for several months. Over the 3-week period we followed this case, the enzyme level was stable at 4–5-fold the normal values. The increased enzyme level thus appears to correlate well with IFN treatment since continued injections result in a relatively constant elevation in enzyme, while interruption of the treatment results in a decrease to the normal values.

Curve 4 of Fig. 2 illustrates the importance of monitoring the patient's response to IFN. This was a case of lymphoproliferative disease in a 21-year-old woman with a septic fever and a severe combined immunodeficiency (after immunosuppresive treatment). When the enzyme was first measured, the values obtained were much lower than normal, as is often observed in such patients (see below). Daily injections of 3×10^6 U of HuIFN-α were started on day 0, but the increase in enzyme was very low. It took 6 days of daily injections to attain the mormal level, and after 17 days she reached a level 3 times higher than the normal, a 15-fold increase over her starting level. The abnormal enzyme response may be related to her disease or to previous treatment, indicating some deficiency in the IFN system. Such information on the response of the patient should be very precious to the physician. There was actually no visible clinical improvement during IFN therapy in the patient.

HuIFN-β

The use of HuIFN-β by systemic injections has been criticized because, after I.M. injections, IFN activity cannot be detected in the serum.[19] Better results are obtained by intravenous (I.V.) infusions, but the half-life of the activity is very short and it disappears from the serum 2 hours after injection.[20] We have recently measured the changes in (2′-5′) oligo A synthetase activity following subcutaneous (perineal) injections of 3×10^6 U of HuIFN-β (in part produced in our laboratory by Drs. D. Gurari-Rotman and L. Chen, and in part obtained from InterYeda Ltd., Rehovot, Israel).

As shown in Table 1, we could detect significant increases in the enzyme level of PBM cells after subcutaneous injections of IFN-β. The increases were smaller than for IFN-α (around 3-fold versus 6–8-fold) but seemed to persist for longer periods of time, sometimes for several days. There may also be a cumulative effects of repeated injections. In the same blood sample we also measured NK activity,[21] which was increased by IFN-β injections, as has been found by others (M. Fellous and E. Falcoff, personal communication). In several cases we also detected significant serum levels of IFN-β, and we could demonstrate that VSV growth in the mononuclear cells is inhibited. These other methods are, however, more elaborate, lengthier, and less precise than the enzyme assay which we feel is best suited for monitoring IFN therapy.

Table 1. (2′–5′) Oligo A synthetase after HuIFN-β injections.

Days	Patient a		Patient b		Patient c	
	IFN-β injections	Enzyme	IFN-β injections	Enzyme	IFN-β injections	Enzyme
0		100		100		100
	I→		I→		I→	
1		170		220		120
2		230		140		80
			II→		II→	
3				170		100
4				230		290
					III→	
5				160		190
			III→			
6				n.d.		n.d.
7				380		190
			IV→		IV→	
8				360		250
11				210		190

Arrows indicate HuIFN-β injections (3×10^6 U subcutaneous). The roman numeral is the number of the injection.

PATHOLOGIC INCREASES IN (2′–5′) OLIGO A SYNTHETASE IN VIRAL AND AUTOIMMUNE DISEASES

Acute Viral Infections

Another application of the enzyme assay is to investigate changes in the IFN system in various pathologic conditions. Some species of IFN are probably produced during the course of viral diseases in man, but this production is often difficult to detect and quantitate. If IFNs are produced, we may expect the (2′–5′) oligo A synthetase to increase. In a study of 40 cases of acute viral diseases, we found, as shown in Table 2, that 95% of the patients had an elevated enzyme activity in PBM cells. In 85% of the cases, the increases were over 2-fold, and Table 3 shows that in some instances 5–10-fold increases were observed. Increases were observed in the 13 different viral diseases studied (Table 3).

Table 2.   (2'–5') Oligo A synthetase levels in various diseases.

Disease[a]	Total number of patients	Number of cases with (2'–5') oligo A synthetase activity			
		lower than 60%	normal 60–140%	increased 140–200%	higher than 200%
Viral infections[b]	41	0	2	4	35
Bacterial infections	13	5	6	1	1
Noninfectious diseases (ischemic heart disease, iron-deficiency anemia)	10	0	10	0	0
Collagen diseases	13	1	0	4	8
EBV-related malignancies	10	0	0	4	6
Breast and G.I. carcinomas	10	0	7	3	0
Lymphoproliferative diseases	10	4	5	0	1[c]

a) Details in text. Further details on individual patients available from A.S.
b) Detailed in Table 3.
c) HB_sAg-positive.

Table 3.   Increased (2'–5') oligo A synthetase in viral diseases.

Clinical diagnosis	Total number of patients	(2'–5') oligo A synthetase activity, % of normal mean value
Viral hepatitis, A	8	550, 520, 470, 350, 330, 260, 200, 150
Viral encephalitis	8	800, 340, 320, 320, 300, 200, 170, 100
Infectious mononucleosis	5	700, 590, 490, 480, 210
Upper respiratory infections	5	670, 370, 300, 230, 180
Viral meningitis	3	740, 240, 100
Herpes zoster	3	1940, 290, 140
Acute myocarditis	2	280, 240
Acute viral gastroenteritis	2	1300, 470
Rubella, congenital	1	1070
Varicella	1	730
Herpangina (Coxsackie)	1	270
Viral pneumonia	1	330
Herpetic keratitis	1	240
Total	41	

It is not clear why some patients had only a 2-fold increase while others showed a much larger increase. This did not seem to be related to the severity of the disease or to the virus involved (Table 3). In 2 cases, diagnosed as viral encephalitis and meningitis, there was no enzyme increase. This could be due to a nonviral etiology or to the blood-brain barrier. There were, however, 7 other cases of encephalitis with elevated enzyme values; among these, 2 were due to herpes virus, one to measles, and one to vaccinia virus, and the rest were unidentified.

The variable increases observed may be related in part to the time course of the disease since our blood samples were obtained at any time from 1 day to 6 weeks after the onset of the clinical symptoms. The time course of the variations in enzyme activity will have to be studied for each viral disease individually. One advantage of the enzyme assay over direct IFN assay in the serum seems to be that the enzyme remains elevated for a prolonged period of time after viral infection. This may explain why we found that the vast majority of patients with acute viral diseases have an elevated enzyme level, while in previous investigations[6,7] circulation IFN was detected in only one-third of the patients. Experiments in mice injected I.P. with viruses showed (Fig. 3) that the (2'-5') oligo A synthetase levels in peripheral white blood cells are increased for over a week after the infection. A single injection of IFN itself produced only a transient increase in the enzyme level (Fig. 3, lower panel).

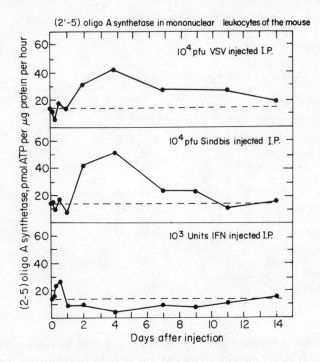

Fig. 3. (2'-5') Oligo A synthetase increases in white blood cells of mice injected with sublethal doses of viruses. VSV: vesicular stomatitis virus; I.P.: intraperitoneally.

Absence of Enzyme Increase in Bacterial and Non-infectious Diseases

Table 2 shows that in 11 out of 13 cases of bacterial infections, the enzyme level was not increased, in contrast to viral diseases. This group of patients included cases of penumococcal pneumonia, gram-negative septicemia, tonsillitis, cholecystitis parotitis, and a rickettsial disease. Two cases of bacterial infections showed, however, elevated values; surprisingly, both were erysipelar infections of the face. It is known that staphylococci and other bacteria can induce some IFNs,[22] but in general we can state that the (2'–5') oligo A synthetase is not significantly increased in bacterial diseases.

We studied another group of 10 patients hospitalized for noninfectious diseases; all of them had normal enzyme levels (Table 2). In yet another group of patients with lymphoproliferative diseases, the only case with a high enzyme level was that of a patient who was HB$_s$Ag-positive.

Enzyme Increase in Chronic Virus-related Diseases and Autoimmune Diseases

Table 2 lists two more groups of diseases in which we observed elevated enzyme values. In a group of 13 patients with autoimmune diseases (collagen diseases including 8 cases of lupus erythematosus, and cases of vasculitis, scleroderma, and dermatomyosis), 60% had high values and another 30% mildly increased values. It is likely that this denotes the presence of circulating IFN-γ, which has been detected in autoimmune diseases.[23]

More surprising was the finding that the (2'–5') oligo A synthetase is also elevated in virus-related malignancies. Among 5 nasopharyngeal carcinomas and 5 Burkitt's lymphomas, both related to Epstein-Barr virus, all the patients had elevated enzyme levels. In one case of juvenile laryngeal papilloma, the level of the enzyme was found to be 270% of the normal value. In comparison, the enzyme levels in patients with breast and G.I. tract carcinomas were not significantly increased.

Finally, we found elevated enzyme levels in a series of neurologic disorders, such as Jacob-Creutzfeldt and amyotrophic lateral sclerosis, which are thought to be of viral etiology (Table 4). The results were less clear for SSPE. In a relatively large group of patients with multiple sclerosis, we can see that a certain number of patients had elevated values while another group had normal values (Table 4). This may suggest a different etiology or different stages in the disease.

Table 4. Other diseases showing increased (2'–5') oligo A synthetase levels.

Disease	Total number of patients	Number of cases with (2'–5') oligo A synthetase activity			
		lower than 60%	normal 60–140%	increased 140–200%	higher than 200%
Jacob-Creutzfeldt	3	0	0	1	2
Slow sclerosing panencephalitis	5	0	3	0	2
Amyotrophic lateral sclerosis	5	0	0	1	4
Multiple sclerosis	27	3	12	5	7

Our test may help clarify the question of whether or not IFN plays any role in multiple sclerosis.[24,25]

Elevated enzyme values seem, therefore, to accompany not only acute viral infections, but also chronic viral diseases and autoimmune diseases. These results represent only a preliminary screening of many different patients. It will be of great interest to determine if the enzyme level varies during the course of these slow diseases and if a prognostic trend can be determined.

DECREASE IN (2'–5') OLIGO A SYNTHETASE AND POSSIBLE "INTERFERON DEFICIENCIES"

Since the level of (2'–5') oligo A synthetase is rather high in mononuclear cells of healthy individuals, we have been particularly interested in the observation that some patients have markedly lowered levels of this enzyme. From a study in mouse T-lymphocytes, it appeared that the level of the enzyme increases with maturation of the T-cells.[14] A low enzyme level could, therefore, be an indication of the presence of immature lymphocytes that are proliferating. Indeed, low (2'–5') oligo A synthetase levels and high 2'-phosphodiesterase (the enzyme which degrades pppA2'p5'A2'p5'A. . .) are characteristics of growing cells.[12] In Friend erythroleukemia we even found that the (2'–5') oligo A synthetase level increases markedly when the cells stop growing exponentially and start to undergo differentiation.[4] The high (2'–5') oligo A synthetase levels which characterize normal PBM cells in humans may result from constant exposure to some IFN spontaneously produced in the organism. In this hypothesis, low synthetase values could indicate some deficiency in the IFN system. Such deficiencies have been previously suggested.[5]

While screening the enzyme level of various patients, we observed that in two diseases there was a particularly large proportion of very low enzyme levels. Table 5 shows that 3 out of 4 non-Hodgkin's lymphomas and more than half of the patients with acute lymphatic leukemias (ALL) had low enzyme values (in general, 10–20% of the normal level). Related leukemias are shown for comparison. Chronic myelogenous leukemia (CML) has a trend to elevated enzyme levels; this may be correlated with the high IFN production observed in cells from these CML patients.[26]

It is obvious that there is much heterogeneity in these groups of patients, but further subclassification of the leukemias could reveal a more consistent picture. There was some correlation between the number of blast cells in ALL and the low level of the enzyme. Most striking are the non-Hodgkins lymphomas, in which there was no histological change in the blood cell population in which the enzyme was measured.

The ability to detect deficiencies in the IFN system by this enzymatic test may have applications in the field of IFN therapy. It may be proposed that

Table 5. Decreases in (2′–5′) oligo A synthetase levels.

Disease	Total number of patients	Number of cases with (2′–5′) oligo A synthetase activity			
		lower than 60%	normal 60–140%	increased 140–200%	higher than 200%
Non-Hodgkin's lymphoma	4	3	1	0	0
Hodgkin's disease	5	1	4	0	0
Acute lymphatic leukemia	25	13	6	2	4
Chronic lymphatic leukemia	24	5	13	6	0
Acute myelogenous leukemia	8	2	2	2	2
Chronic myelogenous leukemia	5	1	0	0	4

patients with low enzyme levels could benefit most from IFN therapy which would bring back their enzyme level to normal. Cancer patients having already high enzyme levels may benefit less from additional IFN injections. It should be recalled that only about one-third of the cancer patients who have received IFN in various studies have responded to IFN therapy by showing some tumor regression.[27] Therefore, there must be some differences among there patients, and our hypothesis is that good responders could be preselected by using the (2′–5′) oligo A synthetase assay. That patients with low enzyme levels actually have some impairment in their IFN systems is further illustrated by one of the patients shown in Fig. 2 (curve 4) who had a very abnormal response to IFN, but in whom prolonged IFN treatment could bring a very low enzyme value back to normal and even elevated levels.

In conclusion, the enzyme assay described here, which is simple and rapid, and which can be applied to large numbers of blood samples, could become a useful tool for monitoring the IFN response of patients and for diagnostic and possibly prognostic purposes.

Acknowledgments

This work was supported in part by NCRD (Israel) and GSF (Munich, Germany). Gifts of HuIFN-α from Dr. H. Rosenberg and T. Bino of the Israel Biological Institute are gratefully acknowledged. A.S. is a recipient of an Israel Ministry of Health fellowship. G.M. is an EMBO fellow.

REFERENCES

1. Gresser, I., Tovey, M. G., Bandu, M. T., Maury, C., and Brouty-Boye, D.: Role of interferon in the pathogenesis of virus diseases in mice as demonstrated by the use of anti-interferon serum. *J. Exp. Med.*, **144**: 1305–1315, 1976.
2. Wheelock, E. F. and Sibley, W.: Interferon in human serum during clinical viral infections. *Lancet*, **2**: 382–385, 1964.

3. Smorodintsev, A. A., Beare, A. S., Bynoe, M. L., Head, B., and Tyrrell, D. A. J.: The formation of interferon during acute respiratory virus infection of volunteers. *Arch. Ges. Virusforsch*, **33**: 9–16, 1971.

4. Petralli, J. K., Merigan, T. C., and Wilbur, J. R.: Circulating interferon after measles vaccination. *New Engl. J. Med.*, **273**: 198–201, 1965.

5. Levin, S. and Hahn, T.: Interferon system in immunodeficiency and deficiency of the interferon system. In: M. Seligman and W. H. Hitzis (eds.), INSERM Symp., No. 16. North Holland Biomed Press, 1980, pp. 465–472.

6. Matthews, T. H. J. and Lawrence, M. K.: Serum interferon assay as a possible test for virus infections of man. *Arch. Virol.*, **59**: 35–38, 1979.

7. Parry, R. P. and Parry, J. V.: Interferon assay as a diagnostic test. *Lancet*, **1**: 506–507, 1981.

8. Merlin, G., Revel, M., and Wallach, D.: The interferon-induced enzyme oligo-isoadenylate synthetase: Rapid determination of its *in vitro* products. *Anal. Biochem.*, **110**: 190–196, 1981.

9. Schattner, A., Merlin, G., Wallach, D., Rosenberg, H., Bino, T., Hahn, T., Levin, A., and Revel, M.: Monitoring of interferon-therapy by assay of (2'–5') oligo-isoadenylate synthetase in human peripheral white blood cells, *J. Interf. Res.*, **1**: 587–594, 1981.

10. Shulman, L. and Revel, M.: Interferon-dependent induction of mRNA activity for (2'–5') oligo-isoadenylate synthetase. *Nature*, **287**: 98–100, 1980.

11. Revel, M.: Molecular mechanisms involved in the antiviral effects of interferon. In: I. Gresser (ed.), Interferon 1. Academic Press, 1979, pp. 101–163.

12. Kimchi, A., Shure, H., and Revel, M.: Anti-mitogenic function of interferon-induced (2'–5') oligo(adenylate) and growth related variations in enzymes that synthesize and degrade this oligonucleotide. *Eur. J. Biochem.*, **114**: 5–10, 1981.

13. Shimizu, N. and Sokawa, Y.: 2'–5' oligo-adenylate synthetase activity in lymphocytes from normal mouse. *J. Biol. Chem.*, **254**, 12034–12037, 1979.

14. Kimchi, A.: Increased levels of interferon-induced (2'–5') oligo-isoadenylate synthetase in mature T-lymphocytes and in differentiated Friend-erythroleukemic cells. *J. Interf. Res.*, **1**: 559–565, 1981.

15. Krishnan, I. and Baglioni, C.: 2'–5' oligo(A) polymerase activity in serum of mice infected with EMC virus or treated with interferon. *Nature*, **285**: 485–488, 1980.

16. Sokawa, Y., Ando, T., and Ishihara, Y.: Induction of 2'–5'-oligo-adenylate synthetase and interferon in mouse trigeminal ganglia infected with Herpes Simplex virus. *Infection and Immunity*, **28**: 719–723, 1980.

17. Hovanessian, A. G. and Riviere, Y.: Interferon-mediated induction of 2–5 A synthetase and protein kinase in the liver and spleen of mice infected with Newcastle disease virus or injected with poly(I): poly(C). *Ann. Virol (Inst. Pasteur)*, **131E**: 501–516, 1980.

18. Cantell, K. and Hirvonen, S.: Preparation of human leukocyte interferon for clinical use. *Tex. Rep. Biol. Med.*, **35**: 138–144, 1977.

19. Edy, F. G., Brillian, A., and De Somer, P.: Non-appearance of injected fibroblast interferon in the circulation. *Lancet*, **1**: 451–452, 1978.

20. Treuner, J., Niethammer, D., Dannecker, G., Hagmann, R., Neef, V., and Hofschneider, P. H.: Successful treatment of nasopharyngeal carcinoma with interferon. *Lancet*, **1**: 817–818, 1980.

21. Huddlestone, J. R., Merigan, T. C., and Oldstone, M. B.: Induction and kinetics of natural killer cells in humans following interferon therapy. *Nature*, **282**: 417–420, 1979.

22. Degre, M. and Dahl, H.: Interferon production and prevention of viral infections in mice by components of a mixed bacterial vaccine. *Acta. Pathol. Microbiol. Scand.*, **82**: 904–910, 1974.

23. Hooks, J. J., Moutsopoulos, H. M., Geis, S., Stahl, N. I., Decker, J. L., and Notkins, A. C.: Immune interferon in the circulation of patients with autoimmune disease. *New Engl. J. Med.*, **301**: 5–8, 1979.
24. Degre, M., Dahl, H., and Vanduick, B.: Interferon in the serum and cerebro-spinal fluid in patients with multiple sclerosis and other neurological disorders. *Acta Neurol. Scand.*, **53**: 152–156, 1976.
25. Neighbour, P. A. and Bloom, B. R.: Absence of virus-induced lymphocyte suppression and interferon production in multiple sclerosis. *Proc. Natl. Acad. Sci. USA*, **76**: 476–480, 1979.
26. Rubinstein, M., Rubinstein, S., Familletti, P. C., Hershberger, R. D., Brink, L. D., Gutterman, J., Hester, J., and Petska, S.: Human leukocyte interferon. Production and purification to homogeneity by HPLC. In: E. Gross and J. Meienhofer (eds.) Proteins: Structure and Biological Functions. Pierce Chemical Company, Rockford, Ill., 1980, pp. 99–103.
27. Gutterman, J. U., Blumenschein, G. R., Alexanian, R., Yap, H. Y., Buzdar, A. U., Cabanillas, F., Hortobagyi, G. N., Hersh, E. M., Rasmussen, S. L., Harmon, M., Kramer, M., and Petska, S.: Leukocyte interferon-induced tumor regression in human metastatic breast cancer, multiple myeloma, and malignant lymphoma. *Ann. Int. Med.*, **93**: 399–406, 1980.

Discussion

Dr. Hopps: This question relates not so much to your beautiful enzyme studies but to the practical application. You showed that in encephalitis compounded disease such as herpes, measles and vaccinia, you do get significant increase. I was wondering if one might apply that technique in terms of looking at milder infection where one has a natural case of measles or perhaps rubella. Has that been looked at?

Dr. Revel: Yes, we have done one case of measles and this was very high. We also had one case of rubella. As I said, 85% of all the viral cases we have looked at, had a more than 2-fold increase. We had only 3% of the viral infections which were normal and the others were intermediate between 130 and 200. If we take, let's say, heart infarct as the control group, 100% fall in the normal class. So I really think that this is a sensitive test for diagnostic purposes.

Dr. Galasso: Since we have returned to the infectious diseases, again I would like to give a word of caution. On a slide there was a rather miraculous cure of herpes excephalitis.

Dr. Revel: I cannot say it was herpes, but herpes antibodies were pound. So maybe it was herpes.

Dr. Galasso: Good, I'm glad you qualified that because herpes is very difficult to diagnose, and without a brain biopsy you cannot say it is herpes encephalitis.

Dr. Revel: I do not make any claim, but I think what was important in this case was that the patient recovered and we could stop interferon and see that the level of the enzyme returns rapidly to normal levels.

Dr. Kojima: What actually happens to enzyme activity in a case of mixed viral and bacterial infection?

Dr. REVEL: I cannot answer the question.

Dr. KUWATA: What is the main cause of the discrepancy between the level of the interferon titer in the serum and the level of 2–5A synthetase in the lymphocytes from the peripheral blood? I understand that yesterday some doctors emphasized the importance of the serum level of interferon. Today you rather emphasized the level of 2–5A synthetase in the lymphocytes of peripheral blood.

Dr. REVEL: What I can say, Dr. Kuwata, is that this work was performed in parallel with studies in Dr. Levine's laboratory at the Kaplan hospital: they measured the serum level and also the antiviral state of the lymphocytes by infecting with VSV. It takes a week to get such results. Our data with synthetase were in good agreement with the antiviral data and were not in such good agreement with the serum levels. Sometimes when you have low serum level you can have a good response; and in one patient who had a very low response there was a high serum level, but the patient did not respond very well. So I think there are discrepancies. My feeling is that we do not have enough data, but it is useful to have a technique which gives results after a few hours. It will be also important to see which method gives the best correlation with clinical results.

Dr. KUWATA: So you would rather emphasize the importance of the level of $2'-5'A$ synthetase.

Dr. REVEL: As you say in Japan, you don't know if you should be Buddhist or Shintoist. I don't know.

Dr. YAMAZAKI: I was very impressed with your results, and I believe many applications are possible. I also believe there remain many questions to be answered, and my question is somewhat related to Dr. Kuwata's. With regard to the relationship with the course of the viral disease, what is the duration that can be detected with the enzyme assay? My second question is concerned with the specificity of this enzyme in viral infections. The enzyme can probably be detected if there are various kinds of lymphokines. Have you seen this in patients with bacterial infections? My third question is related to applicability of this method for diseases of unknown etiology, such as slow virus infections. I think this can be used for etiological study of such diseases, but have you ever tried this method in C-J and other similar diseases?

Dr. REVEL: With respect to the type of virus, I do not think there is a correlation between the level of the enzyme and the severity of the disease. The highest increases that we saw were either in upper respiratory infection—a common cold—or in gastroenteritis, which is very common in Israel. Maybe it relates rather to the reaction of the person; even in a mild disease, you may have a 10-fold increase in enzyme. To the third part of your question: we have looked at quite a few exotic diseases, including neurological disorders, and there is a tendency for a mild increase in the synthetase. It seems statistically significant, but we do not understand it. It was expected that in immune diseases there would be an increase. There are slight increases in multiple sclerosis and amyotrophic lateral sclerosis, but not as much as with viral disease. We have also observed increases in almost all patients with chronic myelogenic leukemia. There is also a tendency for increase in many patients with solid sarcoma. In contrast, non-Hodgkin's lymphomas and acute lymphatic leukemia stand out with very low values. We do not understand, but we think that these studies should be continued.

Dr. YAMAZAKI: What about the relationship with the duration of the infectious disease?

Dr. REVEL: We do not have enough data for the moment, but the enzyme level sometimes comes up before the symptom occurs. We have taken blood from healthy people and seen a high level, and the next morning they had flu or another infection. And the level usually comes down before the end of the disease, rather earlier than the disappearance of the clinical symptoms. But I think this should be studied more carefully in each case. It is not well documented yet.

Human Interferons: Purification of the Proteins and Their Expression in Bacteria

Sidney PESTKA, Shuichiro MAEDA, Russell McCANDLISS, Warren P. LEVY, Philip C. FAMILLETTI, Alan SLOMA, and Donna S. HOBBS

Roche Institute of Molecular Biology, Nutley, NJ 07110, U.S.A.

INTRODUCTION

Basic research has laid the foundation for the clinical use of interferon (IF) and it should be emphasized that it will require much more basic research to bring IF to its optimal clinical use in the years to come.

The human IFs consist of at least three kinds: fibroblast, leukocyte, and immune IFs. These appear to be distinct moieties. Numerous actions have been ascribed to the IFs: antiviral action antitumor activity, as well as general antiproliferative activity on both normal and tumor cells and finally, a number of immunomodulatory activities.

Isolation and Translation of IF Messenger RNA

Messenger RNA was extracted from human cells which were induced to produce IF. The isolated message was placed in a mouse cell-free extract with appropriate components for protein synthesis. After translation, the extract was assayed for human IF activity (Fig. 1). It was shown that the isolated message could code for the synthesis of human IF.[1,2] While our studies were being carried out, similar studies were performed elsewhere.[3,4]

In order to clone IF, it was necessary to have an assay for IF messenger RNA (mRNA). These experiments provided that assay and paved the way for the subsequent cloning of IF.

In addition, it was useful to answer a number of other basic questions. Briefly, these were:

Was the Carbohydrate Moiety Necessary for Activity?

It was shown that under conditions where no carbohydrate was being syn-

369

CELL-FREE INTERFERON SYNTHESIS

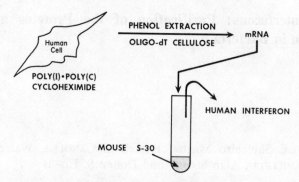

Fig. 1. Schematic illustration of procedures involved in cell-free synthesis of human IF. Human fibroblast monolayers were induced to synthesize IF in the presence of poly I: poly C and cycloheximide as described.[1,2] RNA was extracted from the induced cells and the polyadenylated mRNA was isolated from the total cellular RNA by fractionation on oligo (dT)-cellulose. Translation of the mRNA was performed in an Ehrlich ascites cell-free extract (mouse S-30). The products of translation were assayed directly for IF activity.[1,2]

thesized in the cell-free product, the IF that was made was active. Therefore, it was concluded that carbohydrate was not required for activity.[5] Studies taking a different approach by Bose *et al.*,[6] in which about 80% of the carbohydrate was removed, came to the same conclusion.

Is the Precursor Active?

Under conditions where the precursor polypeptide was synthesized and remained intact,[1,7] it was found that IF activity was generated. It was therefore concluded that the precursor protein was also active.

In terms of cloning, it was important to know that the precursor protein and nonglycosylated protein were, in fact, active; otherwise, it would not have been rewarding to look for activity of recombinants directly.

In order to isolate and purify mRNA and to prepare recombinants from it, it was necessary to use more efficient systems for translation. Cell-free extracts required about 1 to 10 μg of IF message to make an active protein. Although 1 to 10 μg may not seem much, in terms of IF mRNA and the resources that were available to us, it was an enormous amount. So it became critical, if the IF message was to be purified and used for cloning, that more sensitive assays be used. Such an assay was the microinjection of mRNA into frog oocytes.[8] Each oocyte was injected with about 50 nanoliters of material containing between 1 and 50 nanograms of mRNA. With this oocyte assay, it was possible to detect 1 ng of total mRNA from induced cells.[5,9,10] This allowed us to use the mRNA more efficiently and enabled us to purify IF message.[11]

PURIFICATION OF INTERFERONS

While the above studies were proceeding, it was evident that some additional approaches would have to be undertaken to accomplish the ultimate goal of cloning IF because it was necessary to have some information about the amino acid sequences of the IF molecules. In 1974, very little was known about the IF proteins themselves. Accordingly, we began purification of the IFs to learn about their strcuture. Use was made of white blood cells from normal donors. Newcastle disease virus (NDV) was utilized to induce IF and after overnight incubation, IF was found in the medium. This was similar to the procedures reported by Mogensen and Cantell[12] and those of Wheelock[13] with NDV. An additional modification that was incorporated was the substitution of milk casein in the medium instead of serum.[14] It was hoped that the purification would be simpler, that it would be easier to isolate IF from casein than from the huge number of proteins in serum. This method seems to work quite well and is a method that continues to be used in many of the cellular incubations carried out in our laboratory.

To purify IF, a number of routine steps were employed, but it was found that with the small amounts of material that were available, some new technology would have to be tried. We then discovered how to apply high performance liquid chromatography (HPLC) to the purification of proteins.[15,16] Previously, HPLC could not be used to purify proteins, but we (with Menachem Rubinstein and Stanley Stein) discovered and developed the methodology to do this. In each high performance step illustrated in Fig. 2, fraction number is plotted on the abscissa and fluorescence of the protein on the ordinate. A sensitive fluorescence technique was used to detect proteins. Sidney Udenfriend, Stanley Stein, and their coworkers developed these fluorescent detection techniques[17,18] that were used and provided a constant source of support, encouragement, and ideas.

The first HPLC step (top panel, Fig. 2A) involved a column which contained octadecyl groups linked to silica. The IF was eluted and placed directly onto the second column, which was silica to which glycerol groups were attached (Fig. 2B). At this point, it was noticed that the leukocyte IF separated into at least 3 peaks. These peaks were arbitrarily called α, β, and γ leukocyte IF. Occasionally in some preparations, a δ fraction was also observed. Each of these fractions was subsequently purified on the next high performance step, again on an octadecyl silica HPLC column, at a different pH (Fig. 2C, D). The γ fractions were purified to homogeneity. Occasionally a fraction was obtained which has been termed γ_1, but in the case shown little or no γ_1 was seen. The major peak was γ_2, and there were also peaks for γ_3 and γ_4, and relatively less often, a peak was observed for γ_5. It has now been possible to purify 5 γ species. The α and β species have likewise been purified, as well as the δ species.[19]

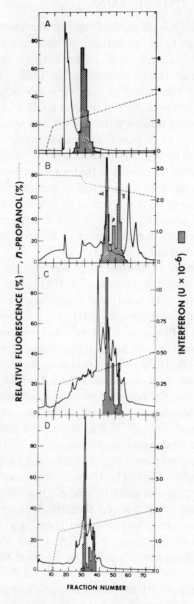

Fig. 2. High performance liquid chromatography of IF.
A: Chromatography on LiChrosorb RP-8 at pH 7.5.
B: Chromatography on LiChrosorb Diol at pH 7.5.
C: Chromatography on LiChrosorb RP-8 at pH 4.
D: Rechromatography on LiChrosorb RP-8 at pH 4.[15]

Multiple species of leukocyte IF have been purified, 8 of these to homogeneity.[19] They exhibit a range of molecular weights, and they appear to represent a number of diffferent amino acid sequences as well. The various species of leukocyte IF have different biological activities. Table 1 shows the activity of the various species on bovine MDBK and human AG-1732 cells. It can be seen that several species exhibit about the same ratio, whereas β_2 has about a 2-fold higher activity on bovine cells than on human cells; and γ_3 and γ_5 exhibit much higher activity on bovine than on human cells.

Table 1. Specific activities of human leukocyte IFs.

Species	Specific activity on bovine MDBK cells (units/mg $\times$ 10^{-6})	Specific activity on human AG-1732 cells (units/mg $\times$ 10^{-6})
α_1	260	260
α_2	400	300
β_1	340	440
β_2	400	200
β_3	400	300
γ_1	260	200
γ_2	400	150
γ_3	350	15
γ_4	350	400
γ_5	90	2

Antiviral activities of the purified human leukocyte IF species (IFL-α_1, α_2, β_1, β_2, β_3, γ_1, γ_2, γ_3, γ_4 and γ_5) were assayed.

It must be pointed out that, whereas a relatively short time ago researchers talked about "human leukocyte interferon," it is now clear that this term represents a family of proteins: leukocyte IF is not one protein, but a protein family.[20] Exactly how many proteins are included in this family is not yet known. As will be discussed later, the recombinants containing the human leukocyte IF sequences also exhibit a multiplicity that confirms that leukocyte IFs represent a family of proteins.

By similar procedures, it has been possible for Stein et al.[21,22] to purify fibroblast IF to homogeneity by two steps, including one single step of HPLC.

Having purified both these IFs, we proceeded to obtain some information about their amino acid composition and sequence. Figure 3 shows the first 19 amino acid residues of human fibroblast IF. The first 13 residues are identical to those reported by Knight et al.[23] as well as Tan et al.[24] The first 22 residues of human leukocyte IF are presented in Fig. 4. Sequences of most tryptic peptides have also been obtained. The sequence reported for the first 20 residues of lymphoblastoid IF by Zoon et al.[25] is similar to the amino terminal analysis shown here, with two differences at positions 14 and 16. This also confirms that the human leukocyte IFs consist of distinct, but homolgous proteins. The sequences obtained for both fibroblast (Fig. 3) and leukocyte (Fig. 4) IFs agree with those coded for by recombinants obtained for fibroblast and leukocyte IFs in our laboratory and others.

```
  1                   5                        10
MET-SER-TYR-ASN-LEU-LEU-GLY-PHE-LEU-GLN-

                     15
ARG-SER-SER-ASN-PHE-  ? -GLN-LYS
```

Fig. 3.   The 19 NH$_2$-terminal amino acids of human fibroblast IF.[21]

```
  1                                          10
SER-ASP-LEU-PRO-GLN-THR-HIS-SER-LEU-GLY-

 11                                          20
ASN-ARG-ARG-THR-LEU-MET-LEU-LEU-ALA-GLN-

 21
MET-ARG
```

Fig. 4.   Amino-terminal sequence of human leukocyte IF. Differences between this sequence (human leukocyte IF species α_1, α_2, and β_1, ref. 20) and that of lymphoblastoid IF (up to position 20, ref. 25) are shown in boldface: Thr-14 instead of Ala-14 and Met-16 instead of Ile-16.

We conclude therefore that the leukocyte IFs represent a family of proteins, whereas fibroblast IF appears to be a single major protein. Some preliminary results from other laboratories (M. Revel and P. Sehgal, personal communications) suggest that there may be multiple fibroblast IFs as well.

Most of the IF that has been used in clinical trials to date has been relatively crude material less than 1 % of which consists of the IF protein.[12] Therefore, determination of the activities of pure IF is of major interest. We have shown that the pure IFs exhibit antiviral activity. A number of additional studies were initiated with the purified IFs to delineate their spectrum of biological activities.

The growth-inhibitory activity of the purified IF species was studied in an assay with a lymphoblastoid cell line, the Daudi cell.[26-29] IF was added to some cultures and not to others. The cells were counted after 3 days. The results for the β fractions (Fig. 5) show both antiviral and antigrowth activity for the species. From these data, we concluded that all the fractions that have antiviral activity also have antigrowth activity. Therefore, the antigrowth activity is an intrinsic property of the IF molecule. In addition, differences in activity profiles between the species are significant. One fraction that shows

Table 2.   Growth-inhibitory activity of human leukocyte IF.

Addition to culture medium	Growth (% of control)
Unfractionated IF	15
Homogeneous leukocyte IF γ_2	12
No additions	100

Unfractionated human leukocyte IF was added to lymphoblastoid (Daudi) cell cultures to a final concentration of 25 and 50 units/ml. Homogeneous human leukocyte IF was added to cultures to a final concentration of 36 units/ml. Growth of cells is expressed as a percentage of the growth of control cells after 3 days. Details of the procedures are described elsewhere.[26-28]

high antiviral activity shows low antigrowth activity. Another shows relatively high antigrowth activity. The ratio of antiviral activity to antigrowth activity for the purified species varies over a range of 50-fold. This observation has immense importance. These results indicate that the species that may be best for antiviral activity may not be the best species for antitumor studies. To determine which IF is the best one for a particular activity will take a great deal of further work. In addition, it is certain that synthetic IFs analogous to the natural species will also have variations in these activities.

These species have also been examined by Ronald Herberman and John Ortaldo for their ability to stimulate natural killer cell activity. These purified fractions do stimulate natural killer cell activity of lymphocytes.[30,31]

MONOCLONAL ANTIBODIES TO IF

Thirteen monoclonal antibodies to human leukocyte IF have been isolated.[32] These have been most useful in studying and purifying IFs[33] as well as in developing a rapid radioimmunoassay[34] for IF.

PLASMID RECOMBINANTS AND BACTERIAL EXPRESSION OF THE HUMAN IFs

Starting with mRNA, recombinants containing the IF nucleic acid sequences were prepared. From these recombinants, specific clones containing human leukocyte and human fibroblast IF sequences were isolated, identified, and characterized. Maeda *et al.*[35] isolated human leukocyte IF recombinants. Colonies were screened for specific hybridization to mRNA from induced cells.[36] Screening yielded three classes of hybridization to colonies: no hybridization, minimal to moderate hybridization, and strong hybridization.[35] IF clones were found in the minimal to moderate hybridization class by screening plasmids from these colonies for specific binding of IF mRNA.[37] The recombinant p104 thus obtained was used as a probe to screen a bank of

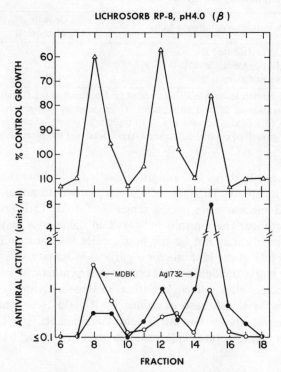

LICHROSORB RP-8, pH4.0 (β)

Fig. 5. The growth-inhibitory and antiviral activities of the β peak of human leukocyte IF. The β species eluting from LiChrosorb Diol was chromatographed on LiChrosorb RP-8, pH 4. The growth-inhibitory activity on Daudi cells (upper panel) and the antiviral activity on human AG-1732 and bovine MDBK cells (lower panel) were determined as described.[26-28]

recombinants prepared from mRNA from induced cells. A number of distinct, but homologous, recombinants were isolated, clearly confirming the multiplicity of the human leukocyte IF gene family. Expression vehicles were made to express the clones and produce IFs in the bacterial recombinants.[38] At this time, we have expressed both human leukocyte[38] and human fibroblast[39] IFs in bacteria. In these recombinant organisms, IF production is controlled by the tryptophan-regulatory region. The leader sequence was removed and a methionine codeword (ATG) added to the 5′-end of the gene (corresponding to the natural amino terminus). The recombinant organism produces approximately 0.5 mg of recombinant leukocyte interferon (IFLrA) per liter of culture. Other groups have cloned human leukocyte[40] as well as fibroblast[41-43] IFs. With the sequences of all these published, it is now relatively easy for anyone to prepare human leukocyte or fibroblast IF recombinants.

The biological activity of our first human leukocyte IF recombinant expressed in bacteria, termed leukocyte IF A (IFLrA), was studied. As shown in Fig. 6, it exhibits antigrowth activity.[44] It aslo stimulates natural killer cell activity.[45] It is active in monkeys in preventing EMC-virus infection,[38] and we all eagerly await to evaluate its activity in humans.

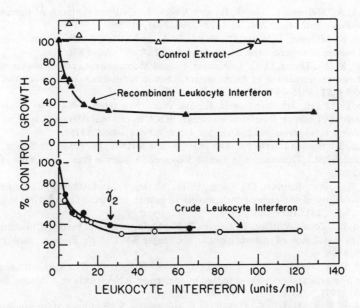

Fig. 6. Comparison of the growth-inhibitory activity of recombinant leukocyte IF with that of crude and purified human leukocyte IFs. The growth inhibitory activity of leukocyte IF was measured with the Daudi cell assay as described.[26-28] Briefly, Daudi cells were cultured in RPMI-1640 medium supplemented with 10% fetal calf serum and 50 ug/ml of gentamicin. A late logarithmic phase culture with a cell density of 2×10^6 cells/ml (98% viability as determined by trypan blue dye exclusion) was diluted with fresh warmed media to a density of 2.1×10^5 cells/ml. After the addition of IF to 1-ml aliquots of cells dispensed in 16-mm wells, the plastic tissue culture plates were sealed with polyester adhesive sheets and incubated at 36°C for 3 days. The number of cells present in IF-treated cultures was then compared to the number of cells in media-treated cultures. This is expressed as the "% control growth" on the ordinate. The amount of IF added per well is indicated on the abscissa as the antiviral titer in reference units/ml, determined on bovine MDBK cells. Each point represents the mean of duplicate determinations; the relative error in this assay is approximately 5%. Control extract was prepared from equivalent numbers of *E. coli*-carrying nonrecombinant plasmid pBR322 ($\triangle-\triangle$). Recombinant leukocyte interferon (IFLrA) ($\blacktriangle-\blacktriangle$) was prepared as described.[38] Crude and homogeneous human leukocyte IFs (IFL-γ_2) were prepared as previously reported[15]; crude leukocyte IF: ($\bigcirc-\bigcirc$); IFL-γ_2: ($\bullet-\bullet$).

It is hoped that it will not only be possible to treat virus infections, but that IF will have many other uses. Although many surprises have already occurred in IF research, many more are still to come. Further basic research will lay the foundations for its proper and most efficient clinical use.

REFERENCES

1. Pestka, S., McInnes, J., Havell, E., and Vilček, J.: Cell-free synthesis of human interferon. *Proc. Natl. Acad. Sci. USA*, **72**: 3898–3901, 1975.
2. Pestka, S., McInnes, J., Weiss, D., Havell, E. A., and Vilček, J.: *De novo* cell-free synthesis of human interferon. *Ann. N. Y. Acad. Sci.*, **284**: 697–702, 1977.
3. Thang, M. N., Thang, D. C., DeMaeyer, E., and Montagnier, L.: Biosynthesis of mouse interferon by translation of its messenger RNA in a cell-free system. *Proc. Natl. Acad. Sci. USA*, **72**: 3975–3977, 1975.
4. Reynolds, F. H., Jr., Premkumar, E., and Pitha, M.: Interferon activity produced by translation of human interferon messenger RNA in cell-free ribosomal systems and in *Xenopus* oocytes. *Proc. Natl. Acad. Sci. USA*, **72**: 4881–4885, 1975.
5. Pestka, S.: Human interferon: The proteins, the mRNA, the genes, the future. In: H. Weissbach (ed.), Dimensions in Health Research. Academic Press, New York, 1978, p. 29.
6. Bose, S., Gurari-Rotman, D., Ruegg, V. Th., Corley, L., and Anfinsen, C. B.: Apparent dispensability of the carbohydrate moiety of human interferon for antiviral activity. *J. Biol. Chem.*, **251**: 1659–1662, 1976.
7. Green, M., Zehavi-Willner, T., Graves, P. N., McInnes, J., and Pestka, S.: Isolation and cell-free translation of immunoglobulin messenger RNA. *Arch. Biochem. Biophys.*, **172**: 74–89, 1976.
8. Moar, V. A., Gurdon, J. B., Lane, C. D., and Marbaix, G.: Translational capacity of living frog eggs and oocytes, as judged by messenger RNA injection. *J. Molec. Biol.*, **61**: 93–103, 1971.
9. Cavalieri, R. L., Havell, E. A., Vilček, J., and Pestka, S.: Synthesis of human interferon by *Xenopus laevis* oocytes: Two structural genes for interferons in human cells. *Proc. Natl. Acad. Sci. USA*, **74**: 3287–3291, 1977.
10. Cavalieri, R. L. and Pestka, S.: Synthesis of interferon in heterologous cells, cell-free extracts, and *Xenopus laevis* oocytes. *Tex. Rep. Biol. Med.*, **35**: 117–125, 1977.
11. McCandliss, R., Sloma, A., and Pestka, S.: Isolation and cell-free translation of human interferon mRNA from fibroblasts and leukocytes. *Methods Enzymol.*, **79**, 51–59, 1981.
12. Mogensen, K. E. and Cantell, K.: Production and preparation of human leukocyte interferon. *Pharmacol. Ther.*, [A] **1**: 369–381, 1977.
13. Wheelock, E. F.: Virus replication and high titered interferon production in human leukocyte cultures inoculated with Newcastle disease virus. *J. Bacteriol.*, **92**: 1415–1421, 1966.
14. Cantell, K. and Tovell, D. R.: Substitution of milk for serum in the production of human leukocyte interferon. *Appl. Microbiol.*, **22**: 625–628, 1971.
15. Rubinstein, M., Rubinstein, S., Familletti, P. C., Miller, R. S., Waldman, A. A., and Pestka, S.: Human leukocyte interferon: Production, purification to homogeneity, and initial characterization. *Proc. Natl. Acad. Sci. USA*, **76**: 640–644, 1979.
16. Pestka, S., Evinger, M., Familletti, P. C., Gross, M., Maeda, S., McCandliss, R., Rubinstein, M., Rubinstein, S., Sloma, A., Tabor, J., and Takeshima, H.: Human interferon: The messenger RNA and the proteins. In: A. L. De Weck, F. Kristensen, and M. Landy (eds.), Biochemical Characterization of Lymphokines. Academic Press, New York, 1980, p. 315.

17. Stein, S., Böhlen, P., Stone, J., Dairman, W., and Udenfriend, S.: Amino acid analysis with fluorescamine at the picomole level. *Arch. Biochem. Biophys.*, **155**: 203–212, 1973.

18. Böhlen, P., Stein, S., Stone, J., and Udenfriend, S.: Automatic monitoring of primary amines in preparative column effluents with fluorescamine. *Anal. Biochem.*, **67**: 438–445, 1975.

19. Rubinstein, M., Levy, W. P., Moschera, J. A., Lai, C.-Y., Hershberg, R. D., Bartlett, R. T., and Pestka, S.: Human leukocyte interferon: Isolation and characterization of several molecular forms. *Arch. Biochem. Biophy,* **210**: 307–318, 1981.

20. Levy, W. P., Shively, J., Rubinstein, M., Del Valle, U., and Pestka, S.: Amino-terminal amino acid sequence of human leukocyte interferon. *Proc. Natl. Acad. Sci. USA,* **77**: 5102–5104, 1980.

21. Stein, S., Kenny, C., Friesen, H.-J., Shively, J., Del Valle, U., and Pestka, S.: NH_2-terminal amino acid sequence of human fibroblast interferon. *Proc. Natl. Acad. Sci. USA,* **77**: 5716–5719, 1980.

22. Kenny, C., Moschera, J., and Stein, S.: Purification of human fibroblast interferon produced in the absence of serum by Cibacron Blue F3GA-agarose and high performance liquid chromatography. *Methods Enzymol.*, **78**: 305–309, 1981.

23. Knight, E., Jr., Hunkapiller, M. W., Korant, B. D., Hardy, R. W. F., and Hood, L. E.: Human fibroblast interferon: Amino acid analysis and amino terminal amino acid sequence. *Science*, **207**: 525–526, 1980.

24. Okamura, H., Berthold, W., Hood, L., Hunkapiller, M., Inoue, M., Smith-Johannsen, H., and Tan, Y. H.: Human fibroblastoid interferon: Immunosorbent column chromatography and N-terminal amino acid sequence. *Biochemistry*, **19**: 3831–3835, 1980.

25. Zoon, K. C., Smith, M. E., Bridgen, P. J., Anfinsen, C. B., Hunkapiller, M. W., and Hood, L. E.: Amino terminal sequence of the major component of human lymphoblastoid interferon. *Science*, **207**: 527–528, 1980.

26. Evinger, M., Rubinstein, M., and Pestka, S.: The growth-inhibitory activity of human leukocyte interferon. In: A. Khan, N. O. Hill and G. L. Dorn (eds.), Interferon: Properties and Clinical Uses. Leland Fikes Foundation Press, Dallas, Texas, 1980, p. 249.

27. Evinger, M., Rubinstein, M., and Pestka, S.: Growth inhibition and antiviral activity of purified leukocyte interferon. *Ann. N. Y. Acad. Sci.*, **350**: 399–404, 1980.

28. Evinger, M., Rubinstein, M., and Pestka, S.: Antiproliferative and antiviral activities of human leukocyte interferons. *Arch. Biochem. Biophy,* **210**: 319–329, 1981.

29. Pestka, S., Evinger, M., McCandliss, R., Sloma, A., and Rubinstein, M.: Human interferon: The messenger RNA and the proteins. In: R. F. Beers, Jr. and E. G. Bassett (eds.), Polypeptide Hormones. Raven Press, New York, 1980, p. 33.

30. Ortaldo, J. R., Pestka, S., Slease, R. B., Rubinstein, M., and Herberman, R. B.: Augmentation of human K-cell activity with interferon. *Scand. J. Immunol.*, **12**: 365–369, 1980.

31. Herberman, R. B., Ortaldo, J. R., Djeu, J. Y., Holden, H. T., Lett, J., Lang, N. P., Rubinstein, M., and Pestka, S.: Role of interferon in regulation of cytotoxicity by natural killer cells and macrophages. *Ann. N. Y. Acad. Sci.*, **350**: 63–71, 1980.

32. Staehelin, T., Durrer, B., Schmidt, J., Takacs, B., Stocker, J., Miggiano, V., Stähli, C., Rubinstein, M., Levy, W. P., and Pestka, S.: Production of hybridomas secreting monoclonal antibodies to the human leukocyte interferons. *Proc. Natl. Acad. Sci. USA,* **78**: 1848–1852, 1981.

33. Staehelin, T., Hobbs, D. S., Kung, H.-F., Lai, C.-Y., and Pestka, S.: Purification of recombinant Human leukocyte interferon (IFLr A) with monoclonal antibodies. *J. Biol. Chem.*, **256**: 9750–9754, 1981.

34. Staehelin, T., Stähli, C., Hobbs, D. S., and Pestka, S.: A rapid quantitative assay of high sensitivity for human leukocyte interferon with monoclonal antibodies. *Methods Enzymol.*, **79**: 589–595, 1981.

35. Maeda, S., McCandliss, R., Gross, M., Sloma, A., Familletti, P. C., Tabor, J. M., Evinger, M., Levy, W. P., and Pestka, S.: Construction and identification of bacterial plasmids containing the nucleotide sequence for human leukocyte interferon. *Proc. Natl. Acad. Sci. USA*, **77**: 7010–7013, 1980; **78**: 4648, 1981.

36. Maeda, S., Gross, M., and Pestka, S.: Screening of colonies by RNA-DNA hybridization with mRNA from induced and uninduced cells. *Methods Enzymol.*, **79**: 613–618, 1981.

37. McCandliss, R., Sloma, A., and Pestka, S.: Use of DNA bound to filters for selection of interferon-specific nucleic acid sequences. *Methods Enzymol.*, **79**: 618–622, 1981.

38. Goeddel, D. V., Yelverton, E., Ullrich, A., Heyneker, H. L., Miozzari, G., Holmes, W., Seeburg, P. H., Dull, T., May, L., Stebbing, N., Crea, R., Maeda, S., McCandliss, R., Sloma, A., Tabor, J. M., Gross, M., Familletti, P. C., and Pestka, S.: A human leukocyte interferon produced by *E. coli* is biologically active. *Nature*, **287**: 411–416, 1980.

39. Goeddel, D. V., Shepard, H. M., Yelverton, E., Leung, D., Crea, R., Sloma, A., and Pestka, S.: Synthesis of human fibroblast interferon by *E. coli. Nucleic Acids Res.*, **8**: 4057–4074, 1980.

40. Nagata, S., Taira, H., Hall, A., Johnsrud, L., Streuli, M., Ecsödi, J., Boll, W., Cantell, K., and Weissman, C.: Synthesis in *E. coli* of a polypeptide with human leukocyte interferon activity. *Nature*, **284**: 316–320, 1980.

41. Houghton, M., Stewart, A. G., Doel, S. M., Emtage, J. S., Eaton, M. A. W., Smith, J. C., Patel, T. P., Lewis, H. M., Porter, A. G., Birch, J. R., Cartwright, T., and Carey, N.H.: The amino-terminal sequence of human fibroblast interferon as deduced from reverse transcripts obtained using synthetic oligonucleotide primers. *Nucleic Acids Res.*, **8**: 1913–1931, 1980.

42. Taniguchi, T., Sakai, M., Fujii-Kuriyama, Y., Muramatsu, M., Kobayashi, S., and Sudo, T.: Construction and identification of a bacterial plasmid containing the human fibroblast interferon gene sequence. *Proc. Jpn. Acad.*, **B55**: 464–469, 1979.

43. Derynck, R., Content, J., DeClercq, E., Volckaert, G., Tavernier, J., Devos, R., and Fiers, W.: Isolation and structure of a human fibroblast interferon gene. *Nature*, **285**: 542–547, 1980.

44. Evinger, M., Maeda, S., and Pestka, S.: Recombinant human leukocyte interferon produced in bacteria has antiproliferative activity. *J. Biol. Chem.*, **256**: 2113–2114, 1981.

45. Herberman, R. B., Ortaldo, J. R., Mantovani, A., Hobbs, D. S., Kung, H.-F., and Pestka, S.: Effect of human recombinant interferon on cytotoxic activity of natural killer (NK) cells and monocytes. *Cellular Immunology*, (in press).

Biological Significance of Interferons

Samuel BARON

Department of Microbiology, University of Texas Medical Branch, Galveston, Texas 77550 U.S.A.

SUMMARY

The IFN system is now known to be composed of a number of interacting components. Some generalizations, although hazardous, may be attempted. Isaacs' concept that a foreign nucleic acid is the inducer of IFN-β may be extended to the possibilities that the foreign cells (procaryotic and eucaryotic) are inducers of IFN-α and foreign antigens are inducers of IFN-γ. The varied actions of IFNs are determined in part by the type of IFN, the target cells, and the overlapping activation of hormonal activities. There is need to correlate causally the various biochemical effects of IFN with the various biological effects. Further complexity of the IFN system comes from the findings that most of the major actions of IFN each have multiple components. This complexity may allow the IFN system to be highly selective in its actions within the body. The complexity may also permit more selective therapeutic application of IFN.

INTRODUCTION

Some of the early concepts of the interferon (IFN) system have been supported by the accumulating evidence. For example, the natural defensive role of IFN during many viral infections is now well supported (Table 1).[1-3] Other concepts of the IFN system have changed markedly since its original discovery. The early model of the IFN mechanism was the simple induction by virus of IFN which interacted with cells to induce intracellular production of antiviral protein(s) which in turn were responsible for the antiviral action of IFN.[3,4] A large body of evidence now supports the view that each of the steps in the IFN

381

system has multiple components (see references in 5). Thus, multiple stimuli may induce multiple types of IFN that may induce multiple biochemical effects in target cells, leading to multiple functional effects in these cells. Some trends and limited generalizations may now be possible to help organize the large body of information. Recognizing that generalizations based on limited data are hazardous, the following comments should be regarded as tentative working hypotheses for further testing. Many of the ideas presented do not necessarily originate here but are derived from the referenced publications.

Table 1.   Evidence supporting the defensive role of IFN during viral infections.

Type of evidence	Example
Time correlations	IFN produced just before and during arrest of virus replication
Place correlations	IFN produced at the site of its action
Transfer	Exogenous IFN controls viral infections
Absence	Deletion of IFN in cell culture, eggs, and animals increases severity of viral infections
Sufficiency of quantity	Concentrations of IFN produced *in vivo* are sufficient to account for defensive action
Specificity of probes	Antibody to IFN, broad antiviral activity of both infected organ and IFN; characterization of IFN produced during infection
Reproducibility	Confirmation in many animal species and humans

Possible Relationships among Inducers, Producer Cells, and Type of IFN

Originally, Isaacs and coworkers[6] proposed that IFN production was a response by body cells to the intracellular presence of a foreign nucleic acid, such as viral nucleic acid. In general terms, this prediction has been supported by the induction of β (fibroblast) interferon (IFN-β) by human fibroblast and epithelial cells exposed to a variety of foreign nucleic acids (Table 2).[7,8]

An analogous induction is that foreign cells may be the major inducer of α

Table 2.   Interferon types.

IFN type	Stimulus for production	Major producer cells
Leukocyte (α)	Viruses Bacteria Foreign cells Mitogens for B-lymphocytes	Null lymphocytes B-lymphocytes Macrophages
Fibroblast (β)	Viruses Polynucleotides	Fibroblasts Epithelial
Immune (γ)	Foreign antigens Mitogens for T-lymphocytes Galactose oxidase Calcium ionophores	T-lymphocytes

(leukocyte) interferon (IFN-α) in unsensitized human leukocytes (B-lymphocytes, NK lymphocytes, and macrophages) (Table 2). The evidence supporting such a possibility is the induction of IFN-α by tumor cells, xenogenic cells, virus infected cells[9-11] and by bacteria (see references in 12). B-cell mitogens may induce IFN-α by mimicking B-lymphocyte induction by foreign cells. A possible exception is the induction of IFN-α by virus infection of leukocytes, but this may in some cases be due to the creation of "foreign" cells by the presence of viral antigen on the surface of infected isologous cells.

Concerning γ (immune or type II) interferon (IFN-γ), the available information indicates that its production may result from stimulation of sensitized T-lymphocytes by specific foreign antigens.[13] This IFN is one of the many lymphokines produced by the reacting T-lymphocyte. T-lymphocyte mitogens can mimic this type of antigen induction.[14]

Biological Actions of IFNs

A variety of biological actions may occur in cells and animals exposed to IFNs. These actions include antiviral effects, inhibition of cell division, immunoregulation, NK lymphocyte activation, protection of normal cells against NK killing, macrophage activation, hormonal activation of sensitized T-cells, transfer of IFN effects among cells, and others (see references in 5). In this manner, IFNs may cause not a single effect but a set of functional effects with one or more of these actions being dominant.

The dominant effect, in some cases, may be determined by the IFN type. For example, IFN-γ has been reported to exert a disproportionately greater anticellular effect[15,16] and also a disporprotionately greater immunoregulatory effect[17] than do IFN-α and -β.

Another determinant of the dominant effect of IFN is the target cell. Examples are: the immunoregulatory action of IFN operates mainly through lymphoid cells (see references in 18); interferon may protect only certain cells against NK killing[11]; macrophages, NK cells, and sensitized T-lymphocytes but not other body cells, are activated for enhanced phagocytosis and cell killing, respectively.[19,20]

Overlapping Activities among IFNs and Hormones

IFN and hormones have a number of similarities.[21] Both are polypeptide chemical messengers, not consumed as they activate cells, directed at a common cell receptor,[22] able to cross-activate each other,[23] and able to cross-transfer cell activation to adjacent cells.[24] Recently, it has been shown that epinephrine can activate the antiviral resistance function of IFN in mouse cardiac cells containing the surface receptor for epinephrine.[23] Conversely, IFN can activate epinephrine effects in these same myocardial cells. Furthermore, the two effects may be transferred by direct contact between treated and untreated cells, as occurs with the antiviral action of the IFN system.[24] Most recently, evidence has been presented that some forms of IFN-α may contain the ACTH- and melanin-stimulating hormone amino acid sequences and induce these hormone activities in target cells.[9]

Each IFN Action May Have Multiple Components

Many of the effects of IFN may have multiple components. For example, the ways IFN may exert an antitumor effect are listed in Table 3. It may be seen that at least 7 separate activities may account for the antitumor action. Recently it has been recognized that partially purified IFN-γ preparations may exert a direct cell killing effect (as opposed to a cytostatic effect) in a few murine tumors,[25] but definitive separation of this activity from lymphotoxin is required. Undetermined is which antitumor mechanism(s) can be the most effective for each tumor. The other effects of IFN (e.g., the antiviral action) may also have multiple mechanisms of action (see references in 5).

Table 3. Antitumor actions of IFN.

Demonstrated	Direct inhibition of cell division
	Activation of: sensitized T-lymphocytes
	NK cells
	ADCC null cells
	Macrophages
Possible	Regulation of immune sensitization
	Hormonal effects
	Direct cell killing

Biochemical Effects

IFN induces a number of biochemical changes in its target cells. These biochemical effects have been well reviewed (see references in 5) and will not be considered here. Importantly, the multiple biochemical effects induced by IFN are not yet correlated with the function effects. Studies are needed to determine which biochemical pathway(s) induced by IFN can cause each of the functional effects.

THE COMPLEXITY MAY PERMIT SPECIFICITY OF THE IFN SYSTEM

The complexity of the IFN system may make possible highly selective (specific) actions within the body. For example, local production of IFN-α or -β at the site of viral infection results in the greatest antiviral activity occurring at that local site, with rapidly diminishing antiviral activity even at short distances away from the site of IFN production.[3] However, during virus infections when viruses reach cells in contact with the circulation, IFN is produced within the circulatory system and is partly disseminated to protect distant organs.[26] A possible selective aspect of IFN-γ is its production and highest concentration at immunologic reaction sites. Thus, IFN-γ may be present in highest concentration at the site of the immune response where the IFN-γ may function as an immunomodulator (see references in 18).

Another mechanism which may lead to specificity is the transfer of the antiviral activity from an IFN-activated cell to cells in contact with that cell.[24] This transfer mechanism has been proposed as a method for local amplification of the IFN effect. Also, when mobile leukocytes become activated by IFN, they are capable of transferring IFN action to cells they contact.[27] In theory, an IFN activated leukocyte could migrate and transfer activity to distant cells. Thus, any selectivity for distant target cells by IFN-activated leukocytes could add to the selective dissemination of IFN's action.

The different types of IFN may influence the dissemination or localization of IFN action. In humans, IFN-α is disseminated through the circulation more readily than is IFN-β. Thus, at least some actions of IFN-β may be more localized than those of IFN-α.[28]

The time required for activation of cells by IFNs may vary greatly, thereby also allowing for selectivity and specificity of action. For example, IFN-α and -β can activate cells after a few minutes of contact while IFN-γ requires many hours—perhaps due to its induction of an intermediary protein before the effector proteins of the IFN system are made.[29] It is possible that *in vivo* the rapidly acting IFN-α or -β. can activate cells while transiently passing through a tissue, while IFN-γ may be required to be present much longer to activate cells.

Strong potentiation of the actions of IFN can occur if IFN is mixed with IFN-α or -β.[30] The antiviral potentiation is approximately 10-fold in human and mouse cells. The antitumor actions of IFN are similarly potentiated in the mouse by such combinations.[31] Thus, any local production of IFN-γ along with either IFN-α or -β at a body site could lead to such potentiation occurring naturally.

Along with production of IFN-γ by T-lymphocytes is the production of other lymphokines. One of these lymphokines is an inhibitor (regulator?) of IFN action.[31] The inhibitor is extremely potent against establishment of antiviral activity by IFN and the inhibitor could serve as an important regulator of IFN action within the body. Studies of the natural occurrence and role of this inhibitor are needed.

Possible Use of IFN's Complexity for Selective Therapy

For selectivity of therapy it may be possible to take advantage of certain of the complex aspects of the IFN system. For example, the strong potentiation of the action of IFN-α and -β by small quantities of IFN-γ may be attempted in humans. Such potentiation may provide greater antitumor or antiviral therapy with available amounts of IFN. However, if the toxicities of IFN are also potentiated, then the use of the mixtures may be limited to reducing the dose of IFN-α and -β and thereby extending the available supplies of IFN.

As even larger quantities of IFN-γ become available, it may be used alone instead of in combination with IFN-α or -β because of its greater antitumor action. Increased activity of IFN-γ in humans may be achieved by elimination of the inhibitor of IFN action which is often produced along with the IFN-γ.

Concentrations of IFN above those currently being applied to humans may further increase the antiviral and antitumor effects. Thus, therapeutic delivery of high concentrations of IFNs to the target site, as occurs naturally, may increase the therapeutic effects in humans while decreasing systemic toxicity.

REFERENCES

1. Baron, S.: Mechanism of recovery from viral infection. *Adv. Virus Res.*, **10**: 39–64, 1963.
2. Baron, S.: The interferon system. *Am. Soc. Microbiol. News*, **45**: 358–366, 1979.
3. Isaacs, A.: Interferon. *Adv. Virus Res.*, **10**: 1–35, 1963.
4. Taylor, J.: Inhibition of interferon action by actinomycin. *Biochem. Biophys. Res. Commun.*, **14**: 447–451, 1964.
5. Baron, S. and Dianzani, F. (eds).: The interferon system: A current review to 1978. *Tex. Rep. Biol. Med.*, **35**: 1–573, 1977.
6. Isaacs, A., Baron, S., and Allison, A. E.: As referenced in Interferon. *Sci. Am.*, **204**: 51, 1961.
7. Baron, S., Bogomolova, N. N., Billiau, A., Levy, H. B., Buckler, C. E., Stern, R., and Naylor, R.: Induction of interferon by preparations of synthetic single-stranded RNA. *Proc. Natl. Acad. Sci. USA*, **64**: 67–74, 1969.
8. Lampson, G. R., Tytell, A. A., Field, A. K., Nemes, M. M., and Hilleman, M. R.: Inducers of interferon and host resistance. I. Double-stranded RNA from extracts of penicillium funiculosum. *Proc. Natl. Acad. Sci. USA*, **58**: 782–789, 1967.
9. Blalock, J. E. and Smith, E. M.: Human leukocyte interferon: Structural and biological relatedness to adrenocorticotropic hormone and endorphins. *Proc. Natl. Acad. Sci. USA*, **77**: 5972–5974, 1980.
10. Svet-Moldavsky, G. J., Nemirovskaya, B. M., and Osipora, T. V.: Interferonogenicity and antigen recognition. *Nature*, **247**: 205–206, 1974.
11. Trinchieri, G. and Santoli, D.: Antiviral activity induced by culturing lymphocyte with tumor-derived or virus-transformed cells. Enhancement of human natural killer cell activity by interferon and antagonistic inhibition of susceptibility of target cells to lysis. *J. Exp. Med.*, **147**: 1314–1333, 1978.
12. Baron, S., Brunell, P. A., and Grossberg, S. E.: Mechanisms of action and pharmacology: The immune and interferon systems. In: G. L. Galasso *et al.* (eds.), Antiviral Agents and Viral Diseases of Man. Raven Press, New York, 1979, pp. 151–208.
13. Youngner, J. S.: Properties of interferon induced by specific antigens. *Tex. Rep. Biol. Med.*, **35**: 17–22, 1977.
14. Wheelock, E. F.: Interferon-like virus-inhibitor induced in human leukocytes by phytohemagglutinin. *Science*, **149**: 310, 1965.

15. Blalock, J. E., Georgiades, J. A., Langford, M. P., and Johnson, H. M.: Purified human immune interferon has more potent anticellular activity than fibroblast or leukocyte interferon. *Cell Immunol.*, **49**: 390–394, 1980.
16. Salvin, S. B., Youngner, J. S., Nishio, J., and Neta, R.: Tumor suppression by a lymphokine released into the circulation of mice with delayed hypersensitivity. *J. Natl. Cancer Inst.*, **55**: 1233–1236, 1975.
17. Sonnenfeld, G., Mandel, A. D., and Merigan, T. C.: The immunosuppressive effect of type II mouse interferon on antibody production. *Cell Immunol.*, **34**: 193–206, 1977.
18. Johnson, H. M. and Baron, S.: Interferon: Effects on the immune response and the mechanism of activation of the cellular response. *CRC Crit. Rev. Biochem.*, 4: 203–227, 1976.
19. Gresser, I.: Antitumor effects of interferon. In: F. Becker (ed.), *Cancer: A comprehensive treatise*, vol. 5. Plenum Press, New York, 1977.
20. Huang, K. Y., Donahoe, R. M., Gordon, F. B., *et al.*: Enhancement of phagocytosis by interferon-containing preparations. *Infect. Immun.*, 4: 581–588, 1971.
21. Baron, S.: The biological significance of the interferon system. In: N. Finter (ed.), Interferon. North Holland Pub. Co., Amsterdam, 1966.
22. Friedman, R. M., Grollman, E. F., Chang, E. H., Kohn, L. D., Lee, G., and Jay, F. T.: Interferon and glycoprotein hormones. *Tex. Rep. Biol. Med.*, **35**: 326–329, 1977.
23. Blalock, J. E. and Stanton, G. J.: Common pathways of interferon and hormonal action. *Nature*, **283**: 406–408, 1980.
24. Blalock, J. E. and Baron, S.: Interferon-induced transfer of viral resistance between animal cells. *Nature (London)*, **269**: 422–425, 1977.
25. Tyring, S., Fleischmann, W. R., Jr., and Baron, S.: Personal communication, 1980.
26. Baron, S.: The biological significance of the interferon system. *Arch. Intern. Med.*, **126**: 84–93, 1970.
27. Stanton, G. J., Weigent, D. A., Langford, M. P., and Blalock, J. E.: Human leukocyte transfer of viral resistance to heterologous cells. In: A. Kahn, N. O. Hill, and G. Dorn (eds.), Interferons: Properties and Clinical Uses. Wadley Institute of Molecular Medicine, Dallas, Texas, 1980.
28. Billiau, A., De Somer, B., Edy, V. G., De Clercq, E., and Heremans, H.: Human fibroblast interferon for clinical traials: Pharmacokinetics and tolerability in human experimental animals and humans. *Antimicrob Agents Chemother.*, **16**: 56–63, 1979.
29. Dianzani, F., Zucca, M., Scupham, A., and Georgiades, J.: Immune virus induced interferons may activate cells by different derepressional mechanisms. *Nature*, **280**: 400–402, 1980.
30. Fleischmann, W. R., Jr.: Potentiation of interferon activity by mixed preparations of fibroblast and immune interferon. *Infect. Immun.*, **26**: 248–253, 1979.
31. Fleischmann, W. R., Jr. Kleyn, K. M., and Baron, S.: Potentiation of antitumor effect of virus-induced interferon by mouse immune interferon preparations. *JNCI*, **65**: 963–966, 1980.
32. Green, J. A., Cooperband, S. R., and Kibrick, S.: Immunespecific induction of interferon production in cultures of human blood lymphocytes. *Science*, **164**: 1415, 1969.
33. Fleischmann, W. R., Jr., Georgiades, J. A., Osborue, L. C., Dianzani, F., and Johnson, H. M.: Induction of an inhibitor of interferon action in a mouse lymphokine preparation. *Infect. Immun.*, **26**: 949–555, 1979.

Discussion

Dr. MACHIDA: In the production of different types of interferon, such as α, β and γ, which is the predominant factor governing production in your opinion, the producing cell type or the type of inducer? The reason I ask this question is because interferon production can be seen in places other than the combinations that you showed in the first slide, and I think it may be possible to imagine or hypothesize which type is being produced.

Dr. BARON: I believe that is an important question, but there is, at least to my knowledge, not enough information to answer it in a general way. It is clear that certain cell types, regardless of the inducer, seem to be able to produce only one type of interferon. For example, fibroblasts do not seem to respond to mitogens, so there clearly the cell type is critical. On the other hand, macrophages seem to be able to produce two types of interferon depending upon the stimulus. And I think that it is a little too early to make generalizations and that work is needed in this area.

Dr. KUWATA: I have one question. Could you explain more about your interferon inhibitor? I am interested to know the mechanism of the interferon inhibitor you just mentioned.

Dr. BARON: Dr. Fleischmann is the scientist who discovered the interferon inhibitor, and he discovered it when Dr. Georgiades in our department was fractionating the lymphokine preparations to purify gamma interferon. One of the fractions separated the immune interferon from a material which, when mixed with other interferons, decreased their activity. In fact, when they purified the gamma interferon, they recovered more interferon activity in he purified interferon than in the original crude preparation. So that suggested an inhibitor which was separable from interferon. The inhibitor, according to Dr. Fleischmann—he hasn't got too far in the studies yet—is active up to several hours after application of interferon to cells, but not thereafter. So a fully established antiviral state cannot be reversed by the inhibitor. But we do know that at 3 hours the antiviral state is beginning to be established, so Dr. Fleischmann believes that the action of the inhibitor occurs during the early stages of the induction of the antiviral state. The other thing he wishes to point out is its great potency, because only four units of this inhibitor was able to prevent the antiviral action of 400 units of interferon. I don't know that he knows the molecular size yet, so I can't comment on that aspect of it. The inhibitor is not produced by normal spleen cells.

Dr. VILČEK: I have a question concerning the mixed cultures of human lymphocytes and mouse L cells. I missed what challenge virus was used; do the lymphocytes support replication of the challenge virus or is it only the L cells that replicate the virus?

Dr. BARON: VSV was used as the challenge virus, and the great bulk of the virus comes from the L cells and not from the lymphocytes. The lymphocytes are poor producers, so that any decrease you see there is due to antiviral activity in the L cells. As you probably know, we used selective virus types in this transfer phenomenon when we combined mouse and human systems. We used poliovirus and have shown that transferring antiviral activity from mouse to human cells can be expressed as inhibition of poliovirus, which only grows in the human cell.

Dr. VILČEK: Since you have quite a large amount of human interferon produced in that system, and there is a component of human alpha interferon that crosses very efficiently into mouse cells, can you rule out the possibility that the resistance is not due to that subspecies of human alpha interferon?

Dr. BARON: Yes, I think that's a very important consideration and one that Drs. Stanton a Blalock addressed themselves to. What they did was to collect the supernatant fluids and apply those directly to L cells, and there was no activity of that material on the L cells.

Production and Characterization of Interferon from Human Leukemic Lymphoblastoid Cells Grown in Hamsters

Jiro IMANISHI,* Chin-Bin PAK,* Haruo KAWAMURA,* Masakazu KITA,[2]* Shigeru SUGINO,* Shoko HOSHINO,* Hidekazu MATSUOKA,* Tadao TANIMOTO,[2]* Kazuo MASUDA,[2]* Koji YOKOBAYASHI,*[2] Masakazu MITSUHASHI,[2]* Yasuichi NAGANO[3]* and Tsunataro KISHIDA*

*Department of Microbiology, Kyoto Prefectural University of Medicine, Kyoto, [2]*Hayashibara Biochemical Laboratories, Inc., Okayama, [3]* National Hospital of Sagamihara, Sagamihara, Japan

INTRODUCTION

Human lymphoblastoid cell interferon (HuIFN-α (Ly)), particularly Namalwa cell IFN can be produced on a large scale[1,2] and has been used for the treatment of some viral and malignant diseases.[3] However, sizable apparatus and large volumes of culture medium, fetal bovine serum, and inducer virus are required for large-scale production. Adams et al.[4] and Miyoshi et al.[5] discussed the possibility of transplanting human lymphoblastoid cells into newborn hamsters treated with antilymphocyte serum. If IFN could be produced from human lymphoblastoid cells grown in hamsters instead of by cultivation in vitro in big spinner vessels, production costs would be very low because a large number of lymphoblastoid cells may be obtained in this way without specialized apparatus or large volumes of medium and serum. The purpose of the present study was to investigate the possibility of producing IFN by human leukemic lymphoblastoid cells grown in hamsters and to characterize the induced IFN both biologically and physicochemically.

MATERIALS AND METHODS

Hamsters: Golden hamsters bred in our laboratory were used in these experiments. Newborn hamsters less than 24 hours old were employed for the implantation of human leukemic lymphoblastoid cells.

391

Cells: Human leukemic lymphoblastoid cells (BALL-1), the characteristics of which have been described in detail elsewhere,[6] were used for the production of IFN. These cells were serially transplanted for passage in newborn hamsters.

FL cells propagated with Eagle's minimum essential medium (MEM) containing 5% calf serum were used for the assay of IFN activity and the propagation of vesicular stomatitis virus (VSV). To determine the spectrum of the species dependence of antiviral activity we used bovine MDBK, rabbit RK-13, mouse L929, and hamster BHK C-25 cell lines, all of which were maintained with Eagle's MEM supplemented with 5 to 10% fetal bovine serum.

Cell growth inhibition was examined by employing human leukemic T-cell line Molt-4 and human Burkitt's lymphoma cell line Namalwa, maintained in RPMI 1640 medium, as well as human sublingual tumor cell line KB and human diploid fibroblast cell line Flow 7000 maintained in Eagle's MEM. HeLa cells in Eagle's MEM were utilized as the target cells of NK cell activity and spontaneous tumor cell growth inhibition by lymphocytes (STGI).

Treatment with antilymphocyte serum: Antilymphocyte serum was prepared by sensitizing rabbits with hamster thymocytes. Immediately after the transplantation, 0.1 ml of this serum was inoculated intraperitoneally (I.P.) and the inoculation was then repeated twice a week.[5]

Viruses: Sendai virus was inoculated into 11-day-old chicken eggs. Two to 3 days later, the chorioallantoic fluid was collected, centrifuged at 20,000 rpm for 1 hour resuspended in human serum, and stored at $-80°C$ until required. For the assay of IFN activity, a New Jersey strain of vesicular stomatitis virus (VSV) propagated in FL cells was used.

IFN assay methods: IFN activity was assayed by the microtiter method and the plaque reduction method using FL cells and VSV as challenge virus. The details of these procedures have been described elsewhere.[7,8] IFN activity was expressed in terms of international units (IU) by comparison with a standard reference IFN preparation (Code 69/19).

For the determination of species dependence, IFN activity was assayed by the microtiter method using various types of cell lines, as noted above.

IFN production: Five to 10×10^6 BALL-1 cells were transplanted subcutaneously into each newborn hamster after treatment with antilymphocyte serum. Three or 4 weeks later, the tumor mass that developed in each newborn hamster was transferred into a dish, minced with scissors, dissociated into single cells by pipetting and filtration through a metal mesh, and washed with Eagle's MEM by centrifugation at 1,300 rpm for 10 min. The cell concentration was adjusted to 5×10^6 cells/ml with RPMI 1640 medium without serum after counting viable cells by the erythrosin B dye exclusion test. BALL-1 cells were infected with 500 HA/ml of Sendai virus after priming with 100 IU/ml of human lymphoblastoid IFN. The medium was harvested after a 20 hour incubation at 37° C in a spinner vessel and centrifuged at 6,000 rpm for 20 min at 4° C. The supernatant solution was acidified to pH 2.0 with 6 N HCl and maintained under these conditions for 24 hours to inactivate residual inducing virus.

Purification of IFN: The method used to purify IFN was a modification of Bodo's method.[9] Crude human lymphoblastoid IFN was adjusted to pH 4.0 by addition of 6 N NaOH. The resulting solution was applied to a column of SP-Sephadex C-25 (Pharmacia Fine Chemicals) equilibrated with 0.1 M glycine-HCl buffer (pH 4.0) containing 0.2 M NaCl and eluted with 0.1 M phosphate buffer (pH 8.0) containing 0.1 M NaCl. The eluate was dialyzed twice against distilled water at 4° C for 2 hours and lyophilized. This product was dissolved in phosphate-buffered saline without Ca^{2+} and Mg^{2+} (PBS(−)), applied to a column of Sephadex G-100 (Pharmacia Fine Chemicals) equilibrated with PBS(−), and eluted with the same buffer. The eluted IFN was concentrated and purified by ion-exchange column chromatography on SP-Sephadex as before. Finally, the purified IFN was dialyzed against PBS(−) and lyophilized.

Human leukocyte IFN: Human leukocyte IFN that had been induced in human peripheral leukocytes using Sendai virus was kindly supplied by Dr. Matsuo of Central Research Institute of Green Cross Company, Osaka, Japan. This preparation was purified by column chromatography on CM-cellulose and DEAE-cellulose and then by gel filtration on a column of Sephadex G-100.[10,11]

Time kinetics of the development of an antiviral state by IFN: FL cells were treated with 300 IU of IFN, and 0.5, 1.0, 4.0, 6.0, 10.0, or 24.0 hours later, medium was removed and 100 $TCID_{50}$ of VSV was added. After 24 hours of incubation, the supernatant was collected and the VSV yield in the supernatant was measured by the microplaque method.

Neutralization of IFN by antihuman leukocyte IFN serum: Antihuman leukocyte IFN serum (25 μl) produced in sheep[12] was serially diluted 2-fold with physiological saline on the transferplate (Nunc). IFN (25 μl containing 100 IU) was added to the wells of the transferplate and incubated at room temperature for 1 hour. The mixtures of IFN and antiserum were then transferred to the wells of a microplate in which FL cells had already been cultivated to a confluent monolayer. Twenty-four hours later, the medium was removed and 0.1 ml of a solution of VSV containing 10–15 $TCID_{50}$ was used for challenge. Forty-eight hours later the cytopathogenic effect (CPE) was observed under a microscope. The maximum dilution of antiserum that completely inhibited the CPE was calculated. The neutralization titer of antiserum was expressed as the maximum dilution that completely neutralized one IU of IFN.

Cell growth inhibition tests: Samples (500 μl) of epithelial tumor (KB cell line) and fibroblast cells (Flow 7000 cell line), adjusted to 5×10^4 cells/ml with Eagle's MEM containing 10% fetal bovine serm, were dispersed into plastic dishes (diameter 3 cm) and a sample (500 μl) of the appropriately diluted IFN solution or control solution was added. After incubation for 1, 2, or 3 days in an atmopshere of 5% CO_2 at 37° C, the cells were dissociated into single cells by treatment with trypsin-Versene solution. The viable cells were counted by using the trypan blue dye exclusion test. For the lymphoblastoid cell lines, Namalwa and Molt-4 cell lines, 0.5 ml of cell suspension adjusted to 2×10^5 cells/ml with RPMI 1640 medium containing 10% fetal bovine serum was dispersed into the wells of a Semi-microplate (FB-16-24-TC, Linbro, Inc.), and diluted IFN solution or control solution (500 μl) was put into the same well. After incubation for 1, 2, or 3 days in an atmosphere of 5% CO_2 at 37° C, the viable cells were counted. Human lymphoblastoid and leukocyte IFNs were tested simultaneously.

NBT reduction test: The method for the NBT reduction test has been described in detail elsewhere.[13]

Spontaneous tumor cell growth inhibition by human peripheral leukocytes (STGI) treated with IFN: Peripheral blood (approximately 20 ml) was drawn from healthy donors, and lymphocytes were isolated by the ficoll-hypaque (Pharmacia Fine Chemicals) density method. Lymphocytes (10^6 cells/ml) were placed in a Lab-Tek chamber (Lab-Tek Products). Cells of human tumor cell line HeLa (10^5 cells) and appropriately diluted human IFN were then added to the Lab-Tek chamber. After incubation at 37° C in an atmosphere of 5% CO_2 for 1, 2, or 3 days, the viable cells were counted by the trypan blue dye exclusion test under the light microscope. The degree of cell growth inhibition was expressed as a cell viability index calculated using the following formula:

$$\text{Cell viability index} = \frac{\text{number of viable cells on day 3 in experimental group}}{\text{number of viable cells on day 3 in control}} \times 100.$$

Natural killer (NK) cell activity: Trinchieri's method[14] was used to determine NK cell activity.

RESULTS

Production of IFN by human leukemic lymphoblastoid cells grown in hamsters: Five to 10×10^6 BALL-1 cells were subcutaneously transplanted into each newborn hamster treated with antilymphocyte serum. During the period of 3 weeks, a tumor mass averaging about 13 gm per hamster developed and 3.5 $\times 10^9$ viable BALL-1 cells were recovered from each tumor mass. By 4 weeks, tumors averaging about 21 gm per hamster had developed and 5.2×10^9

of viable BALL-1 cells could be recovered from each (Table 1). About 17,000 to 20,000 IU/ml IFN was induced in BALL-1 cells infected with Sendai virus; that is, $1.3–1.7 \times 10^7$ IU of IFN was obtained from each hamster (Table 1).

Table 1. Production of IFN in human leukemic lymphoblastoid cell line BALL-1.

Tumor masses grown in newborn hamsters were transferred into dishes, minced by scissors, and dissociated into single cells. These cells were infected with 500 HA/ml of Sendai virus, and the supernatant was harvested, acidified to inactivate residual inducing virus, and assayed by microtiter and plaque reduction methods.

Age	3 weeks old	4 weeks old
No. of hamsters	40	24
Average tumor mass weight (gm/hamster)	13.1	21.9
Average body weight (gm/hamster)	48.9	65.6
Ratio of tumor to body weight (%)	26.8	33.4
No. of viable cells obtained from 1 gm of tumor (cells/gm of tumor)	2.69×10^8	2.38×10^8
No. of viable cells obtained from a hamster (cells/hamster)	3.53×10^9	5.21×10^9
Cell viability (%)	68.4	63.5
Induced IFN (IU/ml)	20,000	17,000
Volume of 5×10^6 cells/ml (ml)	706	1,042
Total of induced IFN per hamster (IU/hamster)	1.4×10^7	1.77×10^7

Purification of lymphoblastoid IFN: The method used to purify IFN was a modification of Bodo's method.[9] Crude IFN was purified by column chromatography on SP-Sephadex C-25. The initial specific activity was 3×10^4 IU/mg protein and SP-Sephadex column chromatography increased this to 1.8×10^5 IU/mg protein with 80% recovery. Further purification by gel filtration on Sephadex G-100 increased the specific activity to 2.1×10^6 IU/mg protein with 55% recovery overall. Finally, the IFN preparation was concentrated and purified by rechromatography on SP-Sephadex C-25. The final specific activity was 5×10^6 IU/mg protein with 37% recovery overall (Table 2).

The biological and physicochemical characteristics of this purified IFN were compared with the corresponding properties of human leukocyte IFN.

Table 2. Crude human lymphoblastoid IFN, adjusted to pH 4 by 6 N NaOH, was applied to a column of SP-Sephadex C-25 equilibrated with 0.1 M glycine-HCl buffer at pH 4.0 and eluted by 0.1 M phosphate buffer at pH 8.0. The eluate was then dialyzed against water at 4°C and lyophilized. After it was dissolved in PBS(−), it was applied to gel filtration of Sephadex G-100 equilibrated with PBS(−) and eluted by PBS(−). It was once more purified by SP-Sephadex C-25 column chromatography.

Purification step	Volume of preparation (ml)	Recovered IFN		Specific activity IU/mg protein
		IU/ml	total (%)	
1. Crude material (pH 2 treated)	17,000	1.90×10^4	3.23×10^8 (100)	3×10^4
2. Sp-Sephadex C-25	469	5.50×10^5	2.58×10^8 (80)	1.8×10^5
3. Lyophilization	43	6.00×10^6	2.58×10^8 (80)	1.8×10^5
4. Sephadex G-100 (fraction pool)	442	4.03×10^5	1.78×10^8 (55)	2.1×10^6
5. Sp-Sephadex conc. & dialysis against PBS (−)	56	2.14×10^6	1.20×10^8 (37)	5×10^6

Species dependence of human lymphoblastoid and human leukocyte IFNs: Human lymphoblastoid and leukocyte IFNs (10,000 IU of both) were assayed using FL cells, MDBK cells, RK-13 cells, L929 cells, and BHK cells to determine the species dependence. Both IFNs showed high antiviral activity with MDBK cells, but no difference was found in antiviral activity between the two IFNs (Table 3). They also showed a slight antiviral activity with RK-13 cells, L929 cells, and BHK cells, and again there was no difference in the antiviral activities of the two IFNs. It was noteworthy that the lymphoblastoid IFN had the same antiviral activity with BHK cells as did the leukocyte IFN which indicated that there was no contamination of the leukemic BALL-1 cells with hamster cells during IFN induction.

Table 3. Species dependence of human lymphoblastoid IFN and human leukocyte IFN. Antiviral activity was assayed by the microtiter methods using various animal cells and VSV as a challenge virus.
HuIFN-α (Ly): human lymphoblastoid IFN.
HuIFN-α (Le): human leukocyte IFN.

Cell	HuIFN-α (Ly) (U/ml)		HuIFN-α (Le) (U/ml)	
FL	10,000[a]		10,000[a]	
MDBK	1,6000,	8,000	13,500,	11,300
RK-13	380,	113	380,	113
L929	95.1,	80	95.1,	160
BHK	33.6,	14	28.2,	24

a) IU/ml.

Time kinetics of the development of the antiviral state by IFN: The antiviral state was induced in FL cells 1 hour after the treatment with IFN, and by 6 hours later the cells had developed a completely antiviral state. The completely antiviral state continued for more than 24 hours. There was no difference in the time kinetics of this development between the human leukocyte IFN and the human lymphoblastoid cell IFN (Fig. 1).

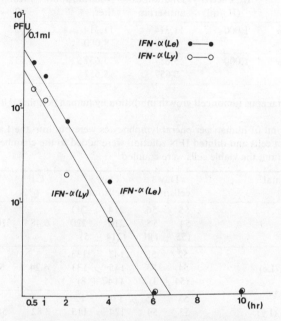

Fig. 1. Time kinetics of the development of an antiviral state by IFN.
Confluently monolayered FL cells were treated with 300 IU/ml of human leukocyte IFN
(●—●) or human lymphoblastoid IFN (○—○).
One-half, 1, 2, 4, 6, 10, or 24 hours later, 100 $TCID_{50}$/ml of VSV were introduced as a challenge and incubated for 24 hours. The supernatant was harvested, and the virus yield in the supernatant was measured by the microplaque method.

Neutralizing activity by antihuman leukocyte IFN serum: As shown in Table 4, the titer required for complete neutralization of one IU of human lymphoblastoid IFN was 9,657 on the average, while that for human leukocyte IFN was 5,657; i.e., human lymphoblastoid IFN was neutralized about 1.7 times more strongly by antihuman leukocyte IFN serum than was human leukocyte IFN.

Cell growth inhibitory activity: Both human lymphoblastoid IFN and human leukocyte IFN markedly inhibited the growth of human leukemic T-cell line Molt-4 and human sublingual tumor cell line KB. There was no difference in cell growth inhibitory effect between the two types of IFN. Both IFNs showed

Table 4. Neutralizing activity of antihuman leukocyte IFN serum.

Antihuman leukocyte IFN serum, diluted on transferplates, and 1,000 IU/0.025 ml of IFN were mixed and incubated for 1 hour, then transferred to the wells of a microplate in which FL cells had been cultivated to a confluent monolayer. Twenty-four hours later, VSV was introduced as a challenge. Forty-eight hours later, CPE was observed and the neutralization titer was calculated.

	IFN activity (IU/ml)	Dilution of antiserum	Neutralization titer	Mean	%
HuIFN-α (Ly)	1,000	11,314 8,000	11,314 8,000	9,657	171
HuIFN-α (Le)	1,000	5,657 5,657	5,657 5,657	5,657	100

Table 5. Spontaneous tumor cell growth inhibition by human peripheral leukocytes treated with IFN.

One $\times$ 10^6 cells/ml of human peripheral lymphocytes were put into the Lab-Tek chamber. One $\times$ 10^5 HeLa cells and diluted IFN solution were added to the chamber. One or 3 days after the incubation, the viable cells were counted.

Experimental group	Day 1 cells/ml		Day 3 cells/ml		GI[b] (%)	Index[c] (%)
Control	55 54 (55 $\pm$ 1)[a]	56 55	214 210 (214 $\pm$ 5)	211 220	6.48	100.0
HuIFN-α (Le) 500 IU	52 54 (54 $\pm$ 3)	58 53	147 145 (140 $\pm$ 8)	133 133	4.24	65.4 $\pm$ 3.7
HuIFN-α (Ly) 500 IU	53 53 (54 $\pm$ 1)	55 54	134 124 (126 $\pm$ 8)	129 115	3.82	58.9 $\pm$ 3.7
PBL	49 58 (55 $\pm$ 4)	55 57	55 60 (56 $\pm$ 3)	52 57	1.70	26.2 $\pm$ 1.4
PBL + HuIFN-α (Le) 500 IU	49 49 (47 $\pm$ 3)	43 46	15 12 (14 $\pm$ 2)	16 14	0.42	6.5 $\pm$ 0.9
PBL + HuIFN-α (Ly) 500 IU	45 46 (47 $\pm$ 3)	52 46	11 13 (12 $\pm$ 1)	10 12	0.36	5.6 $\pm$ 0.5

a) mean $\pm$ standard deviation.

b) GI (growth index) $= \dfrac{\text{Number of target cells on day 3}}{\text{Initial target cell number}} \times 100.$

c) Index $= \dfrac{\text{Number of cells in experimental group}}{\text{Number of cells in control on day 3}} \times 100.$

a similar minimal inhibition of growth of human Burkitt's lymphoma cell line Namalwa and human fibroblast cell line Flow 7000.

Enhancement of spontaneous tumor cell growth inhibition by human peripheral leukocytes (STGI) treated with IFN: HeLa cell growth inhibition by human peripheral leukocytes was enhanced to the same extent by both human lymphoblastoid IFN and human leukocyte IFN (Table 5).

Enhancement of natural killer (NK) cell activity: As shown in Fig 2, when more than 10 IU/ml of either human lymphoblastoid or human leukocyte IFN was added to the coculture of lymphocyte and ^{51}Cr-labeled HeLa cells and incubated at $37°C$ for 22 hours in a humidified 5% CO_2 atmosphere, ^{51}Cr released from the target cells increased. There was no difference in the enhancement of NK cell activity between the two types of IFN.

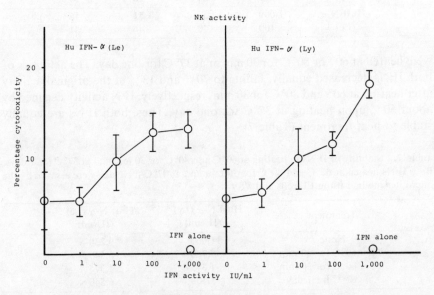

Fig. 2. Enhancement of NK cell activity by IFNs.
^{51}Cr-labeled HeLa cells were seeded into the wells of a microplate at a dose of 1×10^4 cells/well, and 2×10^5 of human lymphocytes and diluted human IFN were added to the wells and incubated at $37°C$ for 22 hours in a humidified 5% CO_2 atmosphere. One-tenth ml of the supernatant fluid was collected from each well for counting in a gamma spectrometer. The percentage cytotoxicity was calculated using the following formula:
$$\text{Percentage cytotoxity} = \frac{\text{Experimental } ^{51}Cr \text{ release} - \text{spontaneous } ^{51}Cr \text{ release}}{\text{Maximal } ^{51}Cr \text{ release} - \text{spontaneous } ^{51}Cr \text{ release}} \times 100.$$

Effect on NBT reduction in human peripheral neutrophils: Human leukocyte IFN enhanced the NBT reduction in peripheral neutrophils in a dose-dependent fashion, but in contrast human lymphoblastoid IFN did not (Table 6). The reason for this difference is not yet clear.

Heat stability: Human lymphoblastoid IFN and human leukocyte IFN

Table 6.   Effect of IFNs on NBT reduction.
Human IFN preparation (0.05 ml) was added to 0.5 ml of heparinized blood and incubated at 37°C for 20 min. NBT solution was then added to the mixture of IFN and blood. The reaction mixture was left for 20 min at room temperature and again mixed. Duplicate smears of this mixture were examined under the light microscope for the dense cytoplasmic inclusion of reduced dye (formazan). The reaction of NBT was expressed as the percentage of neutrophils containing formazan deposits.

IFN prep.	IU/ml	NBT reduction %		
		Exp. 1	Exp. 2	Exp. 3
Control		28	23	9
HuIFN-α	1,000	14	12	10
(Ly)	100	24	16	14
HuIFN-α	1,000	37	51	36
(Le)	100	40	46	31

were heated at 60° or 80°C for 30 min or at 37°C for one day. The activities of both IFNs decreased equally, falling to 70% and 13% of the original activity after heating at 60° and 80°C for 30 min, respectively. IFN activity declined by about 50% upon heating at 37°C for one day. Thus, both IFNs are equally stable to heat treatment (Table 7).

Table 7.   Stability of IFNs to heating at 60°C and 80°C for 30 min and at 37°C for 1 days. Both IFNs heated at 60°C and 80°C for 30 min and at 37°C for 1 day were assayed by the microtiter method using FL cells and VSV.

Treatment	HuIFN-α (Ly) (IU/ml)	HuIFN-α (Le) (IU/ml)
None	11,000	9,250
60°C for 30 min	7,780	6,540
80°C for 30 min	1,375	1,375
37°C for 1 day	5,500	6,540

DISCUSSION

The most important consideration at present in clinical trials with IFN is the difficulty of large-scale production of the substance and its consequent high cost. The work described in this paper demonstrated that a large number of human lymphoblastoid cells could be obtained transplantation into hamsters.

When human lymphoblastoid cells are grown in hamsters, $3-5 \times 10^9$ cells are obtained from one hamster in 3 to 4 weeks. Because the saturated density of lymphoblastoid cells *in vitro* is $2-3 \times 10^6$ cells/ml, about 2,000 ml of RPMI 1640 medium supplemented with 10% fetal bovine serum is needed for the production of the same number of cells. The use of hamsters makes it possible to produce IFN at a very low cost without the need for specialized apparatus or facilities. The lymphoblastoid cells recovered from the tumor mass grown in each hamster produce as much IFN as do cells cultivated *in vitro*. This lymphoblastoid IFN can be purified by the same methods as other lymphoblastoid IFNs such as Namalwa or human leukocyte IFN.[10,15] Chromatography on SP-Sephadex and Sephadex G-100 resulted in a purification of over 100-fold.

The purified lymphoblastoid IFN showed the same spectrum of species dependence as human leukocyte IFN. It is interesting that the human lymphoblastoid IFN displayed a high antiviral activity with bovine MDBK cells; Gresser *et al.*[16] reported that human leukocyte IFN showed high antiviral activity with MDBK cells. The lymphoblastoid IFN used in this experiment did not contain any hamster IFN because both the lymphoblastoid and the leukocyte IFNs showed equal antiviral activity with hamster BHK C-25 cells. The lymphoblastoid IFN produced inhibition of tumor cell growth, enhancement of spontaneous tumor cell growth inhibition by human peripheral leukocytes, and enhancement of NK cell activity. These findings suggest that human lymphoblastoid IFN could be used for the treatment of cancer patients. The authors intend to compare the antitumor activity of lymphoblastoid IFN with that of human leukocyte IFN *in vivo*. The neutralization of lymphoblastoid IFN by antihuman leukocyte IFN serum suggests that this IFN has a similar, but not identical, antigenic structure to that of human leukocyte IFN. This conclusion agrees with the results of Havell *et al.*[17]

In summary, lymphoblastoid IFN shows biological and physicochemical characteristics similar to those of human leukocyte IFN, except in the enhancement of NBT reduction and the slight difference in susceptibility to neutralization by antihuman leukocyte IFN serum. It is concluded that human leukemic lymphoblastoid cell line BALL-1 grown in newborn hamsters can produce large amounts of leukocyte-type IFN at low cost.

Acknowledgments

This work was supported by a Grant-in-Aid for Cancer Research from the Ministry of Education, Science and Culture, Japan.

The authors are grateful to Dr. A. Matsuo, the Central Research Institute of Green Cross Co., for the supply of human leukocyte IFN preparations, and Dr. K. E. Mogensen, Central Public Health Laboratory, Helsinki 28, Finland, for supplying antihuman leukocyte IFN serum.

REFERENCES

1. Klein, F., Ricketts, R. T., Jones, W. I., De Armon, I. A., Temple, M., Zoon, K. T., and Bridgen, P. J.: *Antimicrob. Agents Chemother.*, **15**: 420–427, 1979.

2. Bridgen, P. J., Anfinsen, C. B., Corley, L., Bose, S., Zoon, K. C., and Ruegg, U. T.: *J. Biol. Chem.*, **252**: 6582–6587, 1977.
3. Dunnick, J. K. and Galasso, G. J.: *J. Infect. Dis.*, **139**: 109–123, 1979.
4. Adams, R. A., Pothier, L., Hellerstein, E. E., and Boileau, G.: *Cancer*, **31**: 1397–1407, 1973.
5. Miyoshi, I., Hiraki, S., Kubonishi, I., Matsuda, Y., Kishimoto, H., Nakayama, T., Tanaka, Y., Masuji, H., and Kimura, I.: *Cancer*, **40**: 2999–3003, 1977.
6. Miyoshi, I., Hiraki, S., Tsubota, T., Kubonishi, I., Matsuda, Y., Nakayama, T., Kishimoto, Y., and Kimura, I.: *Nature (London)*, **267**: 843–844, 1977.
7. Imanishi, J.: *Jpn. J. Microbiol.*, **19**: 337–342, 1975.
8. Imanishi, J., Oishi, K., Kishida, T., Negoro, Y., and Iizuka, M.: *Arch. Virol.*, **53**: 157–161, 1977.
9. Bodo, G.: In: Proc. Symp. Preparation, Standardization and Clinical Use of Interferon. Yugoslav Academy of Sciences and Arts, Zagreb, 1977, pp. 49–57.
10. Matsuo, A.: *J. Kyoto Pref. Univ. Med.*, **87**: 79–91, 1978.
11. Matsuo, A., Hayashi, S., and Kishida, T.: *Jpn. J. Microbiol.*, **18**: 21–27, 1974.
12. Mogensen, J. E., Phyhälä, L., and Cantell, K.: *Acta Pathol. Microbiol. Scand.*, **B83**: 443–450, 1975.
13. Pak, C., Imanishi, J., Kishida, T., and Matsuo, A.: *Microbiol. Immunol.*, **24**: 717–723, 1980.
14. Trinchieri, G. and Santoli, D.: *J. Exp. Med.*, **147**: 1314–1333, 1978.
15. Cantell, K. and Hirvonen, S.: *J. Gen. Virol.*, **39**: 541–543, 1978.
16. Gresser, I., Bandu, M. T., Boyé, D., and Tovey, M.: *Nature (London)*, **251**: 543–545, 1974.
17. Havell, E. A., Yip, Y. K., and Vilček, T.: *J. Gen. Virol.*, **38**: 51–59, 1977.

Index of Authors